HEALTH
PROFESSIONAL
AND # PATIENT
INTERACTION

HEALTH PROFESSIONAL
AND PATIENT INTERACTION

EIGHTH EDITION

Ruth Purtilo, PhD, FAPTA

Professor Emerita
MGH Institute of Health Professions
Boston, Massachusetts

Amy Haddad, PhD, RN

Director, Center for Health Policy and Ethics
The Dr. C.C. and Mabel L. Criss Endowed Chair
   in the Health Sciences
Creighton University Medical Center
Omaha, Nebraska

Regina Doherty, OTD, MS, OTR/L

Associate Professor and Director
Occupational Therapy Program
School of Health and Rehabilitation Sciences
MGH Institute of Health Professions
Boston, Massachusetts

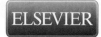

ELSEVIER
SAUNDERS

3251 Riverport Lane
St. Louis, Missouri 63043

HEALTH PROFESSIONAL AND PATIENT INTERACTION ISBN: 978-1-4557-2898-5

Notices

Knowledge and best practice in this field are constantly changing. As new research and experience broaden our understanding, changes in research methods, professional practices, or medical treatment may become necessary.

Practitioners and researchers must always rely on their own experience and knowledge in evaluating and using any information, methods, compounds, or experiments described herein. In using such information or methods they should be mindful of their own safety and the safety of others, including parties for whom they have a professional responsibility.

With respect to any drug or pharmaceutical products identified, readers are advised to check the most current information provided (i) on procedures featured or (ii) by the manufacturer of each product to be administered, to verify the recommended dose or formula, the method and duration of administration, and contraindications. It is the responsibility of practitioners, relying on their own experience and knowledge of their patients, to make diagnoses, to determine dosages and the best treatment for each individual patient, and to take all appropriate safety precautions.

To the fullest extent of the law, neither the Publisher nor the authors, contributors, or editors, assume any liability for any injury and/or damage to persons or property as a matter of products liability, negligence or otherwise, or from any use or operation of any methods, products, instructions, or ideas contained in the material herein.

Library of Congress Cataloging-in-Publication Data or Control Number
Purtilo, Ruth B.
  Health professional and patient interaction / Ruth Purtilo, Amy Haddad, Regina F. Doherty.—8th ed.
    p. ; cm.
  Includes bibliographical references and index.
  ISBN 978-1-4557-2898-5 (pbk. : alk. paper)
  I. Haddad, Amy Marie. II. Doherty, Regina F. III. Title.
  [DNLM: 1. Health Personnel—psychology. 2. Professional-Patient Relations. 3. Attitude of Health Personnel. 4. Communication. 5. Social Values. W 21]
  610.69'6—dc23   2012043274

Vice President and Publisher: Linda Duncan
Content Strategist: Jolynn Gower
Publishing Services Manager: Gayle May
Production Manager: Hemamalini Rajendrababu
Senior Project Manager: Antony Prince
Design Manager: Teresa McBryan

Printed in the United States of America

Last digit is the print number: 9 8 7 6 5 4 3 2 1

Working together to grow
libraries in developing countries

www.elsevier.com | www.bookaid.org | www.sabre.org

ELSEVIER   BOOK AID International   Sabre Foundation

*With gratitude to the patients, professional colleagues, friends,
and students whose stories have enhanced the pages
in this book—and enriched our lives.*

Ruth, Amy, and Regina

Preface

There is a Chinese saying that a trip of a thousand miles begins with the first step. As this eighth edition of *Health Professional and Patient Interaction* goes to press the authors are aware that careers in the health professions continue to expand and the level of education for participation in health care is evolving. This book is a companion for one of the first steps every person embarks on in a journey leading to a career in health care. Everyone must gain a basic understanding of the dynamics of the human relationships in health care environments. The core of these relationships consists of respectful interactions that shape and influence the success of all care delivery and thus is the focus of this book.

Readers will have the opportunity to (1) engage in critical self-reflection, (2) clarify their roles in shaping the health professional and patient relationship, and (3) develop awareness of the larger health care and societal context in which each relationship takes place. Clarification of personal, professional, and societal values sets the stage for exploring the context of interactions and the unique perspective that a health professional and patient each brings to their relationship.

Respect is the thread that weaves together discussions regarding relationships in the health care environment. *Health Professional and Patient Interaction* includes respect-generating resources from the foundational disciplines of the social sciences, humanities, communications, ethics, and current clinical research.

The content is designed to apply to everyday clinical experiences across different disciplines, taking into account the different levels of formal education they may involve, from two year programs to doctoral level preparation. Obviously the autonomy and direct accountability for patient outcomes will differ, but the human-to-human encounter remains constant. Part of the function of this book, therefore, is to show the extent to which the different members of the health care team share common challenges, goals, and opportunities for service as they participate in the delivery of patient- and family-centered care.

In some instances, it is necessary to assign meaning to key terms. We mention three here: (1) *patient*—the recipient of and participant in a health care interaction, (2) *experiential learning*—the portion of formal education that takes place at the type of worksite where a person will practice, and (3) *clinical experience*—the accumulation of actual experiences in one's chosen field.

The names of patients, health professionals, and other persons in the cases and other examples are fictitious. They represent a variety of clinical settings and disciplines to allow the reader to reflect on professional interactions across the lifespan and throughout the wide spectrum of care delivery environments.

When the last word of a manuscript has been written, its life has just begun. In sharing our ideas with you, the reader, we hope that in turn you will be stimulated to share yours with others, thus making us all more knowledgeable and skilled in respectful human interactions in the health care environment.

Ruth Purtilo • Amy Haddad • Regina Doherty

Acknowledgments

One joy of preparing this eighth edition of *Health Professional and Patient Interaction* has been the opportunity for us to work together in its development.

Each of us also has discussed issues examined in the book with students and other readers, as well as clinicians and faculty members around the country and the world. We thank them for their insights. Several persons at Elsevier have been outstanding in their guidance and support. Many people have asked who provided several original drawings which have appeared consistently since the first edition. For this contribution, we gratefully acknowledge Grant Lashbrook.

Finally, we extend our heartfelt thanks to our husbands, Vard, Steve, and Dan, who encourage us in all of our professional projects and enrich our lives, and to Regina's daughter, Olivia, who continues to be a source of inspiration as she grows, develops, and interacts with the world.

Contents

PART ONE

Creating a Context of Respect

As you know from your own life, relationships never take place in a vacuum! They are always challenged by forces that may or may not be in your control. Therefore, as you enter into the pages of this book about the health professional and patient relationship, the first thing we bring to your attention are some features of your personal life, the health care institutional environment, and the diversity of patients you will meet. Each will have a profound impact on that relationship, and you will also help to shape them through your own actions.

Chapter 1 begins with a definition and discussion of values in relation to respect. Respect is so central to a good working relationship between health professionals and patients that you will meet the concept many times in this book. Basic values—your own, those of the health professions, and the institutions in which health professionals work, and society's—constitute a firm ground for respect to take root and grow. Respect in professional and patient relationships is essential in supporting a caring response, the most fundamental goal of that relationship. To get you started we provide a brief description of care in this context. The chapter is optimistic, as are we, about your opportunity to honor and help foster respect in the health professions.

In Chapter 2 we direct your attention to some key elements of the institutions of health care: how physical environments, laws, regulations, and policies factor into respect in your professional relationships. We emphasize areas that we judge to have the most influence on your relationships with patients, their families, and others.

In Chapter 3, the final chapter of Part One, we give you an opportunity to think substantively about the rich diversity of social characteristics that individuals and groups bring to relationships. We ask you to consider ways you can learn to appreciate differences, including those of culture and ethnicity, socioeconomic status, religion, age, and gender, and to show respect for people no matter those characteristics.

CHAPTER 1

Respect: The Difference It Makes

CHAPTER OBJECTIVES

The reader will be able to:

- Give a brief definition of respect
- Describe why respect is so central to the success of the health professional and patient relationship
- Identify three spheres of values that constitute a person's "value system"
- Discuss some reasons why the professions today have become concerned about professionalism
- Distinguish collective professionalism from individual professionalism
- List some values that have been proposed as being shared by all people including "primary goods"
- Distinguish between the core professional value of care and caring in general
- Cite examples of when a person or group may not embrace a fully integrated value system

---

When I was small, there was a week when the whole country knew that every human life is irreplaceable. It was many years ago, but, as I recall, a child somewhere in the Midwest fell down an abandoned well, and for a week rescue teams worked to bring her out. This was a time before television, and radios were playing everywhere—in the stores, in the buses, even at school. Strangers met in the street and asked each other, "any news"? People of all religions prayed together.

As the rescue effort went on, no one asked if that was the child of a professor down there, the child of a cleaning woman, the child of a wealthy family. Was that child black, white, or yellow? Was that child good or naughty, smart or slow? In that week everyone knew that these things did not matter at all. That the importance of a child's life had nothing to do with those things. A person lost touched us all, diminished us all.

R.N. Remen[1]

Chances are you do not recall where you first encountered the idea that there is something about human beings that commands our attention and respect, something that goes beyond the differences that sometimes tend to separate us. The physician who wrote the above quote about her childhood experience goes on to say

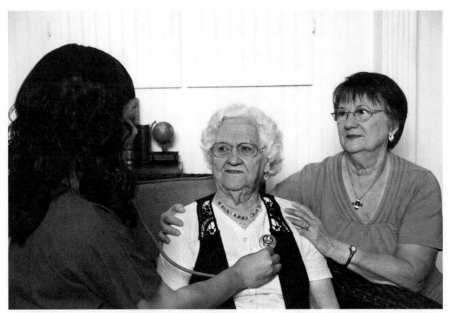

FIGURE 1-1: Health professional with patient and the patient's family. *(©iStockphoto.com.)*

that this experience was important because, as she would learn later, the idea that persons have a basic human dignity deserving of respect is at the heart of the health professional and patient relationship.

To get you started on your exploration of respect as it is expressed in your professional encounters, consider the picture of this health professional and a patient (Figure 1-1).

⊚ REFLECTIONS

What are the clues in this picture that show respect, however you define it, is present? Some things we could draw from this simple example include:
- She looks like she is inviting the patient to express what she is feeling.
- Her body language says she is paying attention to the patient
- The professional has not created an environment where he might feel embarrassed or unworthy due to the compromised condition of her own health at the moment.

You may see other features of this relationship that suggest the health professional basically respects this patient.

Whether you are preparing to enter a profession for the first time or are continuing to seek excellence in it through further study, being able to show and receive respect is a key to the satisfaction you will be able to realize over the course of your career as a professional. You might, in fact, think of respect as a linchpin that holds together your professional identity. Without respect for (and from) others you will almost inevitably find the paths you are choosing in your professional life to be veering off course.

What Is Respect?

Respect comes from the Latin root *respicere,* which means "to look at closely." In common parlance it has come to be interpreted as approaching a person, group, idea, or object with regard or esteem.[2] It says, "you matter," "you are worth the trouble." No matter how extreme our circumstances, we as humans hope that others will not discount our need to be somebody, that we will be sympathetically accompanied through the most difficult and unlikable or threatening aspects of our struggles. And when we rejoice, we hope others will join us in our celebration of accomplishment. In other words, we count on others' respect for who we are in a very fundamental sense that we all are humans. Many writers who have tried to explain that humans have basic worth agree that we share a common essence, which they term *dignity.* Even the ancients, in their myths, described this common essence, a theme also explored in virtually all the world's major religious traditions.[3] The essence is often referred to as the *inherent dignity* of persons to help emphasize that it resides beyond the physical, social, or psychological characteristics that distinguish us from each other.[4]

Inherent dignity is deeply ingrained into the idea of a profession. There have been centuries of attempts to fully explain it, an exploration that continues to this day on the assumption that there is a common thread of humanity that warrants basic regard of a person as such, no matter the variations that distinguishes him or her from others. In your study of this textbook we will help you look for specific expressions of respect through such everyday actions as the tone of your voice when you address a patient, the adaptation of your pace and body language to meet the needs of a child versus an elderly patient, your trustworthy keeping of a patient confidence, your attention to cultural differences, your presence during a crisis, and your willingness to work together with a patient's family and other professionals to reach his or her personal health-related goal.

In the health care setting your show of respect is a response to the fact that patients are vulnerable in ways that do not exist outside of the health care context but they also remain able to participate in decisions directly (or sometimes through a surrogate voice) that protect meaning in their life. Therefore, if you value respect, you will want to protect patients from exploitation or harm and advocate for them in ways that will be to their benefit. A helpful concept to help you understand the deeper relational dynamics that are taking place in respectful communications is care.

Respect and Care

Everyone talks about care as a positive feature of human relationships. It is. But care has a much more serious function in sustaining them than we often acknowledge. It is the link we make with another human being in distress, taking their suffering and well-being into account. Reich associates true caring with what we decide to do in a relationship when the chips are down.[6] Often it is not limited to the warm sentimentality so often expressed on the inside of greeting cards. True caring requires us to choose among our priorities and may become a challenge or even a burden. Our lives and energies are expended on what in reality we care about or value, no matter what we may say to the contrary.[6] This is precisely what distinguishes sentimentality from a motivation to care: Sentimentality stresses the awareness that you feel an emotion which evokes something in you to respond, whereas caring always requires involved concern about the specific barriers to a person's well-being and the action required to relieve them. We introduce it here because it helps to connect the idea of respect more generally with how our actions are outgrowths of core values we hold and are expressed in our roles as a person, professional, and member of society.

Respect and Your Values

Values describe things we hold dear. We say that something is "of value" when we estimate it to be of worth or usefulness to us for an important end. Values can include ideals, principles, attitudes, or actions and are treasured for their power to provide a spiritual, moral, or practical compass for leading a good life and to help us understand what will give life its meaning. Some values are presented as aspirations or duties. Other values are dispositions or traits of character such as love, compassion, honesty, generosity, faithfulness, or a sense of adventure. Yet other values are in the form of rituals or everyday practices and may include leisure, worship, work, and a myriad of other ways we choose to spend our time and energies. Finally, we value objects, too, for their usefulness, beauty, or power to evoke memory or meaning. One criterion of a "true" value is that it has become part of a pattern of a person's life.

Taken together, your values constitute your *value system*. Some values in that system are highly specific to you. Some will be adopted through your cultural and/or professional subgroup. Still others are shared by humans because of our common "human condition." The unique value system for each person creates a profile of his or her idea of "the good life."

Personal Values

Personal values are strictly one's own. We learn our early values from parents and other childhood friends, caregivers, teachers, religious beliefs and traditions, and cultural influences such as TV and the Internet. Values are imparted, taught, reinforced, and internalized. We incorporate many of them into our lives as a personal value system. We also exist in a complex world of bureaucracies and institutions. These influence us, too, so that as we mature our values evolve with us.

Most people cherish more than one personal good, or value. Literature provides striking examples of the exception: Ahab braved the high seas relishing the thought of getting revenge on the great white whale, Moby Dick; Sir Lancelot suffered many grave adversities in his relentless quest for the Holy Grail; and, before his change of heart, Ebenezer Scrooge treasured money. The narrow scope of personal values of Ahabs, Sir Lancelots, and Scrooges are exceptions. Most people have many personal values, some more clearly defined than others, and go through life trying to realize or balance several values simultaneously.

The process of developing self-consciousness about one's values is the focus of values clarification exercises. Values clarification provides the means to discover what values we live by. An individual who can identify his or her own values is able to place worth on actions or objects that lead to personally satisfying choices. Conversely, if unclear about our values or the connection between values and choices, it is likely that there will be poor decision-making and dissatisfaction.[7]

⊚ **REFLECTIONS**

The following values clarification exercise is helpful in identifying personal values and how these values play out in real life.

First, make a list of your 10 most important present values in order of importance.

Next, compare and contrast your own list of personal values with peers' values.

Then, compare the list of your own highest-ranking values with your own behavior.

To what degree is your behavior consistent with your stated values? If there is an inconsistency, why?

What can you go do (if anything) to get your stated values and behaviors in closer alignment?

As we suggested, sometimes your personal values will conflict with each other. An example is the case of a man who is excessively obese. Although there are many factors contributing to obesity, consider the obese person who finds security in consuming food. Unfortunately, his habitual eating eventually causes his body to break down, and his physician tells him that he can expect a shortened life span. At this point his basic value of life itself is endangered by the competing personal value of feeling secure. Because both of these values are essential to good health, treatment often is directed toward helping this person derive security from aspects of life other than eating. Similar examples of clashing values surround challenges related to other life-endangering practices, such as smoking, substance abuse, or lack of exercise or good sleeping habits.

⊚ **REFLECTIONS**

Your choice to make a career in the health professions has come from a desire to act on some of your most cherished values. Can you name some personal values that you recognize as consistent with your commitment to becoming and being a good health professional?

When patients seek your services their own personal values are almost always the motivation. They value being healthy, getting well, or finding comfort during chronic or life-threatening illness. They want you to help them maintain their value of health and optimize their functioning. Because health care is concerned primarily with personal values that are addressed through person-to-person relationships, your professional preparation through the use of this book gives you an opportunity to study and think about the challenges your own personal values pose and to identify many that facilitate your success.

Professional Values and Professionalism

Having chosen to become a health professional requires that you embrace values that are consistent with what being a professional means and what professional practice entails. Fortunately, many of these values overlap with your personal values or at least do not come into conflict with them. The word "professional" itself comes from the root, "to profess" or declare something. When you adopt the values of your profession, as a professing-person you are saying something important to society about your place in the community.

Many health professional organizations have articulated basic values that undergird their identity. The values help explain the reasonable expectations that society can count on regarding what that profession promises to do or not do. For example, seven essential values listed by the American Association of Colleges of Nursing for nurses are altruism, truth, aesthetics, equality, freedom, justice, and human dignity.[8] Another example is the list of values developed by the Education Section of the American Physical Therapy Association. *Professionalism in Physical Therapy: Core Values* lists accountability, altruism, compassion and caring, excellence, integrity, professional duty, and social responsibility.[9] It is worth your effort to identify the values your own professional organization has generated. You will readily see areas of overlap among the professions and begin to observe a general profile of professional values.

▶ These values arise in part from ongoing discussions of what constitutes a profession, making it special and distinct from other lines of work. Some themes appear over and over. For instance, professions have an organized body of specialized knowledge and skills that are prized by society;

▶ Knowledge and skills serve some basic human need. Basic need often renders a person or group vulnerable, so a profession's values of altruism and compassion are its promise to treat the patient's vulnerability with due care; and

▶ A profession has a code of ethics to which its members are expected to conform.

It is not surprising, then, that some of the professional values observed in the literature focus on ethical ideals of selfless conduct, trustworthiness, and accountability.

In recent years professional organizations have devoted growing attention to the idea of *professionalism*. The initiatives geared to professionalism share the common goal of identifying, protecting, and fostering the appropriate focus of the professional's role in society. As one book subtitle summarizes it, the goal is to create and sustain "a culture of humanism" in the health professions.[10] The underlying concern is that forces outside of the professions themselves such as changes in the health care system and pressures from society to conform to its whims may place undue pressure on professionals.

Professional responsibility is a dominant theme in professionalism. It emphasizes that the professions must be responsive to today's societal changes and demands. At the same time, in his probing analysis of the role of the professions in today's society, William Sullivan advises professionals to be careful not to lose their own core values in their attempt to mold themselves to society's expectations.[11] More than ever, he notes, they "have become responsible for key public values." It is this responsibility that sets off professionals from other workers. Although professionals are engaged in generating or applying new ideas and technologies, they are all directly pledged to an ethic of public service.

Of course, reflection by the professions on the values they uphold, and why, is by no means an entirely novel phenomenon unique to the present age. Such reflection has been the focus of lively study and debate since the delineation of three traditional professions (law, medicine, and the clergy) during the Middle Ages. Today many still refer to a profession as a "calling" that requires total devotion, specialized knowledge, and extensive academic preparation. From these root terms and interpretations the professions today are identified as groups whose members have responded to an opportunity to hold a special place in society, differentiated from those who simply hold a job or have an occupation. Their claims derive from society's values and society's beliefs.

Swisher and Page point out that today's emphasis on professionalism is *collective professionalism* because it applies to all members of a professional group. The challenge for you, the individual professional entering today's health care system, is to tailor the guidance from your profession to fit the requirements of your own specific professional practice.[12] In other words, the task is to incorporate appropriate values of professionalism into your personal value system. Sometimes students wonder why so much time is devoted to something like this that seems obvious in many regards, but the authors have found that the preparation is well worth the time because all health care providers will have conflicting claims placed on them and be involved in extremely complex situations. During such times the ability to ground oneself in one's own and the profession's values allows an informed, intentional movement forward.[13]

Care as a Value

The basic idea of care as a component of respect was introduced at the beginning of this chapter. We raise it here through the lens of professional values. The value of care and its active form, caregiving, are pivotal to professional practice. Professionals are judged in large part by whether or not they offer competent care appropriate to their expertise. In that regard care expressed as a professional is different from caring in a relationship with a spouse, child, friend, or colleague. It is shaped according to ethical duties, rights, and character traits that describe the proper place of a professional. But patients are drawn to the idea of care because the term conveys that a high-stakes human story is taking place and for them it always is. Patients have a personal story that holds all their hopes, dreams, and fears, and the health professional's care must reflect that the story is heard.[14] A key question in all health professional and patient interactions, then, is, "What is required of a health professional to fully express 'I care'?"[15] If a health professional does not hold this value as essential in his or her own professional identity or a key to work satisfaction over time, a professional career is not a good fit for this person. As this book unfolds, skills needed for effective care and many examples of care will be explored, both those that fall within the appropriate contours of a health professional and patient relationship and some that challenge those boundaries.

Societal Values

A third set of values that make up your values system derives from the larger society. One well-recognized characteristic of "the human condition" is that we, as human beings, organize ourselves into complex interactions as groups of individuals called *societies.* You belong to many communities within the larger society already. Each subgroup has values that you are aware of and may accept, reject, or question in regard to how they support your attempt to lead a good life.

⊚ REFLECTIONS

Take a minute to name some of the societal subgroups you are most influenced by such as your extended family, neighborhood, ethnic community, the part of the country where you live, school you attend, religious affiliation, and social or civic organizations.
Can you name one or two values you have absorbed from your membership in each of these subgroups? If not, where did your values come from other than from these common sources?

The scope of societal values that influence value choices has expanded greatly in the past few decades. Millions have immediate access to the World Wide Web, radio, and television. We can travel extensively or meet those who do. These broadening circles of access and influence have led some to conclude that we are all indeed members of a global society and to survive must come to grips with the common values that will help all lead a good life. As you will see in Chapter 9, patients have taken advantage of the World Wide Web, TV commercials, travel, and other means of data gathering to gain clinical information not previously available to them.

In spite of the increasing exposure to new and ever-expanding sources of values, some dimensions of our humanity seem to cut a wide swath across subgroups. Starting with the assumptions that we are communicating beings, technologically inclined, historically grounded as a species, and with capacity to try to create order and beauty, humans value:

▶ Being able to share their hopes, fears, thoughts, and ideas with each other
▶ The use of tools to assist in the completion of daily tasks
▶ Building cultures on the basis of wisdom, mistakes, and knowledge of those who lived before us
▶ The design of laws and habits to govern or facilitate a wide range of interactions
▶ Creating nonfunctional objects and cherishing them for their beauty alone

As spiritual beings humans want to perform rituals. As moral beings, they want to enjoy the ability to distinguish between right and wrong and adjust their behavior accordingly.[16] In short, human beings are social beings and therefore rarely find satisfaction outside the social context of living in a society.

All of these values have been proposed to be universal, though the list of such values is much longer. Some sources of these mainstream Western values are laws, philosophical inquiry, and shared experiences. For example, lawmakers in most such

> ## ⑤ REFLECTIONS
>
> Consider whether you believe the following are universally held societal values and what supports your conclusion.
> * Protection of human life
> * Rights and liberties
> * Having power and opportunities
> * Income and wealth
> * Self-respect
> * Health and vigor
> * Intelligence and imagination
> * Character traits such as courage, compassion, a desire to do justice, honesty
> * Faith and hope
> * Love
> * Autonomy, having say-so, self-governance

societies rely on the principle that human life itself is a basic value and therefore ought to be protected and nourished.

Philosophers are an ongoing source of input as well. John Rawls, one of the most influential American philosophers of the 20th century, argued that humans value several primary goods. *Social primary goods* include rights, liberties, powers, opportunities, income, wealth, and self-respect. (Self-respect is necessary for a person to have a sure conviction that his or her life plan is worth carrying out or capable of being fulfilled.) The realization of these goods is at least partially determined by the structure of society itself. *Natural primary goods,* also partly determined by societal structures but not directly under their control, include health, vigor, intelligence, and imagination.[17] Together, he says, these social and natural primary goods provide a sort of "index of welfare" for individuals in any society.

Other writers suggest certain character traits that produce a good life for the larger community; however, there is dispute over which character traits are the central ones. For instance, in ancient Greek thought, the *cardinal virtues* of temperance, prudence, a desire to do justice, courage, and fortitude (or moral strength to do what is right) were considered central to being able to lead a good life in any societal context. Early Christian thinkers argued that these alone were not sufficient for a good life and that faith in God, hope, and love were crucial. Other world religions and schools of philosophical thought have contributed their lists.

Societal values have power to affect well-being positively or negatively. Any time it is impossible to live up to society's expectations and the values it dictates, a person may experience tremendous anxiety (Figure 1-2).

Whatever one's lot in life, the individual's need to be accepted within society and be able to embrace and live by its most basic values influences well-being.

The Good Life and You

In this chapter you have encountered examples of three sets of values—personal, professional, and societal. Their differences have been highlighted, but in everyday

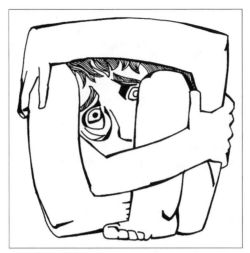

FIGURE 1-2: When a person is placed in a position in which it is impossible to live up to society's expectations, he or she may experience tremendous anxiety and discomfort.

life a person usually adopts a set of personal values that overlap in part and are harmonious with role-related and the larger society's values. Figure 1-3 shows a schematic representation of a person's integrated value system.

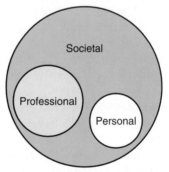

FIGURE 1-3: Integrated personal, professional, and societal values.

This person has internalized societal and role-derived values so that he or she cannot distinguish them from personal. Motivation for doing so usually arises from choosing to live harmoniously in society (and for the health professional, in her or his work role) and valuing personal benefits that derive from it. It is possible to say of anyone who lives according to his or her values system, "That person has a good life." However, when a person's value system includes values that help to uphold and further society as well, we say, "That person *leads* a good life."

Of course, not everyone adopts a set of personal values compatible with societal values or even with those of his or her own social or cultural subgroup. Such a person's value system is represented in Figure 1-4.

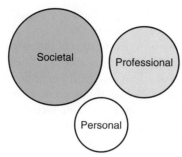

FIGURE 1-4: Values in conflict.

In the extreme form, this person has not internalized any societal or other cultural values. Such a person either desires not to live in harmony with society or more likely believes that there are no benefits to be derived from doing so. Some examples of people whose values clash with societal values are the hermit, the outlaw, and the saint or martyr. The hermit and outlaw reject societal values and replace them with their own; the saint or martyr rejects societal values and replaces them with some "higher" set of values.

There are varying degrees to which such persons divorce themselves from societal values. On the one hand, the woman who drives through a red light to make it to her tennis match on time is replacing a societal value of adherence to traffic rules with the personal value of reaching her tennis game. The conscientious objector who performs alternative service is refusing to accept the societal value of engaging in war to protect one's country on the basis of following the antiwar dictates of a higher law. Most people experience some such conflict from time to time.

This is a serious matter. Humans generally have a tendency not to rock the boat, no matter how unsatisfactory the situation. And so it is jarring when something compels him or her to reflect on his or her values. There is a powerful passage in *Dead Man Walking* when Sister Prejean, the narrator of the book, understands suddenly after hearing a political activist speak that she is going to have to rock the boat, as it were. She becomes convinced that she must speak out against capital punishment in response to data showing that this punishment is administered unfairly to rich and poor offenders. The speaker challenged audience members to reflect on their own values and actions, and Sister Prejean recalls, "She knew her facts and I found myself mentally pitting my arguments against her challenge—we were nuns, not social workers, not political. But it's as if she knew what I was thinking. She pointed out that to claim to be apolitical or neutral in the face of such injustices would be, in actuality, to uphold the status quo—a very political position to take, and on the side of the oppressors."[18]

For the health professional, a disconnect can occur when professional values come into conflict with personal values or what the professional believes are appropriate societal values. Any time a professional does not conform to the norms of his or her profession, it can become a source of discomfort to the majority who accept the status quo. It requires courage and self-knowledge to stand out as a change agent when professional values do not honor the ultimate values the dissenting professional believes are being compromised. At the same time, as in all situations the person who dissents from accepted norms bears the burden of showing why. In the process it may also become clear that the dissent was misplaced.

The ultimate standard by which such conflict can be measured in the health professions context is the extent to which each position honors the widely accepted value in health care that respect for all persons is required, even though a patient's specific values may differ dramatically from one's own. The professional value of respect for persons reminds us that all persons deserve to be treated fairly and in a humane manner.

SUMMARY

Respect for others and reaping the benefits of it yourself are essential ingredients for a successful professional practice. Respect involves both attitudes and behavior that acknowledge your regard for another person's dignity, no matter what his or her attributes and circumstances are. Our values are determinants of whether we will want and be able to express genuine respect for patients, their families, and other professionals. Some values arise from personal preferences, whereas others become internalized over time through the influences of affiliations and societal forces. Professional values are transmitted through the educational, clinical, and research institutions of health care. The core value of competent care will guide you back to the understanding that in your relationships with patients their belief that they are being respected will depend on your ability to convey that you understand the stakes are high for them. You can make good progress on your road to respectful interaction by identifying your own values and developing a genuine interest in others' values.

REFERENCES

1. Remen RN: *My grandfather's blessings: stories of strength, refuge and belonging*, New York, 2000, Riverhead Books.
2. *Webster's New Collegiate Dictionary*, Springfield, MA, 1974, G and C Merriam-Webster.
3. Purtilo RB: Chapter 1: New respect for respect in ethics education. In Purtilo RB, Jensen GM, Royeen CB, editors: *Educating for moral action: a sourcebook in health and rehabilitation ethics*, Philadelphia, 2005, FA Davis.
4. Kilner J: Human dignity. In Post SG, editor: *Encyclopedia of bioethics*, vol 2, ed 3, New York, 2004, Thomson, Gale.
5. Reich WT: Care. In Reich WT, editor: *Encyclopedia of bioethics*, vol 1, ed 2, New York, 1995, MacMillan.
6. Brown D, Grace RK: Values in life role choices and outcomes: a conceptual model, *The Career Development Quarterly* 44:211–223, 1996.
7. *Essentials of college and university education for professional nursing, final report*, Washington, DC, 1995, American Association of Colleges of Nursing.
8. American Physical Therapy Association: *Professionalism in physical therapy: consensus document*, Alexandria, VA, 2003, American Physical Therapy Association.
9. Wear D, Bickel J, editors: *Educating for professionalism: creating a culture of humanism in medical education*, Iowa City, 2000, University of Iowa Press.
10. Sullivan M: *Work and integrity, the crisis and promise of professionalism in America*, ed 2, San Francisco, 2005, Jossey-Bass.
11. Sullivan WM: op cit, pp. 4–9.

12. Swisher LL, Page CG: *Professionalism in physical therapy, history, practice and development*, St Louis, 2005, Elsevier.
13. Doherty RF: Ethical decision-making in occupational therapy practice. In Crepeau ED, Cohn ES, Schell BA, editors: *Willard and Spackman's occupational therapy*, ed 11, New York, 2009, Lippincott, Williams & Wilkins.
14. Purtilo RB: What interprofessional teamwork taught me about an ethics of care, *Physical Therapy Reviews* 17:197, 2012.
15. Purtilo RB, Doherty RF: *Ethical dimensions in the health professions*, ed 5, St Louis, 2011, Elsevier.
16. Adler MJ: *The difference of man and the difference it makes*, ed 2, New York, 1993, Fordham University Press.
17. Rawls J: *A theory of justice*, ed 2, Cambridge, 1971, Belknap Press of Harvard University.
18. Prejean H: *Dead man walking*, New York, 1994, Vintage Books.

Respect in the Institutional Settings of Health Care

CHAPTER OBJECTIVES

The reader will be able to:

- Compare the perspectives of viewing health care from each of Glaser's three realms: individual, institutional, and societal
- List four major forces that have resulted in current structures of health care environments
- Compare public- and private-sector relationships and describe why health professional and patient interactions are public-sector relationships
- Compare relationships within total institutions and partial institutional environments
- Identify two aspects of administration that are likely to have a direct impact on the organizational environment in which you work
- List several types of laws, regulations, and policies that influence the practice of your profession and what you should be able to expect from the institution in which you work
- Discuss the idea of patients' rights documents and the purposes they are designed to serve

The VA Medical Center was wonderful and exactly what I needed, but, as I was repeatedly told while I was there, "This isn't a hotel. You'll have to work here, but this is a good hospital."

M.E. Little[1]

Chapter 1 addressed important aspects of being a professional. This chapter focuses on some key insights regarding where you will exercise your professional skills. You will almost inevitably work in an institutional environment, which exists to provide health care services. Your ability to understand and respect this basic structure and its operations is essential to your work satisfaction and also will determine how you are viewed by patients, colleagues, and others.

Some of you have seen paintings by the French impressionist painter Marc Chagall. He creates a heavenly environment evoking romance, bliss, and promise (Figure 2-1). His work speaks to a deeper meaning: Our environments always create certain expectations and evoke powerful feelings. They influence attitudes and conduct in ways that we are not always consciously aware of or do not fully

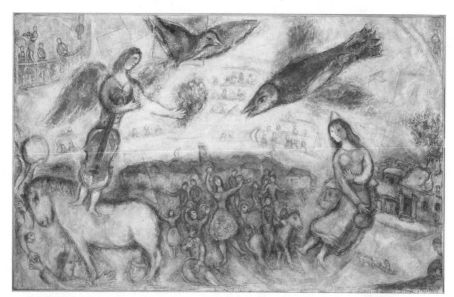

FIGURE 2-1: Chagall, Marc (1887–1985) © ARS, NY. The Journey of the People. 1968. Oil on canvas, 128 × 205 cm. Private Collection. *(Courtesy Scala/Art Resource, NY.)*

understand. It follows that every reader of this book will be influenced by his or her work environment, as well as influence it by participating in its everyday activities. A good starting place for respectful interaction, then, is to become familiar with basic characteristics of such institutions and then address key characteristics of institutional relationships within them. It will also benefit you at this point to become aware of some key policies and practices designed to command respect from all who engage with the institution, whether employees or those seeking goods and services, so we introduce them in a general way in the final sections of this chapter.

Characteristics of Institutions

Glaser describes three realms of social activity—individual, institutional, and societal—each having an impact on the health professional's effectiveness and sense of well-being. Institutions sit at the interface between the individual and the larger society (Figure 2-2).[2]

Ideally, institutional policies and practices reflect deep respect for values that guide individual health professionals personally and professionally but also encourage them to be responsive to the basic societal expectation that patients are the top priority. In turn, health professionals will not only engage in respectful interpersonal relationships with patients and families but also be loyal and respectful of management and administrative policies of the institution. We do not live in an ideal world, thus at times challenges arise among the priorities and values in the three realms.

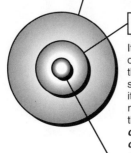

Glaser's Three Realms

Societal **The good and virtuous society**

Its values reflect the common good—the overall and long-term good and goodness of society (city, state, country). It attends to the health, vigor, balance, and equity of society's key systems and structures—political, economic, legal, educational, etc.—so that society increasingly is and continues to be an environment in which persons can be born, grow, labor, love, flourish, age, and die as humanely as possible. *Societal ethics deals primarily with the key systems and structures of society through which it achieves its purpose and in which we read its ethical character.*

Institutional **The good and virtuous institution**

Its values reflect the overall and long-term good and goodness of institutions (families, agencies, corporations). It attends to the health, vigor, balance, and equity of the institution's key systems and structures so that the institution can accomplish its mission, vision, values, and goals while attending to its rights and duties vis-à-vis the individuals who make it up and the larger society in which it exists. *Institutional ethics is concerned primarily with the key systems and structures of an institution through which it achieves its purpose and in which we read its ethical character.*

Individual **The good and virtuous individual**

Its values reflect the good and goodness of individuals. It attends to the balance and the right relationships among various dimensions of a single individual (spiritual, mental, physical, emotional, etc.) as well as the values that support rights and duties that exist between individuals.

FIGURE 2-2: Glaser's Three Realms.

Diversity of Facilities

The institutional realm of health care is a complex web of ideas and values expressed in numerous types of health care facilities. Health professionals work in hospitals, ambulatory care clinics, nursing homes, long-term care facilities, rehabilitation settings, research centers, diagnostic laboratories, schools, hospices, industrial settings, spas, and military first response units; among sports teams; and on cruise ships, to name a few. What is fitting for one type of facility may look quite different from another.

Moreover, the organization of health care is not completely a *rational system*. Rational systems are oriented expressly to the pursuit of one specific goal and have a highly formalized social structure designed to meet that goal.[3] An example is an airport, where the single goal is to move people and goods from place to place. The institutions of health care can be more illustrative of an *open system* in which shifting and sometimes competing interest groups negotiate for their goals to be met. At the same time, some silver threads of commonality among health care institutions will help you understand your work environment. For instance, they share some key values including:

▶ *Efficiency* of operations
▶ *Autonomy*, freedom from undue outside regulation
▶ *Social justice* for underserved populations
▶ *High quality service* in response to health needs of the community
▶ *Loyalty to shareholders* in institutions that operate as a business
▶ *Financial viability*

When you enter a program of professional preparation, the basic type of institutional setting where you will work may be determined in part by the focus of your profession. For example, a focus on maintenance and health promotion may mean you will practice in a health spa, school, industry, or free-standing clinic that provides wellness education. If you are drawn to acute care, rehabilitation, chronic health, or end-of-life care needs, it is likely you will find work in a hospital, rehabilitation center, nursing home, hospice, or in home care.

⊚ REFLECTIONS

- What is the ideal setting of where you would like to go to work each day?
- Take a few minutes to visualize the physical environment. What do the rooms look like? What kind of equipment is in the area? What other functions are served in the same building? Are other types of professionals present? Who are they?
- Where and with whom will you be able to share your professional concerns, relax, and learn on the job?

Multi-Service, Team-Oriented Institutional Environments

Most health care organization in the United States, Canada, Europe and Great Britain today reflect the trend toward comprehensive complexes housing "health plans" and away from institutions with one particular function. This approach represents a move toward more population-based models of care with a defined target population of patients and their health needs (Figure 2-3). Many have commented on this movement in the 20th and 21st centuries, identifying it with the following:

▶ **Industrialization**—The industrial revolution and its compartmentalization of public and private life functions
▶ **Urbanization**—The movement of people to the cities and the resulting potential for increasing efficiency by offering a more centralized site for services
▶ **Specialization**—The emergence of specialized medicine necessitating a centralized site for coordination of care
▶ **Team-oriented management**—The evolution from the single professional and patient to teams of professionals sharing information, equipment, and other institutional resources

Institutional environments have changed and will continue to do so during your professional career. Attention to where you find the best fit for your practice will require attentiveness to changing styles and designs of institutional environments.

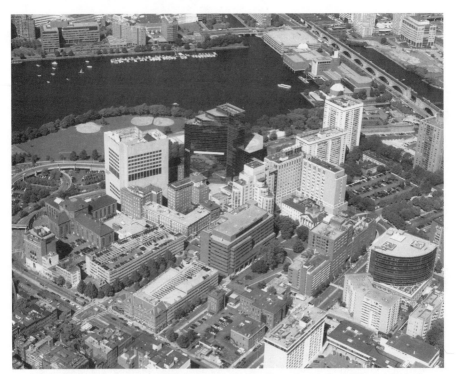

FIGURE 2-3: Aerial view of a large medical center. *(Courtesy Massachusetts General Hospital, Boston.)*

Characteristics of Institutional Relationships

The ability to show and receive respect in the work environment requires an understanding of several characteristics of relationships that take place in health care institutions compared with other types of relationships. To highlight this point we examine two characteristics of health care institutions that distinguish them from some others you participate in, namely their public rather than private nature and the institution's role as a partial rather than a total institution.

Public- and Private-Sector Relationships

Public-sector relationships are interactions reserved for engagements within institutions of public life, whereas private-sector relationships are reserved for the world of family, friends, and other intimates.[3] Individuals generally separate their lives into these two worlds of relationship. Public-sector relationships are designed to serve a useful purpose and then dissolve, whereas private-sector ones are more likely to continue. Student and professor or patient and health professional relationships belong to the world of public-sector relationships. Social boundaries that are maintained in a public-sector relationship permit rapid introduction and rapid separation, promoting cooperation around a common goal. All public-sector relationships are characterized by abrupt changes from extreme remoteness to extreme nearness with the expectation that the relationship will be temporary. Students who become close during their years of formal preparation go their separate ways upon graduation. Professionals in attendance at a conference of their professional organization come from different worksites to learn, share their own research or expertise, enjoy socializing, and then depart back to their own practice settings.

---

⑨ REFLECTIONS

- Think about public-sector relationships you have engaged in during your life. How did they benefit you? Jot them down for further reflection as this chapter unfolds.
- Are your relationships with fellow students or professionals more akin to private- or public-sector relationships? Why?

Opportunities for involvement in each other's lives and well-being and the boundaries of respect that must be honored with patients, families, and peers are addressed throughout this book, especially in Part Five.

The physical structure of an institution helps to enable an effective private- or public-sector relationship. Hospitals or schools, for instance, unmistakably are public buildings. What are some of the clues for this conclusion? Sometimes the environment where health care is administered mingles private- and public-sector environments. For instance, a lounge where patients who are institutionalized for long-term stays can meet often will foster private-sector friendships within the public-sector facility that will last beyond discharge. On a different scale, a home visit to a patient requires that you go to his or her residence, be welcomed in as a guest would be, make your way across the living room among discarded pages of the morning paper, trip over the sleeping dog, and move a bathrobe from a comfortable overstuffed chair to sit down. You have entered a profoundly private-sector environment. However, your presence and professional conduct represent the type of public-sector relationship that takes place within health care institutions and this usually suffices to adequately set the tone for measures that show appropriate respect for a public-sector interaction.

Increasingly computer-generated simulated environments are being added to the physical structures of care, raising interesting questions about what is required when the "institution" is a computer-generated one such as one finds in Second Life. Health professionals and patients interact as avatars but around therapeutic issues that affect them as "real-life" users of this technology. As you read this book reflect on how communications and other aspects of respectful interaction may be influenced and altered by this tool of interaction.

Relationships in Total and Partial Institutions

Another area of consideration about institutional relationships came from a now classic study of how authority is exercised in institutions. More than 50 years ago sociologist Goffman advanced an understanding of institutions on the basis of observations about the participants' relative authority. He noted that the design of institutions enhances the way authority is exercised and by whom, dividing the structural arrangements into "total" and "partial" institutions.[4] To illustrate, recall your experience in a campus dormitory, airport, hospital, or other type of institution. Each has its physical design and function accompanied by certain rules, regulations, policies, and other constraints. We judge such constraints as legitimate if they seem to serve understandable goals of the institution.

Total Institutions

Total institutions are those in which personal autonomy is totally or seriously compromised by the persons who voluntarily or involuntarily are placed in the structure. They are places where, as Goffman describes it, "a large number of like-situated individuals, cut off from the wider society for an appreciable period of time, together lead an enclosed, formally administered round of life."[4] Usually professional and supportive personnel are the sole authority: They "run" the institution, and the assumption is that either the individual or society (and in some cases, both) benefit from the arrangement. Often a ritual act of donning the clothing of the institution (e.g., a nun's habit in a cloistered convent or a prison jumpsuit) further signifies the surrender of identity and autonomy and "the acquisition of a new identity oriented to the authority of the professional staff and to the aims and purposes and the smooth operation of the institution."[4] Although their functions vary, examples of total institutions are many: monasteries, nursing homes, locked Alzheimer's units, long-term care facilities, hospitals for severely mentally ill or developmentally challenged persons, and prisons.

Only a small percentage of health professional and patient interactions take place within the highly codified and rigid structure of a total institution. When they do, the patient's autonomy is lost or diminished by illness, injury, lack of decision-making capacity, or some social factor such as committing a crime. In this situation of uneven authority, every precaution to respect the dignity of the person must be rigorously undertaken. Recognition of the vulnerability of such persons to abuse at the hands of even well-meaning individuals often necessitates writing special precautionary guidelines and policies for health care. For instance, there are especially stringent guidelines for protecting persons in such environments from abuses carried out in the name of clinical research.

At several places in this book, particularly in Part Three, we revisit the idea of turf, those aspects of a personal living space and self-determination that can help to lend dignity in the midst of serious constraints as a result of health-related confinement to an institution.

Partial Institutions

Most health care institutions can be classified as partial institutions because they constrain patients' autonomy in some important ways but also allow for varying degrees of self-determination.

People entering such institutions are concerned about the potential constraints they will face.

ⓢ REFLECTIONS

Suppose you are entering a health care facility for a serious injury that will involve surgery and, possibly, several weeks of inpatient rehabilitation. Of the following questions, which ones do you think would be of concern to you?
- Will I be able to go home from time to time during a long-term institutionalization and, if so, under what conditions?
- Are my children (or spouse, or parents, or friends) allowed to visit?
- May I see my pet?
- What will I be allowed to eat, and what kind of "time off" from a heavy schedule of tests and treatments might I be able to negotiate?
- How much input will I have into changes in my diagnostic or therapeutic regimen?
- May I wear my own clothes?
- May I change doctors or other health care professionals without fear of retribution if there is reason to doubt their competence?

These concerns will vary according to the type of condition and the values system of the individual. However, the important point is that the patient will have concerns about what restrictions the institution will impose.

Your own autonomy in the institution where you work as a professional will also be shaped by the structure and how authority is divided. They may include policies for securing employment, regulations regarding employee conduct, expectations regarding the number of people in your care, and other institutional peculiarities. These will either enable or inhibit your ability to satisfy your professional and personal goals. Obviously a crucial component of your professional choices is to find an institution that is consistent with your personality and values system. As you consider an institutional environment, paying attention to Glaser's three realms should help you to identify areas where your personal, institutional, and societal values overlap and where they may create potential conflicts.

Health professionals are also key sources of institutional change who can help create ways that respect can be expressed in humane and person-centered environments. As people talk about ways in which their autonomy and other values can better be honored within the confines of partial institutions, you can think of ways to help bring about those changes.

Working with the Administration

All employees in institutions have the opportunity and obligation to work well with their administrators. The administration's role is to safeguard the interests of the institution and all of its components. In health care institutions the administration comprises a wide range of groups and individuals, including institutional trustees, boards of directors, and the central administration (including a chief executive officer [CEO] and chief financial officer [CFO], human resources director, and departmental and unit supervisors responsible for operations or services). The range and duties of the administration should reflect the needs of the institution as determined by its mission, goals, and functions. Health care institutions will include at least the following departments:

▶ quality care mechanisms to ensure that patient and family rights are respected,
▶ officers for enforcing legal compliance with federal and other policies and regulations,
▶ accountability mechanisms assuring qualifications of professional employees,
▶ risk management personnel regarding concerns of liability and malpractice, and
▶ means of ensuring that employees get due payment for their services.

Taken together, like other well-working institutions, there will be personnel and mechanisms devoted to oversight, quality assurance, financial solvency, legal compliance and assurances that legal rights are honored, public relations, and efficiency.

These administrative supports should always be designed to allow constructive participation of professionals to ensure their mutually shared goal of good health care. At the same time, differences in the scope of accountabilities determined by their respective roles lead to understandable conflict at times. To illustrate how differently administration and health professionals might look at the same set of challenges, we invite you to consider the following case, first from the point of view of the professional-patient relationship and then from the administrator's point of view.

Mary Jacobs is the coordinator of the large pediatric division of Metro Rehabilitation Center. She is single, the mother of two children. She has mortgage payments and car payments to make, but thanks to her job, she feels quite secure financially.

Mary has worked at the Center for 15 years. The first 12 years she worked as a staff professional in the adolescent unit, with increasing supervisory and student clinical teaching responsibilities. Three years ago she was tapped by the administration for her present position, which involves caring for younger children. Her role includes departmental administrative responsibilities, as well as continuing to treat patients. Although it has many benefits, she realizes her primary concern still lies with the patients and their parents. At the same time she liked the idea of being able to further shape a service with an excellent reputation and took seriously the administration's belief that she was the right person for the job at a time when two competing pediatric rehabilitation units were opening up in the vicinity. She has to admit that the 3 years overall have been both personally and professionally rewarding.

Mary reports directly to the Vice President for Patient Services (Carole Nash), though most of her day-to-day activities revolve around the team, support personnel, and patients. She meets with Carole once a month. She is painfully aware that the pediatric unit has been under increasing financial duress, due to the competition's aggressive tactics to attract private-pay patients. She is not entirely surprised when Carole tells her that due to financial pressures at Metro, Mary must lay off two professional staff and six support staff by the end of the fiscal quarter (within the next 6 weeks). But as she walks back to her unit she begins to resent having to upset such a well-working team and deal with the inevitable crash in morale. Central to her concern is that the upset will have a detrimental effect on patient care quality.

She has to admit that she also resents her unit being asked to make cuts when she is aware that overall the census is down at Metro Rehab.

The next morning Mary calls the Vice President's office to ask if she can discuss this situation with Carole further. Carole's administrative assistant replies that he will check but wants to warn Mary that Carole herself did not make the decision independently, and he believes "the final decision already has been made." About a half hour later Carole drops in to see Mary. She says that she appreciates how difficult this is for Mary and her staff, but adds, "With the present situation in the pediatric unit, there should be no question in your mind, either, what had to be done. As you know, I, too, come from a clinical background, so I'm sure you feel torn. I wish we had the resources to launch an aggressive campaign to counter our competition, but we don't. So I finally agreed with the board that yours is one area we should downsize. Ethically speaking I am torn, but it's the kind of hard decision administrators sometimes have to make. I am sorry."

As is often the case in health care settings, the clinical and administrative roles are not entirely separate, so at some level both Mary Jacobs and Carole Nash can see the other's point of view. Viewed from Mary's perspective as a health professional who identifies with her caregiving role more than her administrative one, reflect on the following:

	Strongly Agree	Agree	Not Sure	Disagree	Strongly Disagree
1. Mary has a right to expect that her concerns be listened to by the higher administration.					
2. If Mary can show that patient care quality in her unit will be decreased by the downsizing, Carole should go back to the board to advocate for finding another place to cut personnel.					
3. Mary's concern that a decrease in team morale might have a detrimental effect on patient care is a legitimate concern.					
4. If Mary does not succeed in making her case, she should resign.					

▶ What values, duties, and other considerations are appropriate for Mary Jacobs to consider in making judgments about the situation she is faced with?

▶ At what point should she share her problem with others, and whom should they be? Why?

▶ What alternatives are open to her other than resigning if she is unsuccessful in reversing Carole's decision?

Viewed from Carole Nash's perspective as an administrator, reflect on the following from the point of view of institutional loyalties:

Continued

	Strongly Agree	Agree	Not Sure	Disagree	Strongly Disagree
1. Carole's major responsibility is to be sure Metro Rehabilitation Center stays financially stable, even though some difficult decisions must be made.					
2. The board's plan to cut personnel to help sustain the financial health of Metro Rehabilitation Center outweighs Mary's concern about the negative effect on team morale.					
3. Carole should meet with the members of Mary's unit before giving Mary the task of laying off personnel.					
4. Administrators in high positions like Carole's would make more rational decisions if they did not have a health professions background. Those who do face a conflict of loyalties between institutional needs overall and what might happen to individual patients or professionals.					

▶ What basic administrative and other values, duties, and other considerations are appropriate for Carole to consider in her position as she responds to this administrative problem?

▶ Should Carole have shared the information with Mary that the decision came from the Metro Board of Directors instead of representing it as being her decision alone? Why or why not?

▶ What, if any, alternatives are open to Carole to help ensure that the positive aspects of the outcome will be optimized and the damage minimal?

This case is just one type of situation in which health professionals and administrators may have to negotiate decisions that are not 100% acceptable to either party. The better the communication channels and the more transparent the policies and processes for mediating difficult decisions, the more likely it is that the highest possible level of satisfaction will be reached.

Respecting the Interface of Institutions and Society

In addition to the constraints and opportunities you, your colleagues, and your patients will experience from the design of the institution and its administrative practices and policies, your daily professional relationships in that institution will be affected by some laws and regulations that govern all types of health care settings. The following pages illustrate some of the most widespread and important categories. They are examples only and not intended to be up to date in all cases because the details may change at any time. As a professional you are responsible for keeping current with all laws and regulations regarding your profession.

Laws and Regulations Requiring Professional Competence

In an effort to protect society from quacks and incompetent practitioners, all health care institutions that want to remain accredited by national and regional accrediting boards must take steps to ensure that their professional staff is well qualified to do the work they say they can do. In the United States, laws of every state include professional licensing, certification, and registration mechanisms whereby a person must pass a test and meet other qualifying characteristics to practice in that state. In other countries, provincial or national laws may be the rule. Some institutions go beyond the minimum requirements established by the government bodies by adding continuing education requirements for their own professional employees. Also, national certifying bodies (such as specialty boards in medicine, nursing, and other professions) have requirements pertaining to specialized and continued competence. Today many health professionals are personally responsible for negligence and other types of conduct that lead to malpractice claims, so institutions increasingly are requiring individuals to maintain personal malpractice insurance. These requirements should not have a negative impact on your work and may even have a positive effect because they have been developed over the years to help ensure that the basic tenets of respect are maintained for all who need your services. However, as is true of all laws and regulations, and as the Gary Larson cartoon on the next page illustrates, having a legal "license" to do something does not alone ensure adherence to society's expectations of what it has given permission for a person to do.

Laws and Regulations to Prevent Discrimination

Several nondiscrimination laws developed in the second half of the 20th century continue to have direct bearing on health care institutions in the United States, and similar ones have been crafted in other countries as well. Consider a few key examples:
- Title VII of the Civil Rights Act (1964) prohibits employers from refusing to hire an employee on the basis of race, color, sex, religion, or national origin.
- The Equal Opportunity Act buttressed and expanded Title VII in 1972.
- The Equal Pay Act of 1963 required that men and women receive equal pay for performing similar work.
- The Age Discrimination and Employment Act prohibiting discrimination against persons 40 to 70 years old was passed in 1967.
- The Rehabilitation Act (Section 504) of 1973 required all employers to have an affirmative action plan that includes hiring impaired persons. Superseding this act was the Americans with Disabilities Act of 1990, which states that institutions with more than 25 employees cannot use a physical examination to deny employment.
Understandably, policies continue to be introduced all the time and older ones evolve.

THE FAR SIDE®   By GARY LARSON

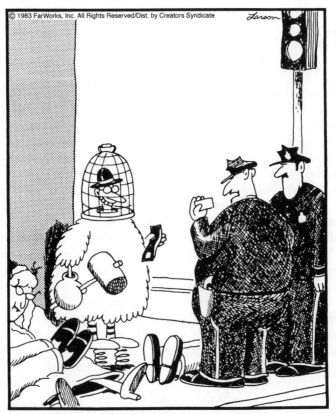

"Well, I'll be darned ... I guess he does have a license to do that."

Other Laws and Regulations

In addition to laws ensuring your professional competence to practice and prohibiting discrimination others have a direct bearing on your relationship with patients. For instance, prohibitions against some types of behavior such as touching a patient without his or her consent or sexual intercourse with patients are often written into licensing laws, as well as being reiterated in institutional policies and the ethical codes of professional organizations.

With the advent of the AIDS epidemic, numerous laws and policies were implemented nationally and within institutions to try to decrease the accidental transmittal of infections through body substances to health professionals, among patients, or to others. The most notable of these in the United States was the *Universal Precautions,* a federal mandate introduced in 1985 and later adjusted to be known as *standard precautions* by 1996. They require all health professionals to protect themselves and others by wearing certain types of protective clothing in treating any patient including gowns and gloves. Goggles or other equipment may have to be added while treating patients with infectious diseases and by adhering to strict methods for handling and disposing of body fluids, bandages, and needles. The requirements for the amount and type of protective devices vary according to the likelihood of body fluids being transferred from patient to health professional or vice versa.[5] For instance, an orthopedic surgery nurse or physician may become splattered from head to toe with blood during surgery and may receive a puncture wound from the slip of a scalpel or from a splintered or protruding bone. A dietitian or an occupational therapist, in comparison, is not likely to be in a situation of direct and extensive contact with body fluids. Some health professionals have worried that the "space capsule" appearance of the protective garb is damaging to health professional and patient rapport, although everyone agrees with the necessity of minimizing transmittal of viruses and other pathogens that reside in body fluids.

Depending on your area of service as a health professional, you may be regulated by other additional laws and regulations. In the United States, if you work in a clinical or laboratory area where blood and other body fluids are handled, you will be subject to an institution's safety standards set out by the Occupational Safety and Health Administration (OSHA). If you work with patients or clients who have sexually transmitted or other infectious diseases, you will be required to report this information to your state's department of health or similar governing body. In some instances this may create an ethical conflict for you if you do not want to break the patient's confidential information entrusted to you.

In the United States, if your patient population falls within reimbursement guidelines established by Medicare and Medicaid regulations, what you may offer in reimbursable services will be governed by those regulations. (Similar concerns of reimbursable services are an issue in almost all settings today.) Laws and regulations regarding the documentation of patient status, patient progress, and other patient information will affect the everyday practice of your profession. The medical record (whether electronic or hard copy) is a legal document, as are many other types of reports and statements you prepare for billings, quality assurance reviews, and other activities requiring data about patients and clients (Figure 2-4). Sometimes professionals treat documentation as a means of protecting their own interests legally. We prefer that you think of your documentation as a kind of travelogue of the journey you and the patient are taking during your professional encounter. Therefore, preparation of your documentation, like all other aspects of your interaction within the institution, should be undertaken first with respect for the patient's dignity and rights and then with respect for the type of professional you want the world to know you are.

Although this sampling of regulations and policies is not intended to be exhaustive, and focuses on situation in the United States, it illustrates that your relationship with society and the institution within which you practice is part and parcel of what you are able to do.

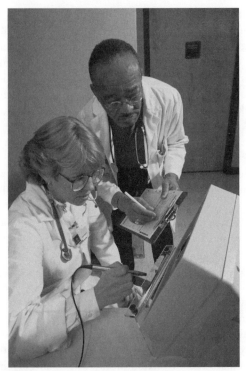

FIGURE 2-4: Health professionals at a computer entering data into electronic medical records. *(© Corbis.)*

Laws, Regulations, and Change

We conclude this section with a short reminder that laws and regulations are always in a state of flux. They deserve to be followed if you judge them to enhance your capacity to be respected and show respect in all your professional interactions. If they present major difficulties for you practically or ethically, you should reflect seriously on how you can help bring about their change. Like every generation of health professionals before you, you have an opportunity throughout your career to help shape a better environment for the health professions by working to change unworkable, unfair, or otherwise inadequate laws, regulations, and other policies. As we introduced in Chapter 1, the professional's freedom to bring about a caring response is the ultimate goal of health professionals, and all institutional activities must reflect that goal.

The process of changing unacceptable laws, regulations, and policy requires willingness, persistence, and courage. Some steps toward that end include the following:

▶ Document problems diligently
▶ Gain an understanding of the informal opinion leaders and formal authorities in the type of situation you want to change
▶ Identify colleagues with whom you can link arms to develop effective strategies for addressing your issue

▶ Be flexible and prepare to negotiate anew as new information comes your way
▶ Stay with the project until change is accomplished or you understand why it cannot be

Patients' Rights Documents

In health care institutions patients, too, have rights and incur responsibilities. Some that are protected by law have been mentioned. However, other rights not addressed by legal guidelines have come to be accepted as important.

Rights often named include the right to:

▶ Considerate and respectful care
▶ Accurate and complete information
▶ Participation (directly or through a legally appointed spokesperson) in health care decisions
▶ Privacy and confidentiality (within constraints of the law). There are rights to information about the institution itself (e.g., who owns it and what its overall services are) and the right to have continuity of care.

All U.S. readers of this book have been—or will be—introduced to the *Health Insurance Portability and Accountability Act (HIPAA) regulations,* which went into effect in 2003. The regulations, called the *New Federal Medical-Privacy Rule,* are designed to help protect patient privacy. They have had a profound effect on health professionals and health care institutions regarding the type of confidential information that can be transmitted into medical records and other information systems. The Rule also contains new requirements regarding information about research subjects. The following types of details are among the most important that may not be photocopied or faxed without specific authorization to do so by the patient: psychotherapy records, counseling about domestic violence, sexual assault counseling, HIV test results, records regarding sexually transmitted diseases, and social work records.[6] Moreover, as a health professional you are not allowed to provide current medical status and information about a patient to third parties, even family members.

◎ REFLECTIONS

> What rights and responsibilities of patients do you think should be included in nationally binding documents in your country of employment?

Grievance Mechanisms

In recent years several professional organizations and institutions have created grievance mechanisms to assist patients who believe their rights or other reasonable expectations are not being honored. Some institutions employ patient representatives, or ombudsmen, whose job is to listen to patients' problems and try to help solve them. Institutional ethics committees bring together health professionals and patients and their families as they try to determine what to do next in complex life-and-death decisions or to help resolve conflicts among various members of the group. The following story illustrates the type of differences that can arise around seemingly straightforward policy decisions affecting patients.

> You work in a long-term care facility that recently experienced an outbreak of scabies (a highly communicable skin disease caused by an arachnid, *Sarcoptes scabiei*, the itch mite). When the usual public health measures fail to prevent new and recurring cases, the decision is made by a committee of senior health professionals in the facility to treat all patients and staff with lindane. One patient, Cora Grosklaus, who is 82 years old, alert, and oriented, refuses the treatment that consists of a prolonged hot bath or shower with a thorough scrubbing followed by the application of the medication, particularly in the pubic area. Regardless of the explanations the staff has provided about the importance of the treatment for her well-being and that of others, Mrs. Grosklaus will have none of it, stating, "I will not submit to such humiliating treatment."[7]
>
> ▶ If you were a member of the team caring for Mrs. Grosklaus, how might you have gone about explaining to her the importance of the application?
>
> ▶ Where might a breakdown in communication have occurred, and what could have been done to possibly prevent this unhappy state of affairs?
>
> ▶ The measure being undertaken is believed by the health providers to benefit Mrs. Grosklaus, as well as be an important public health measure. What should be done if, like the team described earlier, you got nowhere in convincing her?

Sometimes health care institutions feel trapped by patients (or, in this case, long-term care facility residents) who refuse treatments that health professionals believe are necessary. Sometimes individuals do just the opposite of Cora—they insist on treatments that health professionals believe are inappropriate. At other times patients insist on going home before the health professionals believe they are ready. In the latter case, they are said to have left "AMA"—against medical advice. They may be asked to sign a document confirming that they have been informed of the physician's judgment but are choosing to act contrary to his or her advice.

The good news is that great strides have been made toward recognizing and respecting patients' preferences as an integral aspect of decision-making in health care institutions. At the same time, problems do remain. A part of the process of preparing to be a professional is to learn how to recognize, analyze, and help patients move toward an acceptable decision when differences create distress or an ethical dilemma.

Grievance mechanisms for employees are also available. Disputes about policies or practices, salary increases, work hours, and termination of employment are frequent reasons employees seek recourse through institutional processes designed for airing their disapproval and coming to resolution.[8]

An important area of employee protection has been implemented in recent years for personnel whose grievance involves their perception of wrongdoing by others in the institution. They are referred to in business as *whistle-blowers*. In the past the necessity of "blowing the whistle" on an incompetent, unethical, or impaired colleague was often suppressed by the realistic fear of reprisal. Fortunately today many institutions have developed processes and policies to protect the interests of everyone involved until the matter is investigated and resolved.[9] This is consistent with Glaser's statement in the graphic of the three realms that the good and virtuous institution "attends to the health, vigor, balance and equity of the institution's key systems."[2] To uphold this goal, adequate mechanisms must be in place to help ensure that an employee who documents the misconduct or debilitating condition of another employee is protected, as well as the person or unit against which the grievance is made.

SUMMARY

Respect within health care institutional environments requires the cooperation and responsible participation of individuals, institutional leaders, and society as a whole. Professionals' efforts at providing high quality care in a well-working setting will be fruitless without support from institutional leaders. At the same time, respect is so fundamental that you have an opportunity and duty to exercise it at all levels: as an individual professional, as an employee of the institution, and as a citizen. Today numerous legal regulations and guidelines help to shape health care institutions in ways that protect and honor the interests of everyone involved. When institutional policies, practices, or processes threaten to diminish or destroy a respectful environment, a professional's obligation extends to help constructively change the situation.

REFERENCES

1. Little ME: *Stranger in the mirror*, Bloomington, IN, 2006, Author House.
2. Glaser J: *Three realms of ethics*, Kansas City, MO, 1994, Sheed and Ward.
3. Scott WR: *Organizations: rational, natural and open systems*, Englewood Cliffs, NJ, 1981, Prentice Hall.
4. Goffman E: *Asylums*, Garden City, NY, 1961, Anchor Books.
5. U.S. Department of Health and Human Services: Public Health Service, Centers for Disease Control, *Morbidity and Mortality Weekly Report* 36(Suppl 25):55–65, 1987.
6. Federal Register: 67:53182-53273, 2002.
7. Bloche MG: Managing conflict at the end of life, *N Engl J Med* 352(23):2371–2376, 2005.
8. Purtilo R, Doherty R: *Ethical dimensions in the health professions*, St Louis, MO, 2011, Elsevier.
9. Miceli MP, Pollix-Near J, Dworkin TM: *Whistleblowing in organizations*, New York, 2008, Routledge.

Respect in a Diverse Society

Anyway, the patient will die, so what is the use of saying you are going to die of cancer, right? The doctor should say, "You are okay; you will be fine … Just take the medicine, which will get you better." He shouldn't say that you have cancer, so you will die in a few months. Isn't that common sense?

Korean-American Senior Citizen[1]

The first two chapters discussed the value context of individuals, as persons and professionals, and the institutional environment. Respect also involves sensitivity to individual and group differences. Thus, you may discover that, even with deep understanding of your personal values and clarity about the goals and values of the place where you work, respectful interaction still does not result. Yet to be considered is the fact that each person interprets actions, facial expressions, choice of words, and other forms of communication according to his or her cultural conditioning, past experience, and social context. All of these interactions take place within a society that, at least within the United States, has long been described as a "melting pot" in which all of the various cultures and beliefs blend together. The melting pot metaphor hides the negative side effects of such a view of American society that forces assimilation, which strips immigrants and refugees of long-standing cultural traditions and practices. Although some still hold to the melting pot description of the

United States, others claim it is no longer accurate and that it is more like "chunky stew," a stew savored both for the character of the individual ingredients (ethnically derived differences) and for the delicious melding of flavors (social integration).[2] Others countries, such as Canada, have traditionally likened society to a "vertical mosaic" with each person comprising an integral part of a complex but comprehensive picture.[3]

Furthermore, members of cultural groups can individually or collectively adapt to or borrow traits from other cultures, which is quite common when members of diverse cultures are in prolonged contact.[4] The phenomenon of merging cultures is called *acculturation*. In this chapter, we examine some of the cultural and social differences you will encounter in clinical practice and the barriers (e.g., personal and cultural biases, prejudices, discrimination) that get in the way of appreciating differences and inhibit respectful interaction.

Bias, Prejudice, and Discrimination

A *cultural bias* is a tendency to interpret a word or action according to a culturally derived meaning assigned to it. Cultural bias derives from cultural variation, discussed later in this chapter. For example, some cultures view smiles as a deeply personal sign of happiness that is only shared with intimates. Others view smiles as an indication of general friendliness to be shared with any and all. It is quite possible that another can interpret a friendly smile on the part of one person as disingenuous or inappropriate. Regarding health care, attitudes toward pain, methods of conveyance of bad news (such as the seemingly contradictory statement at the outset of this chapter by a Korean-American senior citizen), management of chronic illness and disability, beliefs about the seriousness and causes of illness, and death-related issues vary among different cultures. These different kinds of beliefs about disease and illness have an impact on health care–seeking behavior and acceptance of the advice, status, and intervention of health professionals. Understanding a patient's concept of health and illness is critical to the development of interaction strategies that are clinically sound and acceptable to the patient.

A *personal bias* is a tendency to interpret a word or action in terms of a personal significance assigned to it. It is found largely in what is commonly called *prejudice*. Personal bias can derive from culturally defined interpretations but can also originate from a number of other sources grounded in personal experience. The individual internalizes the cultural attitudes until he or she believes them to be entirely personal. Put another way, a personal bias is an individual's feeling about a particular person or thing that colors his or her interpretation of it. The bias can lead to more favorable or less favorable judgments than are deserved. This process is similar to that of internalizing societal values described in Chapter 1.

Understanding the way personal biases influence us and their effect on our attitudes and conduct are important to the health professional. Whenever bias is present, it affects the type of communication possible between the persons involved and therefore must be recognized as one determining factor in respectful interaction. In some cases, personal bias may produce a positive bias or "halo effect" on certain individuals; that is, a single characteristic or trait leads to positive, global judgments about a person. For example, a patient who is pleasant and cooperative during office visits could also be thought to be compliant with therapy because of the halo effect even though the opposite could be true. Although showing favoritism on the basis of personal bias alone is not permissible in the patient and health professional relationship, common interests can, of course, have legitimate positive effects on the relationship between two persons working together and thus improve the health professional and patient interaction.

Discrimination is negative, different treatment of a person or group. Usually it is derived from prejudice. *Prejudice* is "an aversive or hostile attitude toward a person who belongs to a group, simply because he belongs to that group, and is therefore assumed to have objectionable qualities ascribed to that group."[5] In this way we see how prejudicial attitudes manifest themselves in discriminatory behavior.

In short, every exchange between a patient and health professional undoubtedly will be influenced by cultural differences and other sources of personal bias. Sometimes these feelings will create an attitude of prejudice and a desire to discriminate. In Chapter 2, you were introduced to some of the laws that help define the legal limits to which discrimination can be pushed within the health care environment. However, despite legal guidelines, discrimination occurs craftily and evasively. You must watch for it in yourself and others because both parties involved are inevitably injured by the interaction. Gordon Allport, in his definitive work, *The Nature of Prejudice* (which, although written over 50 years ago, is still widely considered an authoritative study), warns, "It is a serious error to ascribe prejudice and discrimination to any single taproot, reaching into economic exploitation, social structure, the mores, fear, aggression, sex conflict, or any other favored soil. Prejudice and discrimination may draw nourishment from all these conditions and many others."[5] It should be emphasized that treating people differently because of race, religion, ethnicity, gender, or other attributes does not necessarily imply prejudice and discrimination. Respect for differences includes understanding when those differences should count, how they inform the responses of people, and the process of providing patient-centered care.

What can you learn from the previous pages? One thing you can discern is that the cultivation of respectful attitudes and conduct begins with self-examination and consideration of what cultural differences mean to you. This is not as easy as it may seem at first glance. It requires that you enter into a "difficult dialogue" (i.e., you are asked to reconsider long-held assumptions about individuals and groups that raise questions about your values and beliefs). Engagement in this type of activity may lead to feelings of discomfort and uneasiness.[6] These uncomfortable feelings result from the limited experience most of us have in interacting and talking with individuals different from ourselves.

We explore here a variety of differences, both obvious and subtle, that exist between people, such as differences in language, one of the most basic reasons for miscommunication—why, for example, even when we speak the same language, we may hear what a patient says but not understand its true meaning. Once you become aware of your often unconscious biases, you can more easily avoid being controlled by them in your interactions with others. Furthermore, by becoming aware of your hidden biases, you will be less likely to form inappropriate judgments about patients, colleagues, and others and more likely to remain sensitive and open to differences that influence your interactions with them.

Respecting Differences

A cursory look around almost any community in the United States or most other countries would indicate that we live in multicultural societies. Some assert that we are all " ... multi-cultural beings—living in worlds of multiple cultural identities. We are born into one world, and perhaps as adults live in another world where we move between cultural references of family, work, and community."[7] Sensitivity to cultural differences today has increased owing to the various underrepresented minority rights movements over the past several decades and the ever-growing percentage of ethnic minorities in the United States. In fact, in 2011 for the first time in U.S. history, babies born to ethnic minorities outnumbered the number of white toddlers.[8] According to the 2010 census, the national population was approximately 308,745,538; of this total, 16.3% self-identified as Hispanic or Latino; 12.6% as black or African American; 4.8% as Asian; and about 1% as American Indian, Alaskan native, Hawaiian native, or Pacific Islander.[8]

Clearly there is growing diversity on a national basis, but this change in the composition is also felt on the local level within urban and rural communities. Perhaps the shift in the makeup of the population is felt even more strongly in rural areas in which the arrival of refugees and other immigrants seeking jobs has dramatically changed the homogenous nature of communities. This growing diversity also has strong implications for the provision of health care. There is a significant underrepresentation of minorities in the health professions, which contributes to the disparity in the health status of minority groups—African Americans, Hispanics, Asian Americans, American Indians, Alaskan natives, Hawaiian natives, and Pacific Islanders. "A singular challenge facing health care institutions in this century will be assisting an essentially homogeneous group of health care professionals to meet the special needs of a culturally diverse society."[9]

Depending on where you live, you may be more or less aware of the percentage of persons from cultural, ethnic, and racial backgrounds that are different from your own who are living in your community. One way to identify the various cultural groups in your area is to use data from the U.S. Census Bureau, which is organized by state, county, and towns with populations greater than 5000 people. You can access the most recent information by going to the home page of the U.S. Census Bureau (http://quickfacts.census.gov). There you can find the cultures represented, the languages spoken, and other information about where you live and work.

In almost every health care setting, you will interact with patients of backgrounds different from your own. Certain differences are obvious; others are hidden. The iceberg model illustrates how much remains below the surface in our interactions with others (Figure 3-1). For example, we may quickly notice that a young woman is wearing a burka and come to the conclusion that she is Muslim, but we may not as easily know what practices of her faith or her culture could affect health care decisions (Figure 3-2). Health professionals generally believe they know a patient's race or gender merely by interacting with a patient, but, as you will see from further discussion

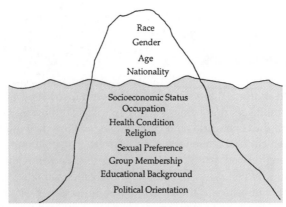

FIGURE 3-1: Iceberg model of multicultural influences on communication. *(From Krepp GL: Effective communication in multicultural health care settings, New York, 1994, Sage Publications. © 1994. Reprinted by permission of Sage Publications, Inc.)*

in this chapter, we may not be as accurate as we think in determining exactly who the person is sitting in front of us. With this limited information about potential differences, a professional can adjust communication patterns and approaches accordingly. However, it is more difficult to assess a patient's socioeconomic status or place of residence, two differences that can have as profound an effect on a patient's health

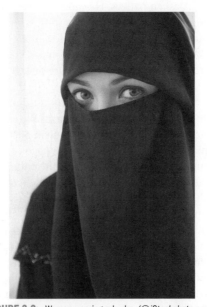

FIGURE 3-2: Woman wearing a burka. *(©iStockphoto.com.)*

beliefs or behavior as do visible attributes such as age and gender. The differences that are hidden may create more stress than those that can more readily be identified.

Even with experience, you may sometimes fail to appreciate significant differences in others with whom you interact. It is a continual challenge to look below the surface at the differences that affect interactions with patients and devise strategies to overcome barriers and facilitate communication. Many such differences have come to be viewed collectively as being characteristics of a person's "*culture*." However, just exactly what "*culture*" is or how the concept is to be used in health care interactions is open to a variety of interpretations. A broad definition of culture is the beliefs, customs, technological achievements, language, and history of a group of similar people.[10] A more nuanced understanding of culture is as follows:

> My position is that culture is a useful analytic category, provided it is understood as ubiquitous and intrinsic to all social arrangements. The concept encompasses local, tacit, largely unquestioned knowledge and practices, but aspects of culture can be debated, disputed, and put to work for political ends.[11]

So you can think of culture in terms of primary characteristics such as race/ethnicity, gender, and age and secondary characteristics such as place of residence, sexual orientation, and socioeconomic status that are all part of the web of social interactions in daily life. Cultural practices and beliefs can have a significant effect on the following health-related issues: diet, family rituals, healing beliefs, understanding of illness and causation, communication process and style, death rituals, spirituality, values, art, and history. Because culture has such a broad impact on health and because of the increasing diversity in the United States, "cultural competence has gained attention as a potential strategy to improve quality and eliminate racial/ethnic disparities in health care."[12] We turn your attention to a difference that is the root of numerous conflicts between social groups—race.

Race

Race is one characteristic of culture almost always mentioned in discussions about cultural differences and is perhaps the characteristic or descriptor most fraught with controversy. However, even the distinctions used by the U.S. Census Bureau constitute a system based on outmoded concepts and dubious assumptions about genetic difference. The 1999 Institute of Medicine Report edited by Haynes and Smedley stated that in all instances race is a social and cultural construct based on perceived differences in biology, physical appearance, and behavior.[13] An editorial in *Nature Genetics* flatly stated, "Scientists have long been saying that at a genetic level there is more variation between two individuals in the same population than between populations and that there is no biological basis for race."[14] If the biological understanding of race seems to have been settled, that is not the case. Postgenomic science has revived the idea of racial categories as proxies for biological differences and with it a revival of controversy and new opportunities for discrimination.[15] At a minimum the present idea of race clearly has social meaning because it assigns status, limits opportunities, and influences interactions between health professionals and patients.[16] Take a moment to reflect on the race categories listed in Box 3-1 that are presently being used to classify people by the U.S. Census Bureau.

BOX 3-1

How are the race categories used in Census 2010 defined?

The standards have five categories for data on race: American Indian or Alaska Native, Asian, Black or African American, Native Hawaiian or Other Pacific Islander, and White. There are two categories for data on ethnicity: "Hispanic or Latino" and "Not Hispanic or Latino."

Categories and Definitions

American Indian or Alaska Native. A person having origins in any of the original peoples of North and South America (including Central America) and who maintains tribal affiliation or community attachment.

Asian. A person having origins in any of the original peoples of the Far East, Southeast Asia, or the Indian subcontinent including, for example, Cambodia, China, India, Japan, Korea, Malaysia, Pakistan, the Philippine Islands, Thailand, and Vietnam.

Black or African American. A person having origins in any of the black racial groups of Africa. Terms such as "Haitian" or "Negro" can be used in addition to "Black or African American."

Native Hawaiian or Other Pacific Islander. A person having origins in any of the original peoples of Hawaii, Guam, Samoa, or other Pacific Islands.

White. A person having origins in any of the original peoples of Europe, the Middle East, or North Africa.

From U.S. Office of Management and Budget, www.whitehouse.gov/imb/fedreg/1997standards.html. Accessed December 2, 2011.

⊙ REFLECTIONS

- Consider the following quote: "The fact that we know what 'race' we are says more about our society than it does about biology."[17]
- What is society's role in the determination of racial categories?
- Would someone meeting you for the first time place you in the same racial category or categories you chose for yourself?

The same difficulty with racial identification can occur with your patients as well.

Although it is generally true that patient treatment and counseling are more effective when obtained from members of one's self-identified racial group, it does not mean that patients must always be treated by members of the same race to receive quality care. First of all, this would not be possible because there are so few health professionals who are underrepresented minorities. Second, it is possible to learn how to appropriately work with patients different from our own racial and ethnic backgrounds through sensitivity, knowledge, and skills in cross-cultural communication.

There are other barriers to be overcome between patients and health professionals that are, unfortunately, deeply tied to notions of race. In a national study conducted by the Institutes of Medicine on disparities in health care, evidence indicated that stereotyping, biases, and uncertainty on the part of health care providers can all contribute to unequal treatment.[18] Additionally, there are ample historical reasons for members of minority populations to mistrust the health care system. For example, in the not-too-distant past, African American patients were refused treatment at "white-only" hospitals. Some were undertreated and deceived in the infamous Tuskegee syphilis study. Mistrust in the health care system on the part of African Americans continues to this day because of these historical events and continuing discriminatory events in health care.[19] Gaining the trust of patients whose racial identity is different from one's own is a challenge but not an insurmountable one if a health professional can show that his or her aim is to be "trustworthy" so as to be able to provide optimal care and minimize and eventually eliminate disparities in care.

One of the first steps in reducing disparities in the health care setting is to be aware that they exist. For example, not long ago one of the authors participated in an ethics consultation regarding an extremely ill newborn. The African American parents of the baby looked around the table of health professionals gathered for the meeting. The father quietly commented, "I'd feel a whole lot better about this if there was one other black face besides the two of us at this table." Although all of the health professionals present were there for the good of the baby and his family, the lack of representation of someone of the parents' self-identified racial group was a significant barrier to the discussion and, ultimately, to the decisions made. If the father had not made the comment, the health professionals involved probably would never have noticed the circle of white faces surrounding the parents.

The preceding example indicates that there may be justifiable reasons to consider social categories of race when making clinical decisions. Another situation in which race (and ethnicity) may be a reason for differential treatment is when certain medications are prescribed because both can, in certain cases, affect disease pathophysiology and drug metabolism.[20,21] "Certain genetic variations may well correlate with groups whose ancestors lived in particular regions (e.g., the sickle-cell trait is found in areas of western Africa, the Mediterranean, and southeast India, where malaria has long been prevalent). These correlations can help in identifying and treating diseases."[22]

Race and ethnic background can also influence dietary habits and other activities of daily living that have a direct impact on health care outcomes. Although different treatment based on race or ethnicity may be justified in special cases such as those mentioned, it is the exception, not the rule. You must remain alert for unjustified differences in care based on race or ethnicity.

Gender

Gender issues interact with other primary and secondary characteristics of culture to shape a person's identity. There are many implications for assessment and treatment of patients based on differences in gender. Gender inequities in health status and health care access exist worldwide and are strongly related to other social determinants of health such as education and economic status. Women in developing countries often lack access to basic health care and suffer from domestic violence and murder at a higher rate than their counterparts in countries with more education and economic resources.[23] However, even in the relatively affluent United States, women have a history of unequal access to sources of economic and political power that impacts access to health care resources.[24] This is especially true for African American women or older women who experience the combined impact of race, gender, and age discrimination. Gender inequities in health care are inexcusable but often subtle and unfortunately widespread. At the same time it is also important to simultaneously acknowledge differences that should be taken into consideration and accommodated in planning and delivering care.

Let us take as an example the preferences of patients regarding the gender of their physician. Numerous studies have documented the fact that 20% to 56% of women explicitly prefer a female physician for women's health problems.[25,26] Because many women feel uncomfortable and perhaps embarrassed during a gynecological examination, they may prefer female physicians because they are familiar with the female body and have firsthand experience with the examination. If women are more comfortable with the examination, then they will be more likely to follow through with checkups and follow the recommendations of the physician. A recent study shows that outside of the specialty of obstetrics and gynecology, communication skills was the most important factor for women patients regarding their interaction with a physician.[27] The challenge for all health professionals is to adopt behaviors and communication styles to compensate for any differences from their patients.

A patient's preference for a health professional of the same gender may not only be a personal but also a cultural or religious one. Many cultural groups are concerned about modesty and may require that only a female health professional examine a female patient's genitalia or be present when the patient is undressed. Gender differences regarding modesty can have direct implications for diagnosis and treatment, as is evident in the following case.

A 50-year-old female peasant from Mexico is seen in the clinic. The patient's 35-year-old son accompanies her. The woman has been coming to the clinic for some time. Her son usually interprets because she does not speak English. An interpreter who is employed by the clinic is called because the son has to leave for work and cannot stay and translate for his mother. Before they enter the room, the physician discloses to the female interpreter that he is concerned about whether the health problems claimed by this woman are real or imagined. She has been in the clinic three times before, each time with different vague and diffuse complaints, none of which make medical sense. The physician learns through the translator that the woman has a fistula in her rectum. In her previous visits, she could not bring herself to reveal her true symptoms in the presence of, and therefore to, her son as he interpreted for her. She was so embarrassed that she invented other symptoms to justify visits to the physician. She wanted someone else to interpret but did not know how she could ask because she would have to speak through her son.[28]

Although some problems in this example occurred because of differences in gender, they were compounded by language barriers. The case offers insight into the problems that can arise when language is a primary barrier. Since 1999, federal and state laws require that full language access to health care services be available in health care institutions receiving federal funds.[29] The concerns and issues related to limited English proficiency and interpreters will be addressed in more detail in Chapter 9.

Age

The particular form of stigma associated with being old is related to the prejudices of an ageist society. The word *ageism* was coined to designate the discriminatory treatment of old people (as sexism was coined to describe the systematic devaluation of one sex on both an individual and a societal basis).

Older adults are constantly confronted with ageist conduct in their day-to-day interactions with others. Unfortunately, ageist conduct occurs in the health care environment as well. Older patients often receive less attention or are denied services on the basis of their age alone. Physical and psychological problems may not be addressed because health professionals assume that they are normal for an older person. Additionally, older patients are highly complex regarding the number and types of health problems they possess, so more time is necessary when diagnosing and treating them. Older patients are prime targets for overmedication and experience the effects of poorly coordinated care. Regardless of his or her state of health or physical ability, an elderly patient is commonly met with a patronizing attitude. Ways in which you can overcome the tendencies to engage in ageist behavior are discussed in more detail in Chapter 15.

Ethnicity

Ethnicity refers to a person's sense of belonging to a group of people sharing a common origin, history, and set of social beliefs. Recall from the broad definition of "culture" earlier in this chapter that ethnicity counts as one of the primary characteristics of culture along with race, age, and gender. Ethnicity may also refer to an individual's place of geographical or national origin. For example, the U.S. Census Bureau states that Hispanics may be of any race.[8]

It used to be easy to identify an ethnicity-based cultural variation because one could readily distinguish among the various ways of doing things in different parts of the world. Frequently, early explorers were stunned by the practices they encountered as norms in cultures, and all too often they used the occasion to demean or diminish the importance of the cultural practices of other societies. The world often seems small today with the movement of large groups of people due to war and famine. Health professionals who encounter these displaced refugees in their own communities may be just as stunned as the early explorers were, as is evident in this excerpt from Anne Fadiman's comprehensive work on the Hmong refugees in *The Spirit Catches You and You Fall Down*:

> When refugees from Laos started settling in Merced County in the early 1980s, none of the doctors at [Merced County Medical Center] MCMC had ever heard of the word "Hmong," and they had no idea what to make of their new patients. They wore strange clothes—often children's clothes, which were approximately the right size—acquired at the Goodwill. When they undressed for examination, the women were sometimes wearing Jockey shorts and the men were sometimes wearing bikini underpants with

little pink butterflies. They wore amulets around their necks and cotton strings around their wrists (the sicker the patient, the more numerous the strings). They smelled of camphor, mentholatum, Tiger Balm, and herbs. When they were admitted to the hospital, they brought their own food and herbs.[30]

Today, in most parts of the world, a large variety of influences such as Internet access and social media, telecommunications, the ease of global travel, and the presence of foreign visitors affect what used to be traditional, homogeneous cultures. Although the United States has a history of immigration from various parts of the world, "Never before has the United States received immigrants from so many countries, from such different social and economic backgrounds, and for so many reasons."[31] A result is that it is often more challenging to sort out and identify specific cultural differences that modify behavior in various ethnic groups.

Sometimes as a health professional you may have a difficult time remembering that members of an ethnic group cannot be expected to be homogeneous. Their ethnicity is only one characteristic of the culture or cultures they bring to their present experience. For example, an outstanding physician and friend of the authors grew up in rural Nigeria; studied as an undergraduate in Scotland; took her medical training at Johns Hopkins University in Baltimore, Maryland; and now practices in the heart of Midwest America. When asked if she had difficulty "adjusting" to the Midwest, she said that she simply brought along to "this new culture" the best of what she had the opportunity to accumulate along the way! At times, each of us becomes aware of cultural beliefs held by an individual that, on the surface, seem to be incongruent. For example, a Chinese American may be highly assimilated into the majority culture and seek mainstream health care for a gastrointestinal disorder yet also seek care from a traditional Chinese healer who might prescribe herbs, teas, or other forms of therapies appropriate for his culture. Because we can identify with individual variations in our own cultural beliefs and the blending of seemingly opposite beliefs that can occur within us as individuals, we must appreciate the profound variability that can exist within cultural groups.

One of the widest cultural gaps you will encounter in your role as a health professional is that created by the "ethnocentrism" of health professionals. (Although separate professions often are not thought of as cultures in themselves, they are.) *Ethnocentrism* is the belief that one's own cultural ways are superior. Health professionals often believe that their way is best and so are guilty of medical ethnocentrism. In fact, while you are a student you are learning and adopting the culture of your chosen health profession. The culture of a health professional encompasses the interrelationships of professional values, beliefs, customs, habits, and symbols. You are learning the cultural meaning that your profession gives to concepts such as pain, disability, disease, and illness. You will find that even within the culture of the health professions, there are different meanings and understandings of identical phenomena. Thus, as an individual you may share the same ethnic origin, race, and gender as the patient you are working with and yet not hold the same beliefs and perspectives about some important values related to what his or her care should involve.

The following poem, used here with the author's permission, demonstrates how difficult it can be to reach across the ethnic and other cultural gaps between health professional and patient. Recall the quote from the Korean-American senior citizen that opened the chapter and how this poem echoes the delicate task of holding truth and hope in balance:

4/2

She came into the room smiling.
"This is the real thing," said the interpreter.
"Sientese," I said, gesturing to the chair, grateful for my limited Spanish.
I asked her questions about cancer and illness.
"Only Americans talk of dying of cancer," she said.
I asked her questions about cancer and illness.
"Look in the eyes, you can tell by the eyes," she said.
I looked in her eyes.
I asked her questions about cancer and illness.
"The curanderas use objects and herbs for healing.
They have their own way of speaking.
No one else understands them."
She looked at me.
"That's all," she said. She stood.
that's all that's all that's all
whispered ancestor spirits
holders of ancient wisdom
written in Aztec
kept in jars and pots
herbs animals
stones
goat's milk
"That's all," she said.
she smiled
she left the room.
                    —Jolene Siemsen

Socioeconomic Status

The vast majority of U.S. and Canadian health professionals are white, with average incomes that are in the upper-middle to high economic range when considered globally. The income level and accompanying higher social status of health professionals tend to create barriers in their relationships with patients. "Ethnic minority groups and economically disadvantaged individuals may have particular difficulty feeling in control within a setting dominated by well-educated professionals."[32] The difference in socioeconomic status may hinder patients from asking you important questions, hinder you from empathizing with patients, and limit your knowledge of the practical everyday obstacles that prevent or facilitate the ability of patients to pursue medication or treatment regimens.[33] The following case highlights the challenges some patients face just getting to a medical appointment.

> A young mother and her two small children, a toddler and a 3-month-old, leave their apartment at 7:00 a.m. for a 9:00 a.m. clinic visit. With the baby in a stroller and the toddler at his mother's side, they head for the bus stop that is four blocks from their home. The first bus is late because of icy conditions. She will have to transfer three times to get to the clinic and walk two blocks to the clinic building. She arrives at the clinic 45 minutes late for her 9:00 a.m. appointment. The medical assistant at the intake desk looks at the clock as the mother signs in and says, "Couldn't you have called if you were going to be late?"

We will address different interpretations of time in Chapter 9, but in this case there is no disagreement between the clinic staff and the patient about what "on time" is. The medical assistant does not understand the complications that arise from having to be dependent on public transportation or the hassle of, let alone finding and using, a pay phone while juggling two small children in the cold. The fact that this patient actually made it to the clinic is testament to her desire to receive care. Yet this fact becomes lost in complaints about the patient's tardiness and lack of consideration for the clinic staff. Health professionals may take for granted owning a car or a cell phone, items that could be completely beyond the financial means of some patients.

The difference in social class and economic status also affects the type and frequency of interaction between patient and health professional outside the health care setting. The informal networks that exist in neighborhoods and communities provide opportunities to establish cooperation, exchange information, and determine appropriate behavior. "For instance, minority patients might be described as 'non-compliant' by clinicians (who mainly have been socialized in a white urban middle-class milieu) when, in fact, the patients are 'following the rules,' but rules that are based on a different set of principles."[34] For example, a patient may be told to "get daily exercise" to improve her health and "just go for a walk," which sounds easy for someone who lives in a safe neighborhood. But in a crime-ridden area, a walk around the block could be seen as foolhardy and dangerous.

Outsiders can make unintentional errors in judgment because they underestimate the effects of ethnicity, age, or class on insiders' responses or actions; that is, the responses and actions of individuals born or socialized into membership of the group. Outsiders must work to "get in," to gain, build, and maintain trust with a group.[35]

Level of education is another difference between health professionals and patients related to socioeconomic status. Although patients may respect education in the abstract, they may also be suspicious that you will use your education to take advantage of them rather than to assist them. Patients may also be too intimidated to admit when they do not understand something. For fear that they will be seen as ignorant or superstitious, patients may neglect to mention that they are also seeking alternative methods of care or providers. Even when patients are well educated, they may not speak the dominant language well enough to adequately express themselves. For example, a French tourist in the United States was in a minor accident that required an emergency department visit. The patient, an attorney, spoke some English, but told the nurse in the triage unit that she would feel better if she could talk to someone in French because, "I lack eloquence in English." You may understand what the French patient means if you have struggled to make yourself understood across a language barrier. It is important to remember that the "language" of health care is often foreign to patients as well. In Chapter 9 we discuss in more detail how language and vocabulary, which are partially a result of education, can facilitate or block what patients perceive as respect from you.

Occupation and Place of Residence

One of the first questions we often ask a new acquaintance in a social setting is, "What do you do?" We deeply identify with our occupations in mainstream American culture. Some would go so far as to say that their occupation defines who they are more than their ethnicity or other primary characteristics. Occupations shape how people see the world and what they value. The importance of a person's occupation is sometimes seen more clearly when injury, illness, or retirement forces a change in occupation. How patients occupy themselves, whether they spend their time in the formal workforce or not, can give important cultural clues that have an impact on health care beliefs and decisions.

We do not often think of place of residence as a cultural variable in our interactions with patients, yet there is increasing evidence that place of residence has an impact on how patients think about health. For example, certain health beliefs and practices sometimes differ between urban and rural patients. Rural patients, because of their environment, must often travel a considerable distance to see a health professional. Thus, rural patients are often more independent regarding the use of health care services than their urban counterparts. Another significant difference between rural and urban dwellers is the way health needs are viewed. Rural dwellers, both male and female, from a variety of locations, tend to determine health needs primarily in relation to work activities.[36] Thus, it is important to consider not only where someone lives but the other cultural values that they bring to their place of residence.

A striking example of the impact values held by rural dwellers can have on health decisions is evident in the following case:

Michael T. is a 61-year-old wheat farmer. He maintains his large and profitable family farm with the help of his wife, three sons, and occasional hired help. He has managed and actively worked on the same farm for almost 40 years. Mr. T. attended the state university for 2 years, studying agribusiness. By his state's standards he is well educated; he is in the middle-income bracket. During the harvesting season, he often works parts of the fields alone with the help of rented heavy farm equipment. Two years ago while working in this way, he caught the middle finger of his right hand in a moving part of his equipment while he was adjusting a machine component. He could not pull his finger free, and the injury was quite painful. Mr. T. realized that it might be some time before anyone would come to his aid. The weather was changing, and he needed to complete the harvesting work in the field to avoid

Continued

damage to the wheat crop and prevent additional equipment rental costs. He decided to pull his hand free, severing his finger at its base. He was able to control the bleeding with a tightly bound handkerchief, and he completed harvesting the field.

When he returned home, his son drove him to the nearest town, 57 miles away, where he sought care in the hospital emergency department.

The physician who saw Mr. T. was distressed that he had not retrieved the digit and sought care immediately. While dressing Mr. T.'s wound, the physician explained that, with prompt action and air ambulance transport to the state's major medical center, it might have been possible for the finger to be reattached.

Fortunately, Mr. T. did not develop an infection or other serious complication after his injury. He was able to manage his farm as usual once he healed. When he tells neighbors about the story of this event, he often comments, "It simply goes to show you that, if you go to those doctors too soon, you end up with lots of unnecessary treatment and bills."[37]

Let us return to the case and see how the health professionals involved responded to the situation.

Before continuing with the rest of the case, consider what your reaction might be if you were the first health professional to interact with Mr. T. when he arrived at the emergency department.

▶ Do you think Mr. T. is brave, stupid, shortsighted, practical, hard-working, frugal, or a combination of these characteristics?
▶ If you had been in his position, what would you have done?
▶ How might these personal values and cultural beliefs affect your ability to interact with Mr. T.?

Mr. T. no doubt shares many of the attitudes and beliefs about health status and health care that his urban counterparts do, but his place of residence introduces additional cultural variables. Rural residents tend to value self-reliance more than urban residents. Rural residents, particularly farmers, often are required to maintain a higher level of physical fitness as they take care of yard work, tend animals, manage the maintenance of and use heavy machinery, etc. Their ability to accomplish all of these tasks is tied to their self-identity and self-worth.[38] None of these underlying values would have been obvious to the health professionals who cared for Mr. T. unless they attempted to understand his background.

Whether a patient lives on a farm, in the inner city, or in the suburbs, you will show respect when you are mindful of the impact place of residence can have on interactions with patients. This is especially true when the patient does not have a permanent place of residence or is homeless. The challenges of working with patients whose only home is the streets include major issues such as ensuring the safety and basic well-being of the patient, but also practical considerations unique to this environment such as the need for access to a bathroom or to a source of clean drinking water. Persons who live on the street either by choice or necessity are part of a subculture that is often hidden from view and require openness and understanding from health professionals.

Religion

Another feature of culture that influences your relationship with patients is religious beliefs. Religion gives meaning to illness, pain, and suffering. Religious beliefs are often most apparent when a patient is seriously injured, critically ill, or dying. For example, the Christian faith, with its valuing of human life and belief in eternal life, states that whereas a struggle for health can be meaningful, a struggle against death at all costs to the point that the effort becomes a torment is nonsense.[39] The Christian cultural view of the dying process and death itself influences treatment decisions and may promote requests for symbolically meaningful activities such as receiving the sacraments.

A different view of illness is evident with believers in Islam. "The word *Islam* means to submit; that is, to submit their lives to the will of God (Allah). A fatalistic worldview is common whereby the person attributes the incidence and outcome of a health condition to "inshallah." This belief can make preventive health behaviors or self-care programs difficult to institute. Because God is perceived to be in control of the outcome, what can humans do?[40] However, what may appear to be "fatalistic" could also be shaped by another Muslim duty regarding stewardship of one's body and health. This duty prescribes clear responsibility for one's health. Thus, once again, there is more to culture and beliefs than appears on the surface.

Christian, Jewish and Muslim beliefs are widespread and relatively well known; therefore, health professionals may not find much difficulty in recognizing them. Religious beliefs that are far removed from mainstream religious traditions may challenge health care professionals' understanding, tolerance, and willingness to make accommodations.

Sexual Orientation

In modern society, sexual orientation is yet another characteristic of culture that may elicit biased responses to a person. Gay, lesbian, bisexual, and transgender patients are often treated differently because of sexual orientation. One commonality among gay men and lesbians is that they may hide their lifestyle for fear of prejudicial attitudes and discrimination. Thus, the sexual orientation of patients may be somewhat invisible. However, given the number of men and women who report being homosexual (and that number is probably an underestimate of the actual total), it is highly likely that most health professionals provide care to gay, lesbian, bisexual, or transgender patients.

In an interesting study, undergraduate health professions students focused on their discomfort with a variety of persons from differing cultural groups. The students reported the most consistently negative attitudes toward lesbian, gay, and bisexual people.[41] Because of unexamined homophobia, many health professionals react with shock or thinly veiled unease when they learn that a patient is not heterosexual. This discomfort is evidence that these health professionals view "normal" as being heterosexual.

In addition to the negative attitudes expressed by health professionals toward patients with a sexual orientation different from their own, gay, lesbian, bisexual, and transgender patients find themselves in a health care system that is built on heterosexual assumptions to the extent that women who seek gynecological or obstetrical care may not even be asked about their sexual history. Lesbian and gay patients' partners may not be formally acknowledged. Providing sensitive, culturally appropriate care requires taking the patient's sexual orientation fully into account and ensuring that the information is used to optimize his or her quality of care.

Cultural Sensitivity, Competence, and Humility

The overall lesson to be gleaned from the preceding description of various cultural characteristics is that the atmosphere in health care must rest on fully appreciating what each culture brings to the richness of our society and on acceptance, not on fear and misunderstanding.

What is needed is an approach to each patient, client, and colleague that takes into account cultural differences and that begins with cultural sensitivity (i.e., appreciating that you are a multicultural being, as are others). *Cultural sensitivity* is a necessary foundation for becoming culturally competent. *Cultural competence* is " ... an ongoing process in which the health care professional continually strives to achieve the ability and availability to work effectively within the cultural context of the patient (individual, family, and community)."[42] An important component of becoming culturally competent is the ability to conduct a cultural assessment when interacting with patients. Among numerous cultural assessment tools in the literature, one set of questions developed by Kleinman stands out because the questions focus on the patient's perspective regarding illness:

◗ What do you call your problem? What name does it have?
◗ What do you think has caused your problem? Why do you think it started when it did?
◗ What do you think your sickness does to you? How does it work?
◗ How severe is it? Will it have a short or long course?
◗ What do you fear the most about your sickness?
◗ What are the chief problems your sickness has caused for you?
◗ What kind of treatment do you think you should receive? What are the most important results you hope to receive from this treatment?[43]

Regardless of the patient's cultural background, the preceding questions are a logical and respectful place to start in trying to understand what brought the patient to the health care encounter.

Finally, cultural humility is a component of becoming culturally competent but requires more than knowledge about cultural practices. Cultural humility requires commitment to ongoing self-reflection and self-critique, particularly identifying and examining one's own patterns of unintentional and intentional racism.[44] In Chapter 1, you were reminded to approach each patient with respect. This means, among other things, consciously avoiding unfair judgments about other people's traditions, values, and beliefs. We are much more likely to respect a patient's decision or action if we understand its rationale. Misunderstandings can result in harm to the patient in that he or she may hesitate to seek medical attention or follow the advice of someone so out of touch with his or her beliefs.

One barrier to respectful interaction is the tendency for health professionals to adopt stereotypes and expect certain behaviors from patients from a particular culture simply because they are from that culture. Avoid scripted remarks such as "Jewish patients believe … " or "All Chinese patients practice … " because it is impossible to generalize from one patient to an entire culture. "Although some behaviors may appear similar within an identified cultural group, the astute health provider must assess for differences both within and between groups to plan appropriate care."[45]

In the face of cultural differences you will need basic negotiation skills. This means finding a place where you can feel confident in the exercise of your professional judgment yet incorporate the beliefs and values of patients into their treatment plan to achieve mutually desirable outcomes. The goal of cultural humility is to provide care characterized by respect. Such care is meaningful and fits with cultural beliefs and ways of life for those involved. Beause diversity in society is likely to increase rather than decrease in the coming years, access to the most current statistics regarding demography and tools to assist in providing culturally appropriate care is vitally important. Box 3-2 provides a list of web resources to assist you in obtaining the most current information.

BOX 3-2

Web Resources for Delivering Culturally Appropriate Care

National Center for Cultural Competence	http://gucchd.georgetown.edu/nccc
U.S. Administration on Aging	www.aoa.gov
Stanford Geriatric Education Center	http://sgec.stanford.edu
American Society on Aging	www.asaging.org
Center for Applied Linguistics	www.cal.org
ALTA Language Services	www.altalang.com
The Cross Cultural Health Program	www.xculture.org
Culture Clues	http://depts.washington.edu/pfes/CultureClues.htm
Culture, Language and Health Literacy	www.hrsa.gov/culturalcompetence/index.html
Ethnogeriatrics and Cultural Competence for Nursing Practice	http://bit.ly/rpaTzu

All accessed January 31, 2012.

SUMMARY

The issues relevant to showing respect in the midst of diversity must continually be examined and reflected on. The only constructive approach to evaluating human differences with the goal of showing respect is to take each experience as an opportunity to learn more about the rich diversity of the human condition and to take what one learns as a gift that will enrich one's own life.

REFERENCES

1. Blackhall L, Frank G, Murphy S, Michel V: Bioethics in a different tongue: the case of truth-telling, *J Urban Health Bull NY Acad Med* 78(1):59–71, 2001. (quote p. 64).
2. Spencer M, Markstrom-Adams C: Identity processes among racial and ethnic minority children in America, *Child Dev* 61:290–310, 1990.

3. Porter J: *Vertical mosaic: an analysis of social class and power in Canada*, Toronto, 1965, University of Toronto Press.
4. National Health Service Corps: *Bridging the cultural divide in health care settings: the essential role of cultural broker programs*, Rockville, MD, 2004, U.S. Department of Health and Human Services. (quote p. vii.).
5. Allport G: *The nature of prejudice*, Reading, MA, 1954, Addison-Wesley.
6. Baldwin D, Nelms T: Difficult dialogues: impact on nursing education curricula, *J Prof Nurs* 9(6):343–346, 1993.
7. Marshall P, Koenig B: 2004. Accounting for culture in a globalized society, *J Law Med Ethics* 32:252–266, 2004. (quote p. 259.).
8. U.S. Department of Commerce: *U.S. Census Bureau, Population Division, Population Projections Branch.* Washington, DC, 2010 (website) http://2010census.com.
9. Jones ME, Cason CL, Bond ML: Cultural attitudes, knowledge and skills of a health workforce, *J Transcult Nurs* 15(4):283–290, 2004.
10. Johnson FA: Contributions of anthropology to psychiatry. In Goldman H, editor: *Review of psychiatry*, ed 2, Norwalk, CT, 1988, Appleton & Lange.
11. Lock M: Situated ethics, culture, and the brain death "problem" in Japan. In Hoffmater B, editor: *Bioethics in social context*, Philadelphia, 2001, Temple University Press, pp 39–68. (quote p. 43).
12. Betancourt JR, Green AR, Carrillo JE, Park ER: Cultural competence and health care disparities: key perspectives and trends, *Health Affairs* 24:499–505, 2005.
13. Haynes MA, Smedley BD, editors: *The unequal burden of cancer: an assessment of NIH research and programs for ethnic minorities and the medically underserved. Institute of Medicine*, Washington DC, 1999, National Academies Press.
14. Editorial, Genes, drugs and race, *Nature Genetics* 29:239–240, 2001.
15. Koenig BA, Lee SJ, Richardson SS, editors: *Revisiting race in a genomic age*, New Brunswick, NJ, 2008, Rutgers University Press, p 1.
16. Pinderhughes E: *Understanding race, ethnicity, and power*, New York, 1989, Free Press.
17. Kreiger N, Bassett M: The health of black folk: disease, class and ideology in science, *Mon Rev* 38:74–85, 1986.
18. Smedley B, Stith A, Nelson A, editors: *Committee on understanding and eliminating racial and ethnic disparities in health care, Institutes of Medicine,* Unequal treatment: confronting racial and ethnic disparities in healthcare, Washington, DC, 2003, The National Academies Press, p 1.
19. Scharf DP, Matthews KJ, Jackson P, et al: More than Tuskegee: understanding mistrust about research participation, *J Health Care Poor Underserved* 21(3):879–897, 2010.
20. Hines SE: Caring for diverse populations: intelligent prescribing in diverse populations, *Patient Care* 34(9):135–136, 2000. 139–140, 142.
21. Lin KM, Smith MW: Psychopharmacotherapy in the context of culture and ethnicity. In Ruiz P, editor: *Ethnicity and psychopharmacology,* vol 19(4), review of psychiatry, Washington, DC, American Psychiatric Press, 2000.
22. Kahn J: Getting the numbers right: statistical mischief and racial profiling in heart failure research, *Perspect Biol Med* 46(4):473–483, 2003.
23. Diaz-Granados N, Pitzul KB, Dorado LM et al: Monitoring gender equity in health using gender sensitive indicators: a cross national study, *J Womens Health* 20(1):145–153, 2011.
24. Conway-Turner K: Older women of color: a feminist exploration of the intersections of personal, familial and community life, *J Women Aging* 11(2/3):115–130, 1999.
25. Kerssens JJ, Bensing JM, Andela MG: Patient preferences for genders of health professionals, *Soc Sci Med* 44:1531–1540, 1997.
26. Delgado A, Lopez-Fernandez LA, Luna JD: Influence of the doctor's gender in the satisfaction of users, *Med Care* 31:795–800, 1993.
27. Mavis B, Vasilenko P, Schnuth R et al: Female patients' preferences related to interpersonal communications, clinical competence, and gender when selecting a physician, *Acad Med* 80(12):1159–1165, 2005.

28. Haffner L: Translation is not enough: interpreting in a medical setting, *West J Med* 157(3):256, 1992.
29. Executive Order 13166, "Improving Access to Services for Persons with Limited English Proficiency," August 16, 2000; 65 Fed Reg 50121.
30. Fadiman A: *The spirit catches you and you fall down*, New York, 1997, The Noon Day Press. (quote p. 64).
31. Portes A, Rumbaut R: *Immigrant America: a portrait*, ed 2, Berkeley, 1997, University of California Press.
32. Ramer L, Richardson JL, Cohen MZ et al: Multimeasure pain assessment in an ethnically diverse group of patients with cancer, *J Transcult Nurs* 10(2):94–101, 1999.
33. Waitzkin H: *The politics of medical encounters: how patients and doctors deal with social problems*, New Haven, CT, 1991, Yale University Press.
34. Fineman N: The social construction of non-compliance: implications for cross-cultural geriatric practice, *J Cross Cult Gerontol* 6:219–228, 1991.
35. Kauffman KS: The insider/outsider dilemma: field experience of a white researcher "getting in" a poor black community, *Nurs Res* 43(3):179–183, 1994.
36. Bushy A: Rural determinants in family health: considerations for community nurses. In Bushy A, editor: *Rural nursing*, Vol 23, Newbury Park, NY, 1991, Sage.
37. Long KA: The concept of health: rural perspectives, *Nurs Clin North Am* 28(1):123–130, 1993.
38. Nelson JA, Gingerich BS: Rural health: access to care and services, *Home Health Care Manage Pract* 22(3):339–343, 2010.
39. *Care of the dying: a Catholic perspective*, St Louis, 1993, The Catholic Health Association of the United States.
40. Haddad LG, Hoeman SP: Home healthcare and the Arab-American client, *Home Healthcare Nurse* 18(3):189–197, 2000.
41. Eliason MJ, Raheim S: Experiences and comfort with culturally diverse groups in undergraduate pre-nursing students, *J Nurs Educ* 39(4):161–165, 2000.
42. Campinha-Bacote J: Patient-centered care in the midst of a cultural conflict: the role of cultural competence, *Online J Issues Nursing* 16(2):1, 2011.
43. Kleinman A: *Patients and healers in the context of culture*CA, 1980, University of California Press. (quote on p. 106).
44. Tervalon M, Murray-Garcia J: Cultural humility versus cultural competence: a critical distinction in defining physician training outcomes in multicultural education, *J Health Care Poor Underserved* 9(2):117–125, 1998.
45. Bechtel GA, Davidhizar RE: Integrating cultural diversity in patient education, *Semin Nurse Manag* 7(4):193–197, 1999.

PART ONE

Questions for Thought and Discussion

1. In what important ways is an education preparing you for work in the health professions similar to and different from other types of formal education you could choose?

2. You are the supervisor of an ambulatory clinic. You recognize an increase in the number of Mayan immigrants in your patient population. You are also surprised to learn that English is actually their third language and that they speak Spanish as a second language. What should you do to prepare your staff to care for these patients?

3. An 8-year-old girl presents at the emergency department with her mother. Both are recent immigrants from Afghanistan. The child has several unusual neurological symptoms, but when the physician recommends a lumbar puncture to rule out encephalitis, the child's mother refuses. When asked why, she explains that a "djinn" (a spirit in Islamic folk belief) is involved and the lumbar puncture will upset the djinn and her daughter will become more ill.[1] As a health professional involved in her care, how should you proceed?

4. You are treating a 24-year-old woman whose diagnosis is cervical cancer. You do not know if she is aware of her diagnosis. One day she asks you to get her medical chart for her from the nursing desk. "The 'Bill of Rights for Patients' in this hospital says that I have a right to accurate information, and I figure this is the only way I will get it." You think about what the most caring response is to her and how to respect her dignity in this awkward situation. What will you say to her? What will you do? Why?

REFERENCES

1   C. Seelman, J. Suuromond, K. Stronks, Cultural competence: a conceptual framework for teaching and learning, Med Educ 434 (2009) 229–37.

PART TWO

Respect for Yourself

Part Two focuses on you as an individual because a key to all respectful human interaction lies in respecting yourself. When you and your colleagues enter the health professions, you bring with you your own unique combination of abilities, needs, values, and dreams. Understandably, you expect to incorporate these into the work positions you assume.

Chapter 4 focuses on your student experiences and the opportunity to cultivate self-respect during this period. Questions include: "What habits reflecting respect for myself can I cultivate as a student that will serve me well throughout my professional career?" "What is professional education and how does it differ from other types of education?" "What is expected of me during this period of professional preparation?" "How does it affect me as a person?"

Chapter 5 focuses on respect for yourself in your role in the health professions. Of prime importance for your well-being is to take to heart the suggestions for how to use and contribute to your support communities: family, friends, and colleagues and what to look for in the setting where you choose to work.

Although not all health professions place people in the role of direct patient contact, some of the most challenging aspects of this work are in the clinical setting. Attitudes toward and understanding of the clinical setting and the types of relationships that are appropriate influence the effectiveness of interaction with patients. The role of being one of a whole matrix of persons caring for a patient is examined with attention to the importance of interprofessional health care teams and being able to decide when and why to refer a patient to someone else. By the end of Part Two, you should be better able to view yourself as respectfully as others will in your several roles in the health professions.

CHAPTER 4

Respect for Yourself during the Student Years

CHAPTER OBJECTIVES

The reader will be able to:

- List some positive goals related to self-respect that can be realized by caringly attending to one's own needs and healthful habits.
- Describe some reasons why striking a balance between socializing and solitude is important during the student years.
- Explain what competence involves as a criterion for becoming and remaining a qualified practitioner.
- Discuss three kinds of learning that must take place during professional preparation and why each is essential.
- Identify four types of skills associated with professional practice that students must master.
- Name eight steps in acquiring skills needed for work in the health professions.
- Explain similarities and differences between classroom and worksite settings of professional preparation and what is gained in each environment.
- List five procedures that should assist the student in adjusting to the worksite education phase of professional preparation.
- Evaluate several sources of student anxiety and some methods of addressing it effectively.

"I'm a student nurse," I began by way of introduction. "Could we sit down somewhere and talk?"

Ann led the way with shaky steps to a small table and two chairs. Ruth followed us and stood behind her mother and played with her necklaces.

I asked Ann, "How long have you had this shakiness?"

"Started 2 days ago," Ann replied.

"Has this happened before?"

"Sometimes, but not this bad."

I had seen a few patients react to antipsychotic drugs this way, but not this severely. At least I thought it was a reaction to the medication. Maybe Ann drank as well—I didn't know how to ask her if she did. ...

—A. Haddad[1]

Health professionals throughout their careers are faced with unexpected questions that arise in the course of treating patients. In the above anecdote the student nurse has the added test of being a student with limited hands-on experience in interviewing situations and also in confronting the range of symptoms a patient may have during an antipsychotic drug reaction. In this chapter we take the opportunity to focus on a special portion of a professional's life span, the student years of formal professional preparation, noting some special issues and challenges that arise by virtue of being in that phase of professional development. At the same time we are quick to remind readers that a professional career is one of lifelong learning, so some challenges first encountered in formal professional preparation arise again and again during the course of a professional's career. The need for practitioners to remain on top of ever-changing developments in health care is a compelling reason that most health professions organizations and licensing bodies require evidence that a practitioner has participated in continuing education activities.

We begin this chapter by standing back from some specific aspects of your educational process to first examining the more fundamental question of how you can be caring of yourself during the student years and make physical and psychological space for your optimal functioning. Both are examples of how nurturing yourself will support self-respect that will serve you well throughout your career.

Sustaining Self-Respect through Nurturing Yourself

Nurturing comes from root words meaning *feeding, taking loving care of,* and *bringing into full bloom.* So nurturing yourself is not limited to addressing worrisome problems such as anxiety. In Chapter 1 you were introduced to the idea that a life guided by respect depends in part on the ability to identify and shape one's own life according to personal values and those that help to build a stronger community. The basic question we ask for your reflection is, "What kinds of attitudes and activities can you cultivate during your student years to stay authentically you—healthy, happy, satisfied with your job, and able to integrate your professional and personal values and goals?"

There is the basic question of who is responsible for your well-being. Today the general consensus is that individuals ultimately are responsible for their own health. Do you agree? It certainly is the case that people feel better, look better, and are able to function more fully when nurturing their own sense of well-being, seeking balance in their lives, and mapping a life course that has opportunity for changing priorities. None of these goals ever comes easily! For example, studying for your professional degree means giving up other patterns and pleasures, as well as dealing with competing responsibilities.

The positive results of keeping life-affirming habits, practices, and goals in the forefront of your life plan as new situations arise seem obvious. However, if you are among the millions who make New Year's resolutions each year, you know that acknowledging the benefits of staying healthy physically, mentally, and spiritually and actually being successful in doing so are not the same. In this section, we offer insights and suggestions to help you succeed in staying happy and healthy.

Self-Respect and Self-Care

Here is that idea of care again! You were introduced to it in Chapter 1 in the following paragraph related to values needed in your professional practice:

> … Everyone talks about care as a positive feature of human relationships. It is. But care has a much more serious function in sustaining them than often we acknowledge. It is the link we make with another human being in distress, taking their suffering and well-being into account. Reich associates true caring with what we decide to do when the chips are down. Often it is not limited to the warm sentimentality so often expressed on the inside of greeting cards. True caring requires us to choose among our priorities and may become a challenge or even a burden. Caring always requires involved concern about the specific barriers to the other person's well-being and the action required to relieve them.

What do you notice about this statement? It is about care of *others*. Not surprising, is it, because a core value of the profession is caregiving, searching for how to provide a caring response to a patient's plight. At the same time this emphasis on caring for others points to a deeper issue in the formation of a professional identity. The emphasis on caring for others is so deeply rooted in your professional formation that the care of oneself can easily get left out of the equation. In fact, many health professionals are so attuned to being care *givers* or care *providers* that they perceive themselves as immune to needing care themselves. This illusion begins in student years when pressures of study and achievement increase. Goethe, in his *Elective Affinities,* illustrates that everyone has a potential for organizing a world that fits his or her illusions: "And so they all, each in his own way, reflectingly or unreflectingly, go on with their daily lives; everything seems to have its accustomed course, for indeed, even in desperate situations where everything hangs in the balance, one goes on living as though nothing were wrong."[2]

The illusion that in caring for others one need not pay attention to one's own needs and life-affirming instincts can lead to deep wounds over time, distorting what it means to place the patient first. For instance, to override feelings of deep distress, the need for relaxation or other healthy activities may set a pattern that engenders inappropriate guilt when a decision honoring care of oneself is made. Medical historians tell us that the physician Galen suffered nightmares for the rest of his life owing to his feelings of guilt after he fled his inevitably dying patients during the plague of Rome to protect his own life and that of his family. The health professions have been slow to incorporate the importance of taking good care of yourself as a value, even though you are obviously in a better position to serve others well when you are acting from a position of personal strength gained through the self-respect that comes from taking good care of yourself.

---

⑨ REFLECTIONS

The benefit that can come from respecting your own limits seems to be a blind spot in most writings guiding professionals. If you have chosen a profession, find and review the code of ethics in that field.
Does it include this important aspect of professional life?
If so, what is the wording that encourages you to remain true to your own healthful habits and needs?
If not, write a statement that does include it.

In a word, self-care is part and parcel of good care giving. By looking at the statement again from Chapter 1, but this time thinking of it in terms of self care, you can get a fuller picture of what is at stake:

… Everyone talks about care as a positive feature of human relationships. It is. But *self* care has a much more serious function in sustaining me than often *I* acknowledge. It is the link each *of us* makes with *our own inner selves* in distress, taking suffering and wellbeing into account. Reich associates true caring with what we decide to do when the chips are down. Often it is not limited to the warm sentimentality so often expressed on the inside of greeting cards. True caring requires *me* to choose among *my* priorities and may become a challenge or even a burden. Caring always requires involved concern about the specific barriers to well-being and the action required to relieve them.

Note that none of this attention to the self deflects from the realization that being in a professional relationship with patients means putting their specific health-related needs at the center of your professional deliberation. At the same time, this self-care gives you a measuring rod of qualities that allow you to fully engage without being in a constant state of alert self-protection. To bring these ideas right down to your situation, take a minute to complete the following simple exercise.

---

⑨ REFLECTIONS

In a few words try to describe a couple of things that give you a feeling of personal happiness and well-being more than anything else you can think of. Why do you think this is the case?
In the circle write the name of the most important person (or persons) to you in the center. Add those who are in a second tier. Finally, add those around the periphery but in the mix.

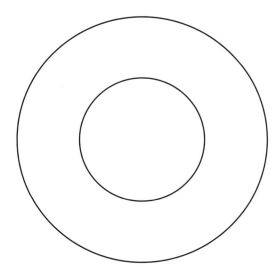

This is a great start. However, we also stated the caveat earlier in this section that most good ideas remain in the realm of dreams or even "resolutions" that fall away. Starting with right now, take a few minutes to follow up on what you have just listed as some what's and who's that will help keep you in a healthful state during your student years.

⊚ REFLECTIONS

Given how pressed I know I am for time and in light of my other priorities, when push comes to shove, one thing I will do during the coming 6 months … to help nourish my personal well-being is:

_____

My strengths and most promising resources for keeping this resolve are:

_____

Self-respect in the student years, then, requires self-care both at the level of identifying what is important to you and finding ways to follow it through into your everyday choices.

Striking a Balance between Socializing and Solitude

Following through on choices that demonstrate self-care requires setting a balance between being with others and having time to yourself for self-reflection. To fail to strike such a balance undermines the self-respect that you assiduously have honored in making choices that show you care about yourself. Most classroom and laboratory learning in educational institutions is accomplished in group situations including face-to-face or on-line discussion, and therefore invite socializing. E-mails, texting, and Twitter create apt opportunities for continuous interaction with others in and outside of the student environment. An important aspect of nurturing yourself includes an awareness of this fact of student life and what you can do to strike a healthful balance between it and the silence of solitude.

Socializing does of course yield both professional and important personal benefits. Of the former, the language often used in the description of what happens in the process of becoming a professional is that the person becomes *socialized* into this identity. Obviously "socializing" (i.e., prolonged, engaged exchanges) with teachers, other students, and the whole environment of health care all are integral parts of *socialization* and distinguish the study of the professions from that of, say, philosophy or literature. From the get-go the professions are preparing students to do something with others. The study of the humanities can be undertaken as an end in itself.

In addition, it goes almost without saying that personal benefits gained from informal socializing as leisure and relaxation activities are for most readers an essential component of their self-care.

Why, then, be concerned with the importance of striking a balance between constant interactions and reflective aloneness as a criterion of self-care during the student years? One compelling reason is that learning in the professions must prepare you for *reflective practice*, not just direct application of material you have absorbed. You will learn more about this in your studies, but basically the processes by which your classroom and initial clinical learning experiences are refined are through additional mechanisms of integration. Benner[3] and others have shown that this process of going from being a *clinical novice* to becoming a *clinical expert* is a self-reflective dimension of learning. In self-reflection you fly solo and need time and open space to do so.

Moreover, personalities differ in their need for internal "quiet time" to grasp and integrate material.[4] If you have not taken a personality inventory like the Myers-Briggs to help you become more aware of your problem-solving styles and strengths, it is a step of self-care you can take because so much of learning to become a competent professional involves aspects of problem solving. Even the most extroverted person needs some solitude if fulsome learning is to take place. In short, a vital strategy for flourishing during the student years and beyond is to strike a balance that includes both interaction and solitude. Because little is said in the health professions education about solitude as a resource for self-care and effective learning, we share these few thoughts about it with you.

Solitude is a positive, active state of being, although the experience of solitude is not identical to happiness and may even be "bittersweet" (accompanied by sorrow or anger); nonetheless, it is sought out as a need in itself, not foisted on one as a result of feeling rejected or "out of contact." It is a form of self-respect realized by embracing the necessity of not always responding to other people whenever they need or want it. As one popular student commented when he began to turn off his cell phone for an hour each day, "I realized over time that I had been acting like a service organization by always interrupting what I needed to do to link up with someone else!" Unlike loneliness, which is a form of suffering, solitude can be wonderful.

⟲ REFLECTIONS

List here the things you most like to do by yourself. If you do not currently make or have enough time for these activities, make two columns, one listing the reasons you do not do them, the other making some suggestions to yourself about how you might make more opportunities to enjoy them.

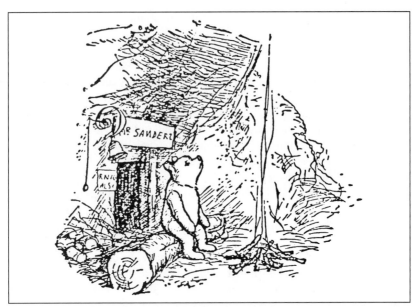

FIGURE 4-1: "And He sits and thinks of the things they know; He and the Forest, alone together ..." *(From Winnie-The-Pooh by AA Milne, illustrated by EH Shepard, copyright 1926 by EP Dutton, renewed 1954 by AA Milne. Used by permission of Dutton Children's Books, an imprint of Penguin Books for Young Readers, a division of Penguin Putnam Inc.)*

Pooh Bear, the most reflective member of Winnie-the-Pooh's community, sought solitude often (Figure 4-1). He understood that solitude is a time to be *with yourself only,* not with others, and to engage in reflections and activities that can better prepare you for relationships. Some people are active in their solitude, finding walking, jogging, biking, reading, or other solitary activities a time for reflection. Others prefer the stillness of meditation or just sitting quietly Pooh Bear style. Some ideas to help you make time for yourself include the following:

▶ Set a time and place and rigorously adhere to it.
▶ Become bold in identifying to others what you are doing.
▶ Take notes on your reflections or keep a log of your activities.
▶ Remind yourself often that a basic minimum requirement on which many other health-supporting activities depend is to take time to be with yourself.

In addition, you can help others to have their own time alone by learning to recognize this need in fellow students and encouraging it.

With this backdrop of self-care and some aspects of your environment you need to help realize it, we turn to other issues in your student years that could challenge your respect for yourself and offer suggestions for ways to support and enrich it.

Self-Respect and the Motivation to Contribute

Most students know that they would like to be able to make a contribution to others in society. It is a motivator for applying to an education program in the health

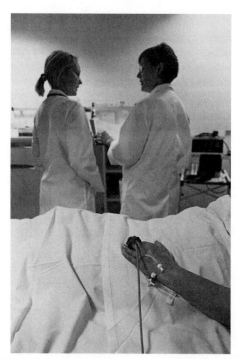

FIGURE 4-2: Identifying a professional role model can enable a student to remain true to his or her course of studies. *(© Corbis.)*

professions and in itself a good reason for self-respect. Many psychologists, philosophers, and others have demonstrated that a life of satisfaction for most adults includes making a contribution that has benefit to others whether it is to one's children and spouse, as a volunteer, or in the public workplace. We address this later in the book from the standpoint of your encounters with adult patients whose difficulties preclude them from performing their adult roles and the self-deprecation they can feel. Often, though not always, the choice of a professional career arises from a student's experience of illness or injury and how he or she was helped by a professional whom he or she came to admire, or a friend or loved one was ill and dying and health professionals showed able assistance and compassion in caring for the person. Sometimes the desire to become a professional is based on a student's recognition that he or she has a talent for being a good listener or a capacity for helping friends when they are in trouble.

The desire to help others is not always the primary or only factor that leads people to choose a career as a health professional. Love of science, the desire to be in a "people-oriented" line of work, the desire for status, and a career that promises to provide a good salary and high satisfaction are other important and understandable motivators. However, the desire to make a significant contribution in life is important in helping you stay true to your course of study when the going gets rough. One good approach is to identify early on a teacher or other professional role model who manifests attributes you admire (Figure 4-2).

⊚ REFLECTIONS

Have you identified classroom or clinical educators whose manner, conduct, attitudes, or skills you admire? What, specifically, are the traits that caught your attention?

How Do I Become Competent in My Field?

Students also have moments when they will feel uncertain of how to proceed to make the kind of professional contribution they have admired in others. The phrase you will hear dozens of times during your preparation for your role in the health professions is that you must become competent in your field. Without it your caring cannot be distinguished from what the person may receive from a friend or someone else who claims to be able to help him. *Competence* means that you are prepared to be and do what reasonably is expected of you in your role insofar as your formal education, licensing, and other requirements placed on you can prepare you. To help you know when you are achieving this ultimate goal, you will be introduced to "competencies" that have been developed by the leaders in your field in response to your profession's own and society's expectations of every member of your field.

You will gradually become aware that preparation for work in the health professions is different from that for other fields. Although students in other programs of study are partying on Friday afternoon, the health professions student may be at the clinic or laboratory carrying out an education internship or field work requirement; while roommates are still trying to get out of bed in the morning, it is not unusual for the health professions student to be on the way out the door; and, although most careers do not require students to adopt a set of professional attitudes, behaviors, and ethical guidelines, the health professions do.

Education in the health professions prepares you to competently carry out a lifelong commitment and realize a certain type of lifestyle. You have already learned that your identity as a health professional carries with it expectations on the part of society, as well as privileges and responsibilities. You will be considered an "expert" in your field, but as a professional you will be looked on as a person whose special knowledge, skills, and attitudes can make the world a better place and improve individuals' lives. In choosing to be a health professional, you are accepting that competence involves not only what you will do but also who you will become in your own eyes and in the eyes of patients and others.

What can you expect during your years of formal education? On the following pages we discuss three types of learning experiences that will predominate: the acquisition of basic concepts and theories (knowledge), the mastery of professional skills, and the attainment of attitudes appropriate to your role as a health professional. Each will support your self-respect for your choice of profession, preparing you for effective and respectful interaction with patients, colleagues, and society.

Knowledge (Theories, Concepts, and Methods)

Traditionally, education in the health professions required knowledge of the classics and, as the scientific age developed, basic sciences. Today, the foundation of required knowledge is much broader.

What knowledge do you need to become a competent health professional?

▶ The physical sciences provide a foundation for understanding the body and the natural forces acting on it.

▶ Behavioral sciences of psychology, sociology, and anthropology provide understanding of people's needs and behaviors and of how these needs and behaviors affect interaction.

▶ The liberal arts expose you to the great political, religious, and philosophical ideas and establish your own and patients' link with history.

▶ Economic and legal concepts prepare you to understand how delivery of health care is financed today and some basic guidelines governing the activities of health care institutions.

▶ Statistics and information technology furnish baseline knowledge for research design, data analysis, and communication functions.

▶ Policy and administration courses help you to understand the links between practice and the larger social context in which you will work.

Depending on the level of your professional preparation you will be exposed to all or most of these areas.

Theoretical knowledge regarding the techniques relevant to your profession explains the rationale for adopting practices consistent with evidence-based information. If the only type of learning for professional competence were acquisition and integration of knowledge, there would be no need to include laboratory experience or clinical education in the preparation of health care providers. Already you begin to see that education for the health professions differs from the formal preparation for most other careers.

Skills

At the time you enter your professional curriculum, it is highly likely you have been more accustomed to classroom learning than to laboratory and clinical learning. The acquisition of skill often requires long, tedious hours of practice. This is where your instructor's skill as an educator and your willingness to persevere really count.

The frustration that often accompanies mastering a skill was illustrated recently when one of the authors decided to learn to fly fish. She read several books, watched a video, and studied the types of flies and equipment, then hired a guide to take her to a trout stream in northern Maine.

The first half-day was spent far from the water, in a field, learning to cast the fly out. At least half the time the fly caught in trees, bushes, and other overhanging obstructions. After lunch, finally in the water, she learned that the coordination required to lay the line flat and cast the fly out far enough from her hook to attract anything other than shore line weeds was a far cry from the pictures in the video. That night, nursing a sore shoulder and wrist, she remembered her instructor's encouragement to rest up and "with practice you'll see yourself improving day-by-day." She wondered. Hundreds of casts later it still wasn't perfect, but the fly more often landed in the stream where she was trying to set it.

Consider four basic skills needed for competence in a health profession:

Technical Skill

Technical skill is the ability to safely and effectively apply technology using highly specialized techniques to secure a diagnosis, conduct an evaluation, or provide a treatment intervention. Your role may be on the front lines of achieving the required result or you may have a role as part of a team of workers in accomplishing the desired end. Among health professionals technical skills cover a broad bandwidth of activities from analyzing the contents of a blood sample to conducting a gait analysis to performing tests using sophisticated computerized instruments. In each case, technical expertise includes an intricate coordination of mind and body, as well as the exercise of sound informed judgment.

Skill in Interpersonal Relationships and Communication

You will interact with a wide variety of people during the course of a day: other health care and support personnel, patients and their families, students, visitors, administrators, and business contacts such as equipment salespersons. This activity demands that you understand appropriate conduct in different types of relationships. It means being able to accept responsibility as a supervisor and constructive criticism when supervised. It involves learning how caring is expressed in the professional role and demands tact, diplomacy, consistency, and forthrightness. Many areas of this book describe means whereby you can express respect through good communications skills, and Part Four focuses specifically on it.

Teaching and Administrative Skill

Education of individual patients or clients and the larger public is essential in every health field. Whatever your choice of a profession, you will be required to engage in educational activities geared to others. This may involve patients, families, students, other professionals, support personnel, and the public. Administrative skills also are essential requiring you to organize and implement workable solutions to potential problems; set reasonable short- and long-term goals in your workplace; engage in fair, objective evaluation of yourself and others; and do your share to maintain a cost-effective operation.

Research Skill

Research advances the knowledge and skills of your and relevant other fields. Skill in quantitative research approaches requires that you develop a research question, design a project, formulate a hypothesis, and collect and analyze data to determine whether your hypothesis is correct. Qualitative research methods include in-depth interviews or other narratives designed to highlight important areas of understanding about a type of problem or phenomenon. Honest, accurate reporting of findings is imperative. As today's students enter practice, their work will be remunerated on evidence-based practices (i.e., those confirmed by research to be effective).

To understand better how students acquire these four types of skills, consider the following steps your educational program will guide you through. You will:

1. Acquire knowledge related to the skill
2. Experience the skill applied to yourself
3. Apply the skill to a classmate
4. Observe a professional person using the skill
5. Assist the professional person in using the skill
6. Be closely supervised in the first attempts to apply the skill yourself
7. Satisfactorily use the skill in a variety of situations, with decreasing amounts of direct supervision
8. Be tested for basic competence in applying the skill

Note the progression from classroom to work setting in this process. Step 1 can easily take place in a classroom or online, while steps 2 and 3 usually must take place in the skills laboratory except in rare circumstances where simulations are able to provide the same learning opportunities for step 3. Steps 4 through 8 take place in the workplace setting, where a variety of situations are available, sometimes initially in simulated patient situations and then with real patients and decreasing amounts of direct supervision. Thus, only part of your learning to assume eventual mastery of professional skills can take place in a real or virtual classroom setting.

As a student, you have a right to expect the faculty's commitment to your learning, adopting appropriate teaching styles to student needs and determining the optimal type and amount of supervision and guidance during the various steps of your professional preparation. The greatest challenge to educators is to shape their approaches to guarantee that you have an opportunity to acquire the skills you will need, but it is their moral and legal obligation to do so.

Attitudes and Character

During your student years, your professors are expected to teach and reinforce attitudes and character traits consistent with respect in your professional role.

Your attitudes toward caring for others, responses to persons who may be different from yourself and the qualities that you believe make life worth living, will be a part of how you respond in time to the challenges of the health professions environment. In most instances your intuitive responses are a great resource as almost all students have some idea in advance of the types of situations they will encounter. Attitudes that seem to keep you at a distance from being able to engage wholeheartedly warrant deep reflection on your part. During your student preparation years there will be opportunities for you to face, discuss, and further form attitudes appropriate for this line of work to help enssure a good fit with one's choice of career.

One important attitude to acquire or cultivate during your student years is a love of learning; it is best planted during this period if it is to flourish in later years. This attitude can actually have a strong bearing on your success in the workplace, where creativity and problem solving are so essential to accomplishing your tasks.[5] We began this chapter saying that lifelong learning is essential. Epstein points out that the competence gained through your knowledge, skills, and attitudes is not a fixed entity once and for all achieved by the time you graduate. Rather it is a dynamic process that changes over the course of your career with changes in health care and the context in which you work.[6] Thus, learning to love learning provides the attitude toward it that can transform this demand on you from a dreaded necessity to an enlivening aspect of the type of work you have chosen.

You have now been exposed to three kinds of learning that take place during formal educational preparation for a career in the health professions: knowledge, skills, and attitude/character formation. In addition, you know the environments in which each kind of learning most efficiently and effectively takes place, though to make a sharp division between them also is artificial. All the while you are learning, absorbing, integrating. With this baseline, you are ready to explore the same basic features of classroom learning versus the learning that takes place in the work environment.

Clinical Education: Situated Learning

Clinical education is situated learning. *Situated learning* refers to learning that takes place in the actual work setting. It is called by different names in different professions: *clinical education, fieldwork, clerkships, rotations,* or *internships,* to name some. This aspect of your education provides you with an opportunity to demonstrate that you will succeed in your future work environment and thus warrant the respect from those who come for your services. The quality and quantity of teaching that occur are determined by wide-ranging and unpredictable variables such as the availability of patient types. New smells, sounds, and sights combine with new tasks to present an exciting challenge, and almost all students find it the most stimulating part of their educational preparation. As one experienced faculty educator put it:

"We know that as soon as students are back from a clinical experience the influence of the academic community seems to pale. Students are energized as they have made connections from declarative knowledge (information, facts, tradition knowledge) to procedural knowledge (the knowhow and practical application of that knowledge). Practice is where it happens."[7]

Refinement and synthesis are important functions of clinical education. Refinement implies that you now have the basic materials with which to work and must begin to learn how to use them optimally. Synthesis is the work of putting together, in a meaningful way, the many details you have learned in your professional preparation up to this time. At this juncture you encounter:

- Large numbers of patients with different problems
- Several manifestations of a single clinical condition
- Time limitations
- Multiple professional responsibilities related to the work environment (e.g., documentation and participating in staff meetings)
- Work with members of various health care teams
- Your role in making the technique you apply into a real life evaluation or treatment procedure

    The desired result is a person competent to enter practice.

Getting Situated Personally

There is inherent wisdom in getting off to a good start in any new venture, and a few practical guidelines apply to beginning your new venture into education that takes place on site in the workplace. A general rule is to acknowledge that you are entering an environment that has its own players with their peculiarities and habits. Some of the personnel may have been working in this setting for years, and you are a newcomer. Respect for the fact that you are in someone else's territory is key. Fortunately, most educators and others in this setting extend themselves to try to help students feel accepted, but you may find the situation initially awkward anyway. Anyone who has started a new job knows the feeling. It is rather like going into someone else's home and being told to "make yourself at home." It takes time to be able to "feel at home" no matter what the host or hostess says. We remember a medical student telling us about her awkwardness at the nurse's station in her first rotation, which happened to be in pediatrics: She had received a thorough orientation from her physician supervisor, who then left.

> I just stood at the nurse's station waiting for someone to ask me what I wanted or tell me what to do. Nobody paid any attention to me. My supervisor was nowhere to be seen. I felt like I was at the grocery store waiting to check out but nobody noticed that I was there. It was awful.

Fortunately, she eventually became more at ease and enjoyed it so much that upon graduation she returned there to do her residency. This student could have been helped over her initial unease by following a few simple suggestions:

- Always introduce yourself to the key players, even those who do not seem to be "important" or particularly interested in who you are.
- Try to assess in advance the usual protocols and ways of doing things in this setting.
- Ask explicit questions about the expectations of your supervisor.
- Assume that occasionally someone may be suspicious of or perplexed by a newcomer in "their" environment, and prepare to respond to their questions or comments in a nondefensive and instructive manner.

- Assume that everyone basically wants to assist in your learning. If you have any reason to believe otherwise, you should discuss it with your faculty advisor.

⊚ REFLECTIONS

If you have already begun or completed this phase of your education, reflect on what you felt and found in this new environment when you first arrived, and what, if anything, had changed by the time you left. Do you have insight into why the changes took place?

Try to recall any situation in your life where you felt awkward in a new environment. In retrospect, what things could you have done to make the situation more pleasant for yourself? Jot them down here.

Busy staff do notice when someone shows genuine interest in their work, their professional challenges, and especially in the patients' well-being. Politely but firmly hold your clinical educators to high standards of their instructional tasks so that they will succeed as educators and you as the learner. In this phase of your education, you are gaining the self-confidence and self-respect for your role that will enable you to proceed deftly toward full professional participation in your chosen workplace.

Staying Alert to Opportunity

No matter how good a student you are or how committed and excellent your faculty, you will not arrive fully prepared to take advantage of every situation you will encounter. But every novel or unexpected happening in the workplace is a learning opportunity and should be grasped enthusiastically. Years ago a mentor gave one of the authors two general pieces of advice that served her well in her situated learning experience:

▶ Give yourself time to "get the drift" of what's going on. With so much new happening in the workplace setting, it is crucial to take time to think about it. Initially, you might find that your mind is quite undisciplined and jumps from one idea to the next with little pattern or coherence. After a while, it is possible to identify familiar themes. This creative work counters the common misconception that merely thinking is wasting time.

▶ Stay neutral toward a specific situation at the outset. This does not mean that you are disinterested. It means that you are willing to view the place and people in a situation with a caring objectivity and withhold passing either positive or negative judgment while taking in the whole of the experience. Keen observation and attuned listening will move you from first reactions to a more considered conclusion and enhance what is to be learned from it.

Finding Meaning in the Student Role

No matter how many of the previously mentioned strategies you use to become accepted in the environment, the fact remains that you are not yet fully one of them. Moreover, you are going to be coming in and leaving in short order. The key is that the situated learning environment has meaning solely as an integral aspect of your education. In trying to find your exact function on the health care team, you will usually be welcomed as a student member. Sometimes because you are a student, you are seen as "up on the latest" and a patient may express that he or she trusts you more than the older, more experienced personnel providing care for those reasons. These moments are gratifying, and when you hear the patient or others treating you in ways beyond what you are prepared to competently handle on your own you can remind them that you are still in training and that you will take up the issue with your supervisor.

Patients sometimes feel it is safe to share delicate information with you. Sometimes you end up spending more time with them than anyone else on the team because your supervisor understands that your education requires such additional time. On occasion this leads to a patient, family member, or someone else sharing something that they do not want you to tell anyone else on the team. This can be a good faith effort reflecting their trust in you. However, there is no room for this type of secret between you and if you hear the conversation going down that direction, it is best to "nip it in the bud" by saying you are professionally bound in your student role to share it with your supervisor. You cannot be put in the untenable position of having to share it and the one giving you the information feeling betrayed.

You may also occasionally find that you are "put in your place" by patients and professionals alike. A case in point involves a clinical imaging student who mustered the courage to call a physician to clarify a referral because she had some questions about it. Although the student had identified herself at the outset of the call, the physician listened intently. When she finished sharing her concerns the physician responded, "Okay dear, you have had your say. Now put a real professional on the line and let me talk with her." That kind of put-down response hurts, no matter how confident she might have felt when she made the call.

⊙ REFLECTIONS

Put yourself in this student's place. What are the steps she could have taken to avoid or diminish this type of response from the physician?

Presumably your response reflects that the better path would have been to raise it with her supervisor, and they could have worked it through together such as you may have done in determining actual steps that would lead to a resolution of this student's concern.

This student role gray zone of being "betwixt and between" usually does not cause undue difficulty as long as everyone in the setting is clear that you are there to learn. At times it does give rise to some sources of anxiety that we explore next though not all anxieties are related to the in-transition nature of the student role in the worksite setting.

Why Do I Feel Anxious?

This chapter has focused on several tools and some key information that should help you maintain a healthy relationship to yourself during your student years. Still, we have been there, both as students and later as faculty advisors, and know that some stresses directly arising from the pressures of student life are difficult to avoid completely because nothing that presents worthwhile challenges comes without some burdens. The good news is that the anxiety which is due strictly to the transitory role of being a student will pass eventually. However, for many students at least three serious questions may be the focus of anxiety or worry, and each is worth attending to.

"Am I/Can I get prepared well enough to pass the courses and complete the degree requirements?" This type of insecurity is most evident just before an exam, and when you can attach your feeling of being stressed out to something as concrete as an exam, it is possible to deal with it. It also sometimes surfaces in early situated learning experiences. Fortunately, many institutions provide counseling services for persons who experience sufficient anxiety over exams or facing new environments such as the worksite for it to interfere dramatically with their preparation and success. If you experience this anxiety, it is well worth the effort of seeking such assistance.

"Do I have what it takes to be in this field?" This worry is rather like the first but is more fundamental. It may arise from the troublesome suspicion that other students and your professional models have qualities that you seem to lack or from the fact that you have responsibilities that compete for your attention. It raises self-doubts regarding your intellectual or moral capacities, as well as your physical or emotional limits. They are questions often asked by students who fail an exam or experience the rather common reaction of feeling faint the first time they see a badly injured patient, observe surgery, or are unexpectedly overwhelmed by a noxious odor. Again there is professional help available for serious anxiety arising from these sources of self-doubt.

At another level, the troublesome feeling may be pointing to something deeper in yourself. The word *education* comes from two Latin terms, *ek* and *ducere. Ek* means "out," and *ducere* means "to draw." Therefore, education means to draw out from within. The process of professional education includes a lot of material coming in from outside, but if you take the time for solitude and reflection, you may realize the educational process itself has freed you to hear that inner voice saying, "You do not want to be in this type of work." Not everyone is cut out for what the professions demand, and maintaining self-respect must not hinge on trying to do the impossible for whatever reason or force oneself into believing that because you began this line of study, or were encouraged to do so, you must stick it out no matter what. At the same time dropping out prematurely would be a tragedy if the anxiety is temporary and there is a way through the difficult time.

"Can I afford to stay in school?" Many students are burdened by the financial demands that an education places on them and their families. Stress related to having to take another loan or find a job or the possibility of having to drop out of school altogether is more common than is sometimes supposed. This is a growing problem as public funds seem to be becoming scarcer, but again the possibilities of financial assistance should be explored before this becomes a reason for giving up on completing your education.

These are just three sources of stress directly related to being a student. However, anxieties arising from nonstudent issues also can impinge on student well-being. An impending divorce, either one's own or that of one's parents or child, an unexpected or unwanted pregnancy, the news that a loved one is seriously ill—these and many other problems can influence a person's feeling of well-being and performance dramatically.

Age-related concerns can also combine with one or more of the above sources of anxiety. Pressures on young people to decide what they are going to be lead many to choose a career early in life, sometimes as early as junior high school. As we suggested earlier, in rare cases this early decision pressure may have been made without enough information to know what really is the right fit for them. At the same time, a growing number of students who have raised children or spent many years in another career are also choosing formal education in the health professions. The latter's concerns often spring from the belief that they are acting on their last chance to realize a dream, are desperately retooling to find a job when another line of work dried up, may be too old to compete competitively in a job market apparently geared to the young, or are not giving enough time to other obligations of midlife.

Responding Constructively to Anxiety?

Most students do go through a skeptical, questioning phase, but if anxiety persists it should be addressed. We provide some suggestions here about what you can do to respond well and go on to enjoy your choice of life's work.

Identify the Source

One of the most important steps in dissipating the destructive tension associated with anxiety is to identify its source if you can do so on your own. Is it directly school-related? Is there some other obvious reason that anxiety has descended on you, or is the source too diffuse to identify? Are there times when you are free from it, and if so, when? What activities seem to help allay it?

Share Feelings with a Friend or Trustworthy Classmate

The sting of anxiety is that it can alienate you from others who know that something is wrong but do not know what or why and lead you to behaviors you know are not healthful (Figure 4-3).

They may even think it is something they have done. In sharing your anxiety with a trusted person, you have overcome the isolation of the experience and in most cases have gained an ally who can help you address it. An unintended side effect of this process is that you may find out how common your feelings are. By knowing that others, too, are feeling stressed, you feel less "out of joint" with the rest of the world.

Seek Professional Help

As we suggested earlier, when talking with a friend is not adequate, you deserve the benefit of help from a professional. In such cases, an instructor or counselor can help you discover why you feel anxious. In other instances, the treatment for stress may require an extended course of intervention over weeks or months. Your well-being is at stake, and this is an area of caring for yourself that, when acted on, will help foster your self-respect for what you took the time to do.

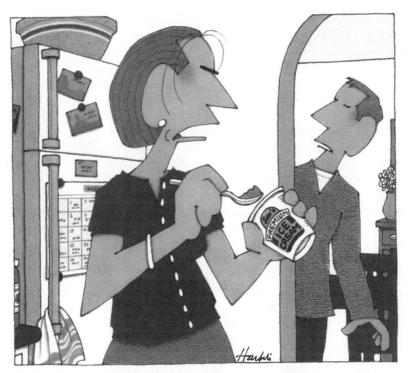

"I'm not eating. I'm self-medicating."

FIGURE 4-3: *(© The New Yorker Collection 2001. William Haefeli from cartoonbank.com. All rights reserved.)*

In all of these methods, the key to decreasing anxiety, once its source is identified, is to attend to it so that it does not ruin what would otherwise be the exciting adventure of professional preparation.

Reaping the Rewards of Perseverance

This chapter would be incomplete without a short note to you on the rewards of persevering.

The health professions continue to rank among the most rewarding and challenging careers available today. Most educational programs select from a large pool of applicants, ensuring that you will spend your career with other highly qualified and interesting colleagues. The opportunity for personal growth and professional advancement is high in almost all health fields.

The daily work is varied and engaging. When you complete your formal study, there will be an awareness of how you can contribute to making the life of another person, indeed the lives of many other persons, better. Fortunately, students usually do learn how to celebrate the successful completion of various aspects of their journey by end-of-term parties, post-exam indulgences, and other markers. The educational programs themselves help mark your milestone through such events as celebrations after board exams, pinning or "white coat" ceremonies, honors convocations and, of course, commencement activities. Because the rewards of persevering to the end are many, the remaining chapters are designed to assist you in maximizing the wealth of experiences open to persons in the health professions. Read on, and plan for a fine future.

SUMMARY

This chapter highlights how self-respect for your choice of profession and your movement through your student years can be cultivated. All along, your self-respect and the caring it generates are cherished resources that can be called on. Both socializing and taking time for reflection and solitude are required. You will understandably face some challenges, anxieties, and anticipations, and this chapter provides guidelines for helping to recognize and address them when the going gets rough. The emphasis on preparedness through the acquisition of knowledge, skills, and ennobling attitudes should help you remain focused on why you are here reading this book in the first place. Our goals for you are to enjoy the student role, be prepared for its challenges when they come, understand them, and then leave the student years respectfully behind for your new career life.

REFERENCES

1. Haddad A: Spring semester. In Haddad AM, Brown KH, editors: *The arduous touch: women's voices in health care*, West Lafayette, IN, 1999, NotaBell Books/Purdue University Press.
2. Goethe JW: *Elective affinities, New York*, 1978, Penguin Books.
3. Benner P: *From novice to expert: excellence and power in clinical nursing practice. commemorative edition*, Upper Saddle River, NJ, 2005, Prentice-Hall.
4. Myers-Briggs Type Indicator: *See Myers and Briggs Foundation*, www.myersbriggs.org.
5. Sullivan WM, Rosin MS: *A new agenda for higher education: shaping a life of the mind for practice*, San Francisco, 2008, Jossey-Bass.
6. Epstein R, Hundert E: Defining and assessing professional competence, *JAMA* 287:2, 2002.
7. Jensen G: 42nd Mary McMillan Lecture. Learning what matters most, *Phys Ther* 91: 1674–1679, 2011.

Respect for Yourself in Your Professional Capacity

CHAPTER OBJECTIVES

The reader will be able to:

- Discuss some benefits of putting family and friends high on one's priorities.
- Name two types of bonds that can develop among work colleagues to help create a network of support and mutual respect.
- Describe guidelines to make an assessment of how supportive an employer and future colleagues are likely to be.
- List some questions that highlight whether future or current colleagues will contribute to enjoying one another in the workplace.
- Distinguish between the characteristics of being an intimate and a personal caregiver in the health professions.
- Compare important aspects of social and therapeutic relationships, describing why maintaining this distinction in everyday practice affects self-respect and respect for others in a professional environment.
- Identify and discuss two respect-enhancing goals that the interprofessional health care team approach is designed to meet.
- Compare key values realized through team decisions that are hierarchy derived and those that are community derived.
- List four criteria for referral of patients.
- Discuss how a health professions career allows one to participate in increasing goodness in the world.

There were a few things that helped to restore my sense of equilibrium. The first was to make a conscious effort to spend time with my wife. . . . A second source of balance came from getting together with other people who were facing similar pressures at work. . . . Another thing that helped was to take 10 or 15 minutes during my morning commute to sit quietly, reflect about my life, and say a few prayers. This helped center me for the day. It gave me a sense of perspective . . . Together these small things helped bring my life and my work back into balance.

J. Allegretti[1]

This chapter continues on the course of moving from your role as a student to thriving in your lifelong career in the health professions. We introduce you to several specific capacities that, if nurtured, will serve you well in this setting. First and foremost is to build on the confidence you gained through attitudes and activities that honor care of yourself. As you recall, we urged that only through self-respect are you in a position to show care well for others. Additional emphases in this chapter prepare you to engage in skilled activities that distinguish your everyday relationships from your professional ones and pointers on the strengths of working as a member of an interprofessional health care team whatever your level of professional preparation.

Together these capacities will help ensure that you will experience deep satisfaction and self-respect throughout your work life.

Showing Respect for Yourself while Enjoying Support

In Chapter 4 you were introduced to some ways to engender and preserve self-respect that are particularly relevant to the unique situation of being a student. We also emphasized that many of the general themes in that chapter continue to be relevant throughout your professional career. We turn now to several considerations that you can add to what you learned, among the most important the necessity of being willing to graciously accept support when you need it and set priorities that keep the most important people in your close circle of your caring. Family and friends are at the top of the list. Professional colleagues are close behind.

Putting Family and Friends First

Because professional life can be so involving, family and friends outside of your work environment are at risk of being left out of your life in important ways unless you make conscious efforts to include them (Figure 5-1). Often they are taken for granted and may get the leftover part of your days, the majority of the best hours having been spent in workplace activities. This excerpt from a day in the life of a health

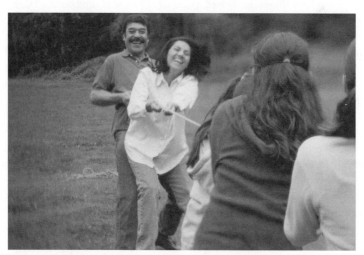

FIGURE 5-1: Health professionals should remember to make time for family and friends. (© *Getty Images/100069.*)

professional reflects a routine that many in health care positions can identify with regarding the amount and quality of time spent with their families:

It is now 7 o'clock. I drive home. The day of work is finished. I know that I shall not have any more calls as I sign my phone out to the telephone answering service. I sit down to dinner with my wife and three school-age children. I listen to the children recount the activities of the day. It is March, and my wife and I begin to talk about possible vacation sites for this summer. After dinner I go to my study and take a journal from a pile of unread periodicals. I thumb through it, unable to concentrate enough to get interested in any one article. I turn on the television and begin to watch an NBA game. Later, my wife wakens me.[2]

⊙ REFLECTIONS

- What do you find encouraging about this scene as you think about your own work life? What is troubling about this scenario?
- What habits do you have that will serve you well in terms of nurturing your most important relationships over the long haul? (You may want to go back to Chapter 4 to the exercise regarding your priorities and how to honor them.)

Your challenge is to establish habits early that will reflect the rhythms needed for your family members and friends to be *able* to support you when you need it. A young lawyer quoted at the outset of the chapter has this further comment as he recounts the choices he began to exercise when he felt himself being consumed by his work:

There were a few things that helped to restore my sense of equilibrium. The first was to make a conscious effort to spend time with my wife. In the beginning, I resisted when my wife would plead, cajole, and sometimes push me out the door of our apartment so that we could spend a few hours watching a movie or going to dinner. Eventually, I realized how important this time was. It strengthened our relationship by keeping the lines of communication open between us. Not only that, it also made me a better worker by giving my anxious mind a much-needed rest.

A second source of balance came from getting together with other people who were facing similar pressures at work. Two or three times a month I would meet with a few friends from law school who were working in other firms around town. Our get-togethers were combination lunches and b.s. sessions. These meetings did wonders for my perspective. I found myself becoming less anxious and self-absorbed as I discovered that my friends were dealing with the same worries and concerns I was facing. We helped ourselves by helping each other.

Another thing that helped was to take 10 or 15 minutes during my morning commute to sit quietly, reflect about my life, and say a few prayers. This helped center me for the day. It gave me a sense of perspective. It allowed me to see the ways in which my work was an integral part of my spiritual life. . . .

Together, these small things helped bring my life and my work back into balance. They let me see my work more realistically. They stopped me from investing too much of myself in my work. And they reminded me that I was more than a worker and that my work was only work.[1]

In short, this young professional used the resources of family, colleagues, and his own form of spiritual reflection to create the balance he felt slipping from him. In the process he created a support network that not only benefited his work but helped him maintain a balance that showed respect for himself and those closest to him. He just mentions in passing that he realized his immediate professional colleagues also were a resource. It is so important that we examine this in more detail.

Honor Bonds with Colleagues

One source of support is that persons working in a health care situation have several common bonds, all of which help to establish rapport and support among them.

Bond of Shared Concerns

Care can be enhanced through having a place to air common concerns about a patient's problems, prognosis, or progress; about the department; about what is happening in their field; and about health services in general. You voluntarily place yourself in the mainstream of human suffering, thereby showing that you care. No one commits you to this role. You choose to be there because you care enough about human well-being to want to effect certain changes by the use of your professional skills.

But this life you chose makes intense demands on you, and an essential resource is to know there is a trusted group with whom to share your common worries, uncertainties, and questions.

Bond of Shared Care and Gratitude

In the crush of everyday work, colleagues take less time telling one another directly that they appreciate and care about them than they do sharing their concerns. Creating a generous atmosphere of such expression helps transform a workplace from a work site only to a true community. Gratitude, too, is expressed too seldom by persons working together. A simple word of thanks can create more good will than months of competent work together, during which neither person makes an effort to express appreciation to the other. There are many ways to say "thank you" or "you are appreciated."

⊚ REFLECTIONS

- What are some ways in previous jobs you have held that you and your colleagues have shown appreciation for each other's contributions?
- What ideas do you have for helping to create a happy and supportive workplace for yourself and your colleagues?

Remembering another person's birthday or the anniversary of a special event and performing other "random acts of kindness" creates a general environment of congeniality in which the language of mutual respect for the efforts and gifts of one another's skills and presence can flourish.

Seek Supportive Institutional Environments

The bonds of shared concern and shared caring and gratitude work together to encourage the realization of mutually shared goals and values. However, as you learned in Chapter 2, it is not enough for individuals alone to desire to create a respectful environment—respect must also be reflected in the structure and values of those who have policy authority. As one group of health care administrators working to contribute to organizational structures that meet the requirement noted: "Optimally there is full alignment among (1) the moral identity of individuals, which informs and shapes their behavior as they work in an organization; (2) the implicit values of the organization as embodied in the organizational culture and stated and unstated practices; and (3) the organization's explicit social purpose and stated mission.[3]

It is a good idea, then, when you look for a position in a new setting, to seek at least one person who appears to be a potential source of support. If no one promises to be such a resource, it is better to look elsewhere. In addition, you should be bold in asking questions that will allow you to gain some understanding of how support is expressed within the department and larger institution. To make an assessment, the following guidelines may be useful:

▶ Inquire of your future employer whether there are meetings or other sessions where problems associated with the everyday workplace stresses of health care delivery are discussed.

▶ Ask potential colleagues what they believe to be the sources of the most intense stress in that environment and how the group handles them.

▶ Make a mental note of those who appear to be potential sources of support, or if no one appears to be. If everyone denies that problems exist or becomes defensive about such questions when they are tactfully posed, this probably signals a setting in which stresses are dealt with alone, without the support of one's colleagues, or the institution.[4]

Fortunately, only in rare situations are no support mechanisms available. In fact, being a support to others is often the key to finding support from them when it is needed. The adage "To have a friend is to be one" holds true in the workplace.

Play: Enjoy One Another's Company

No one could—or should—keep their self-respect if they unnecessarily put up with or contribute to an atmosphere of doom and gloom. Persons in health professions fields are fortunate to be in a line of work in which they know they are usually making a positive difference in patients' lives. That in itself is reason to enjoy their work.

But there's more. Shortchanging the joy that can come from remembering to put some levity and fun into the environment is doing yourself a disfavor. It does not take much—a cartoon, a good joke, a lighthearted story that a colleague or patient is trying to tell, or some other type of pleasure can do the job. One author, himself a health professional, observes:

> Joy is only possible for persons who are attentive to the present. One cannot be happy if one is continually ruminating about what might have been or fretting over whether wishes will come to pass. Americans have a tough time with real joy. Americans are oriented toward outcomes, expectations, and the future; toward ever more competition in proving that they deliver the best results, and anxiously pondering how things might have turned out if only they had chosen differently. This makes it hard to be happy. In health care, these tendencies are exaggerated. Worries about what will happen next to the patient and worries about their own future careers blot out the possibility of joy for many health care professionals. Joy is a present tense phenomenon. It is possible only if one attends to the moment.[5]

Sometimes activities outside of work hours enhance the ability to enjoy one another in a more relaxed environment. There are the usual afternoon coffees or parties or sports teams, but the activities need not stop there. For instance, two of the authors were part of a writing group some time ago. We met regularly with several other health professions colleagues after work. We wrote about our work experiences in the form of short stories, poetry, and essays. At first all of us were scared to share anything, believing it would not be good enough. However, as we became more comfortable with one another, we started looking forward to hearing one another's stories. In addition to writing about some serious problems, we found our gathering to be a great vehicle for laughing at ourselves and good-naturedly at one another, as well as an "excuse" to get to know one another better. One delightful outcome was that we were able to publish some of our work for others to share, too.

In your own search for finding a congenial group, or whether you should stay in your current position or move on, you can use some of the same approaches that we suggested earlier to assess the type of situation you are getting into. Ask yourself:

▶ Does everyone look like they have just heard the worst news of their lives as they rush around?

▶ Are there cartoons, lighthearted comments, and funny pictures anywhere?

▶ Are there bulletin boards or other areas where staff gather with photos of the group having a good time together at a picnic, some other event, or celebrating one of the group?

▶ Is there a congenial place away from the patient care or other professional areas for conversation, relaxation, or a snack?

Obviously the professional or team who substitutes a good time for good work is not one who will, or should, last long in a position. However, finding and helping to further create a positive work environment can do much to generate an enriched, respectful environment for everyone involved, and not the least important, for you.

Refining Your Capacity to Provide Care Professionally

As we described in Chapter 4, the development of your capacity as a caregiver, or as it is often referred to in health care settings, *care provider*, begins as a student. This process will continue throughout your work life if you make yourself available to your continued growth and flourishing. Much rides on this decision because your self-respect and ability to realize full satisfaction depends on it. Some steps toward this laudable goal are to learn to distinguish between intimate and personal modes of caregiving and to recognize important differences between strictly social and therapeutic relationships. The former focuses on the depth of the relationship and the latter on the avenues of expression. We will address each for your consideration.

Intimate versus Personal Relationships

Acts of caregiving, intimate and personal ones, depend on the depth of involvement in which the persons engage in each other's lives. *Intimate care* is what you offer to someone you love or for whom you are willing to do a big favor out of deep gratitude or even duty. Most often that inner circle of intimate relationships is limited to a few—family members, or beloved friends. One test is that the offer of intimate forms of assistance in its most extreme form means that you would be willing to risk personal danger to yourself for this person. In contrast, *personal care* is what you are willing to offer colleagues, friends, acquaintances, or strangers whose human needs you see you can respond to without getting more personally entwined in their lives. It takes many forms in everyday interactions from giving directions, assisting a person physically, or donating money to a good cause. Random acts of kindness express care of this sort. Both types of relationship demand an investment in the well-being of others, and the boundaries are not always hard and fast between the two. For example, in a group of acquaintances you may over time become close to one and find yourselves more and more engaged in each other's lives.

Professional caring belongs to the category of personal rather than intimate relationships. Maintaining the respectful conduct that characterizes personal helping in the health professional and patient interaction is the focus of this book. A more in-depth description of its characteristics is the focus of Part Three.

⟳ REFLECTIONS

Reflect on the past couple days of your encounters with family, friends, and others with whom you have come into contact.
- Which of the encounters would you say were intimate?
- Which ones met the general criteria of personal caring conduct toward the other(s)?
- Why?

Social versus Therapeutic Relationships

A related way to view your relationships from the perspective of your being a care provider concentrates on the type of activities rather than degree of involvement with the other person. Any care you provide in which your resources are not prescribed by specific, well-defined professional skills that maintain boundaries specific to the professional-patient relationship are examples of *social relationships*.

Social caregiving takes many forms because the numbers of resources you can use are as numerous as your imagination and your willingness to extend yourself for someone else's benefit. One helps a child cross the street, one lessens an old man's loneliness by paying him a visit, or lends $5 to a neighbor in need. This type of caring stems from wanting to benefit someone else. Offers of the social help variety are not always welcomed by the recipient and in fact may not be interpreted as showing genuine care at all. This seems especially true if the recipient perceives the offer as being motivated solely by the person supposedly offering care but really wanting only to fulfill his or her own needs.[6] Persons with functional impairments are often victims of this displaced motive. Consider the following case recounted by a student.

> On weekends, the student cared for a 13-year-old boy with paraplegia who ambulated with the help of a wheelchair. One Saturday, the student and boy were shopping in a large department store and paused at a vending machine for a coke. First the student bought a soft drink for his young friend and then turned to buy one for himself. The boy had just taken the first sip and was resting the can on the arm of his wheelchair when a woman laden with bundles rushed up and dropped a dollar in his lap. She patted the astonished boy on the head and exclaimed, "Poor, poor boy. I hope that helps you get better." She then gathered up her packages and scurried away.

⊚ REFLECTIONS

What seems not to be caring behavior in this woman's actions? Why?
Supposing her motives were indeed to show personal care toward this young man, what could she have done that would have made a difference?

It seems to us that a self-reflection on the part of the woman would have quickly exposed her conduct as being inappropriate and maybe even a source of belittlement and bewilderment to the recipient (Figure 5-2).

In short, the helper in the social relationship may use any available means to offer assistance rather than depending on special skills, but how the offer of care is perceived by the recipient will be determined in part by what the motive seems to be and how sensitive the caregiver is to the effects of the offer of some kind of aid. There is another kind of care available and when put into the relational context is recognized as a therapeutic relationship.

A *therapeutic relationship* develops when the professional caregiver performs professionally competent acts designed to benefit the person who needs his or her services. Therapeutic caring is personal but not intimate. At times this is a difficult difference to grasp because often there are aspects of the therapeutic relationship that involve the patient's sharing of deeply intimate details of his or her life and that impinge on usual physical boundaries of propriety. Terms such as *therapeutic*

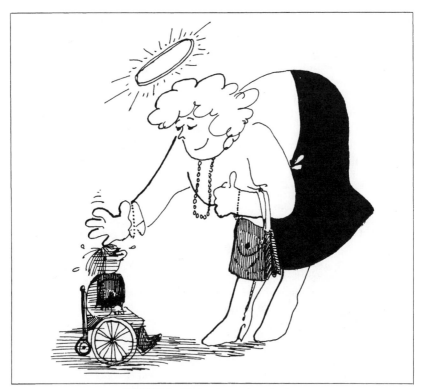

FIGURE 5-2: Misplaced expressions of caring.

use of the self and *therapeutic touch* point to how your primary resources of specific, well-defined skills may involve psychological or physical contact: The prosthetist may massage the stump of a patient's bare thigh in order to be sure the muscles are relaxed sufficiently for a prosthesis mold to fit accurately; a dietitian may interview a patient about deeply personal eating habits to evaluate nutritional status and plan the dietary regimen; nurses, assistants of all kinds, therapists, and others regularly touch, probe, hold, and stroke patients. More details about maintaining respect in these situations are taken up later. The common denominator is that the context determines what is permitted for competent, professionally appropriate care to be provided.

⊚ REFLECTIONS

- If you have chosen a health care field you want to be a part of, name some unique therapeutic activities that you may engage in during your interactions with patients that would not be considered appropriate in other societal environments.
- Name some that are not necessarily unique to this field but fall within the boundaries of a therapeutic relationship as it has been described earlier.

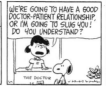

FIGURE 5-3: How not to create an effective therapeutic relationship! *(Peanuts: © United Feature Syndicate, Inc. Reprinted by permission.)*

The therapeutic relationship, although special, obviously includes polite consideration of another consistent with common decency. The importance of including common expressions of human caring is illustrated by its absence in the Peanuts cartoon (Figure 5-3). The following story illustrates a member of the health care team exhibiting this kind of decency within his professional role.

> When Eddy Underhill was admitted to the Veterans Affairs Medical Center again, no one was surprised. He was well known to the staff in the emergency department and to most of the personnel who had been there for any length of time, and none of them were glad to see him. Eddy lived in a furnished room in the poorest section of town, where his veteran's pension was enough to cover his rent plus enough alcohol to keep him drunk almost all the time. Occasionally, he would spend money on food, but never if it meant going without booze.
>
> This time he was admitted with impending delirium tremens, a life-threatening condition resulting from alcohol withdrawal. Often such admissions would occur toward the end of the month when his money ran out, and scavenging could not net him enough money to keep him drinking. Other times he was admitted for pneumonia, contracted after spending a winter night unconscious in the gutter; bleeding from esophageal varices; or trauma from falling on the street or being beaten up by thugs.
>
> Jesse Sampson, a young chaplain who had recently begun working at the hospital, started to visit Eddy after his acute withdrawal symptoms had subsided. Eddy had some degree of brain damage from chronic alcohol abuse but was garrulous and enjoyed "shooting the breeze" with this young man who came to see him every day. Chaplain Sampson was different from the doctors and nurses at the hospital, who spent as little time as possible with Eddy. The chaplain would sit down in a chair next to the bed as if he were not in a hurry to be somewhere else. He would ask Eddy questions about himself and his life as if he really cared about the answers. Eddy told Jesse that booze was his only friend and that his life was lonely, but he seemed warmer and more convivial when he was drunk. He had no family. His friends were the other people on skid row. He had no ambitions. Life was hard and pretty senseless, and he just wanted to get through it as easily as he could. He appreciated being brought to the hospital when he was in really bad shape. There it was warm, and he got decent food, but most of the people treated him with thinly veiled disgust. This often made him angry. "I'm a gomer (get out of

Continued

my emergency room), you know. They hate my kind, but they can't come right out and say so, so they try to ignore me. They wish I would die, and some time I will. Would serve 'em right. But they won't care—they'll just keep on goin' about their prissy and proud ways. They think they are so good-hearted, but they don't know what it's like to live on the street. To be alone with your only friend, the bottle. It's my life, and I got a right to do what I want. I served my time in the war, and I got a right to be in this hospital, to come in here and get dried out and get a little food. I'm an old man. I got a right."[4]

Mr. Underhill is the type of patient who can cause much consternation for health professionals. His diagnosis of acute reaction to alcohol addiction is embedded in a social history that makes it difficult for most health professionals to treat him like everyone else. He is homeless; he does not fit the picture of a patient in many ways, and he keeps coming back again and again. He is not the kind of patient that most care providers welcome. The example set by the chaplain is not always easy to follow, although most would applaud the chaplain's caring approach to providing a therapeutic presence, which most would agree is a health-supporting presence for Eddy Underhill.

⊙ REFLECTIONS

- How many sources of potential negative bias toward a patient can you identify in this story?
- What would you do to try to show care for this patient?
- What things about him would you find difficult to accept?

This dramatic instance is not the only type of challenge you will encounter. For example, some patients who initially seek your services seem to resist any kind of help, even though you judge that the services offered should benefit them. For these patients, receiving help may be seen as a sign of weakness, even though their suffering or troubling condition has driven them to your door. Other types of patients might surprise you. Sometimes people who are lonely do not comply with your efforts because if they do, they will lose the benefit of your company. (For some major challenges that patients face, see Chapter 6.) These and other examples highlight the fact that the appropriate goals of a therapeutic relationship are not always easily accomplished with full respect intact. Doing your job well under even the most challenging circumstance is closely tied to feelings of self-respect, so making sure you are in a situation in which your best self can be expressed in a therapeutic relationship is extremely important.[7] The differences between care as a social relationship and a therapeutic relationship are summarized in Box 5-1.

Sharing Responsibility for Optimal Care

In the next few pages you will examine two mechanisms that will help you succeed in providing optimal care under the wide range of circumstances you will encounter over our career. The first is teamwork, and the second is patient referral.

BOX 5-1

COMPARISON BETWEEN CARING IN A SOCIAL AND THERAPEUTIC RELATIONSHIP

Caring in a Social Relationship
May be an intimate or personal act
Helper uses a wide variety of resources

Caring in a Therapeutic Relationship
Is a personal but not an intimate act
Helper primarily uses well-defined, specialized professional skills

---

These mechanisms have arisen because of the complexity of the health care system and also the knowledge that so much of patient care cannot optimally be offered solely by you as a stand-alone clinician; rather, other competencies of your colleagues are also required to achieve the optimal outcome consistent with a caring response.

Teams and Teamwork

Almost all health care today is provided through interprofessional teams. You will have an opportunity to consider some ways that you can learn to show respect to patients, other members of your team, and what you can expect in terms of their respect for you.

⊚ REFLECTIONS

Take a minute to think about the different types of teams you have participated on.
* What were the criteria for being chosen to be on the team?
* Was it designed to cooperate with other teams or compete against them?
* What were the goals of the team?
* What activities were required of team members to meet these goals?

By referring to your previous experience, you may get a better idea of how your participation as a member of interprofessional health care teams will be similar or different from those situations.

Interprofessional health care teams arose during the middle of the past century to effect two important goals in patient care:

▶ Ensure coordinated and comprehensive care and guard against the fragmentation of services that could result from more specialization

▶ Ensure that the patient's many needs are met in a manner that shows respect for the whole person as a unique individual by using different perspectives to tailor care

Most interprofessional teams include care providers with more than one level of formal education. Some hold doctoral degrees or other university degrees and become qualified legally as professionals in the more traditional sense, whereas many

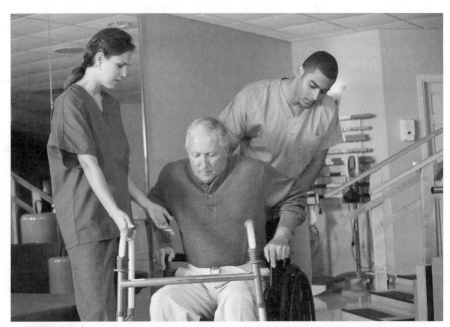

FIGURE 5-4: Physical therapist and physical therapy assistant with patient. (©iStockphoto.com)

other teams include assistants. The *assistant* is someone who works together with a professional to help accomplish the patient's goals. The term itself sometimes adds confusion because some assistants, such as physicians' assistants, are fully qualified professionals themselves and may enjoy the benefit of assistants who aid them. Other assistants are trained in programs to become a part of the support staff for nurse practitioners, therapists, technologists, or other professionals. Professional assistant programs were introduced to help provide lower-cost optimal care and to alleviate serious personnel shortages in many health fields (Figure 5-4).

This multifaceted perspective is an advantage because it can not only expand the range of technical skills available but also allow the patient's caregivers to consider several points of view regarding the larger picture of what is best for the patient. Consider the following case.

> Jack came back from military duty with one arm, the result of a mine explosion that killed four of his buddies with whom he was on the mission. Being one of only three survivors in the incident, he said over and over again that he felt lucky to be alive and planned to live life to its fullest. Following his shoulder disarticulation amputation, he was sent back to the United States to recover and begin rehabilitation. He seemed determined to prove that he was ready to take life on as he participated with vigor in his rehabilitation regimen.

So it came as a surprise when, some weeks into his rehabilitation program, he abruptly announced that he was now leaving the hospital, having decided not to wear an upper extremity prosthesis after all. He said that he had been online talking to various people with amputations, and many of them did not wear their prostheses. He himself had just begun to be fitted and could "tell" it was going to be cumbersome. "I'll do better without that thing," he said.

Most of the therapists involved in his care were convinced that this 23-year-old man was absolutely doing the wrong thing whether from the point of view of reduced function, poorer trunk balance, or aesthetics. But some of the other health professionals, especially some of the nurses, a resident physician, and his social worker were not so sure he was making the wrong decision. A physical therapy assistant who had been working with him for almost the whole duration of his stay sided with those who felt he was making a decision consistent with his personality. For one thing, they believed that he had the psychological makeup to fall into the group of patients most likely to discard their prostheses after a while. The social worker reflected on a discussion with Jack in which he said he felt that going through life with one arm would give him a greater opportunity to tell others how he lost it. That way people would know he believed in the United States and "was proud of losing his arm for his country." The physical therapy assistant conveyed that he had said on one or more occasion, "Those artificial arms aren't real. It wouldn't be me to have one of those things."

To tell the truth, none of the team members were 100% comfortable with his decision. Their interprofessional team meeting lasted longer than usual with the result being that they decided on the following courses of action: First, the physical therapist (whom Jack seemed to like) would probe further as to the reasons Jack made this decision. Second, the staff liaison psychiatrist would talk with him to determine if he had issues that he did not want to raise with the other team members or if this was a result of depression. Third, the social worker would ask his permission to talk with other family members, none of whom could afford to visit him in a state more than 1000 miles from their home, though they talked with him often by phone. His mom and brother had even talked to the social worker a couple of times. Finally, everyone would continue to show him as much support as possible while trying to keep him from bolting right away and also find other areas of his life at the rehabilitation center, where he could exercise his say-so.

This health care team was honoring that a good intervention must fit within the context of the patient's needs, hopes, and fears. Some would have had experience in amputee care and would know that, following a shoulder disarticulation, a person who is well qualified medically to be fitted with an upper extremity prosthesis may be opposed to it on aesthetic, financial, or religious grounds. Assuming that the patient understands the ramifications of each of the options, withholding the prosthesis would be judged a morally permissible course of action despite the technical advantages of the prosthesis. Thus, Jack's well-being became the reference point for deciding what steps could be taken individually and collectively to be sure he was making the right decision.

What happened in Jack's situation? After doing their homework, the team met again. The social worker said that her call to Jack's mom and brother had concerned them enough that they decided to borrow money to come out to visit him. The others agreed that they would urge Jack to hang in there until the family visit had taken place. The visit seemed to turn him around, and he decided to remain in the program. This convinced the team members who had had doubts about encouraging him to try the prosthesis that they should support such a trial.

In addition to the patient-oriented goals that interprofessional health care teams serve, the team approach has been welcomed by institutions because teams can help meet the goals of efficient health care delivery while enjoying a sense of equality and mutuality among themselves. Health care institutions are made up of two broad categories of actions: actions flowing from hierarchy-derived decisions and those flowing from community-derived decisions.

In a hierarchical pattern of decision-making, decisions flow from very few persons to affect very many. The authority and responsibility weigh heaviest at the top. A value realized by this mode of functioning is institutional efficiency. Health care teams implement policies and other decisions made by the administration.

In a community pattern of decision-making, decisions arise more equally throughout the institution. This "bottom-up" approach has gained in recognition in recent years. Authority and accountability are shared across the institution by its various constituents. Power differentials are less obvious. Caregivers with different skills function together with mutual support and as task-sharers. Values realized by this approach are equality and mutuality. Interprofessional health care teams not only help to implement policies and practices created by others but also may generate them.

Looking back at the patient-oriented goals realized through interprofessional teamwork and an understanding of how teams help contribute to an institution's goals, it should be easy to see how the team environment helps each member contribute to optimum care, thereby also enhancing one's own self-respect as a competent caregiver in complex situations.

Patient Referral

Patient referral is another method of ensuring that a person who seeks professional services will receive optimal care while not having to depend completely on one professional's capabilities and resources. It acknowledges that you cannot always single-handedly manage a person's health care needs, even those that warrant skills that fall within the scope of what your profession offers. Sometimes health care providers are reticent to refer a patient to someone else, even though she or he can do the job more effectively and it is in the patient's best interest. Reasons are that health care providers take their jobs seriously, become attached to patients with whom they have been working, and find it painful to admit what feels like failure. None of these reasons justify holding on to a patient who would benefit more from the help of another colleague.

You should take steps to implement referral when the patient's progress is at risk of being hindered because:

▶ you are not experienced in appropriate techniques,
▶ you do not have adequate equipment for providing proper services to that particular person,
▶ you and the patient have a serious and irresolvable personality conflict,

▶ you experience a negative bias toward the person (or group to which the person belongs) to the extent that you believe it may interfere with providing competent care, or

▶ your attachment to the patient is resulting in conduct more akin to intimacy than the conduct appropriate in a therapeutic relationship.

Optimal care, then, entails using the time-honored referral system to extend your professional resources. It requires self-knowledge: knowing when and where to refer the patient for further evaluation or treatment. In this manner, your professional integrity can be maintained, and your self-respect will be enhanced because of your good judgment.

It is to this larger context of resources that the last section of this chapter points you.

Participating in Goodness

This chapter on respect for yourself in your professional capacity understandably includes ways that you can be supported sufficiently to provide a foundation for patients to have confidence in you (Figure 5-5).

Attention to these suggestions will allow you to shift from being a caregiver following the must do's and must not do's to the joy of experiencing the goodness that your role allows you to share with others in the everyday practice of your profession. What is goodness? Everyone's experience of it will vary somewhat. We like this

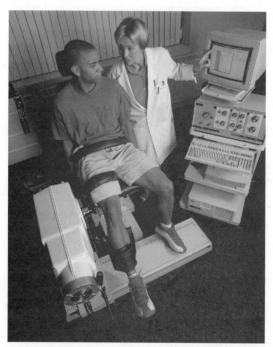

FIGURE 5-5: When the health professional works with the patient, it inspires confidence. *(© Corbis.)*

businessman's reflection on goodness after he had a reverse in his company's success and rebuilt the company on a values-based ethic similar to the ethic one finds in health professions writings. He found that he and his employees were infused with a new passion for their work. They felt they were participating in something wonderful that went beyond the everyday routine of their particular tasks:

> Everyone has experienced a version of goodness, and you don't have to be pushed to the wall, like me, to find it: When you enjoy a work of art, thrill to a piece of music, feel that tingle in your spine when you read a passage in a novel . . . you have been touched by something outside of yourself. Remember when you fell in love? When things of this world grab you like this, in a way that we are inclined to think of as "deep," then you have been touched by goodness.[8]

Although we do not often think of being in love with our work or experiencing and sharing goodness through our daily conduct, there is the potential for that type of richness. Physical and emotional healthfulness is a cherished value in every culture. We participate in promoting that goodness as caregivers in health professions settings. Continuing to find work satisfaction year after year requires striving for the most value one can be in the role and the most value one can contribute and receive. Patients and families respond positively to that ideal, making them more willing to be participants in the process of their own healing and healthfulness.

SUMMARY

Your career in the health professions requires you to assume many roles. Self-respect is an essential component of satisfaction over the course of that career, and to maintain and nurture it requires several capacities. Showing respect to and support for family, friends, and the people you work with daily is in itself a resource: Their support of you is essential to break your fall should you ever feel like you are losing your footing. Understanding that the appropriate nature of your relationships with patients is personal and therapeutic is essential. Your participation on interprofessional teams and honoring when patient referrals are warranted will focus your attention on your own competence and skills. And remembering to enjoy the benefits of this type of work including the opportunity to participate in a basic type of goodness is in large part its own reward.

REFERENCES

1. Allegretti J: *Loving your job, finding your passion: work and the spiritual life*, Mahwah, NJ, 2000, Paulist Press.
2. Reynolds RC, Stone J, editors: *On doctoring: stories, poems, essays*, New York, 1995, Simon and Schuster.
3. Rambur R, Vallett C, Cohen JA, Tarule J: The moral cascade: distress, eustress, and the virtuous organization, *J Org Moral Psych* 1(1):41–54, 2010.
4. Purtilo R, Doherty R: *Ethical dimensions in the health professions*, ed 5, Philadelphia, St. Louis, MO, 2010, WB Saunders.
5. Sulmasy DP: *The healer's calling: a spirituality for physicians and other health care professionals*, Mahwah, NJ, 1997, Paulist Press.

6. Dugatkin LA: *The altruism equation: seven scientists search for the meaning of altruism*, Princeton, NJ, 2006, Princeton University Press.

7. Purtilo R: New respect for respect in ethics education. In Purtilo R, Jensen G, Royeen CB, editors: *Educating for moral action: a sourcebook in health and rehabilitation ethics*, Philadelphia, 2005, FA Davis.

8. Chappell T: *Managing upside down*, New York, 1999, William Morrow.

PART TWO

Questions for Thought and Discussion

1. You have been asked by members of your class to run for office in the national student organization of your profession. You are already busy with schoolwork and your personal commitments, and still you are tempted and honored to be recognized by your classmates. List your most important priorities and decide what would be compromised the most by taking on this new position. What values will determine whether you will choose to run for this office?

2. You have just begun your final situated learning assignment before graduation. You are excited about continuing to refine your skills in this setting because it is one similar to the type of place you imagine applying for a position. The supervisor to whom you are assigned tells you that she has heard you are an outstanding student. She goes on to say that due to an unexpected emergency in her family she is asking you to go in to Ms. Krabowski's room on your own to perform a procedure you have never before performed. You tell her of your lack of experience, and she questions you about how you think it should be done. When she hears your responses, she says reassuringly, "You will be fine.'" You can see that in her mind the discussion is finished. What should you do?

3. Ms. Yeo is a newly graduated professional. Mr. Kazantikis is an effusive patient whom she has treated four times before today. They have always warmly greeted each other, and he said at the end of the last treatment, "You are a honey." He has arrived for treatment, and Ms. Yeo takes him into the treatment area. He hugs her with a quick bear hug. She asks him about his health, how he has responded to his last treatment, about his family. As usual they are now sitting facing each other. He tells her a joke and, laughing at himself, puts his hand on her knee. She moves so as to release his hand and tells him what the treatment today will involve. She asks him to slip off his shirt. He does so slowly, smiling at her.

   What more would you like to know, if anything, about this situation to judge whether Ms. Yeo is in a situation where either she or the patient is confusing intimate and personal relational behaviors appropriate for a therapeutic relationship?

   If you were Ms. Yeo, how would you respond to Mr. Kazantikis's conduct toward you?

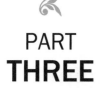

PART THREE

Respect for the Patient's Situation

Part Three examines closely the person who seeks professional services—the patient. Almost everyone becomes a patient at some time, and you can undoubtedly recall some fears and problems you have experienced as one, as well as the sympathy and special attention you received in that situation. Obviously, your understanding of a patient's predicament is a resource that can help you respond more effectively and respectfully.

In most cases, a person's role in society during a period of illness and its accompanying incapacity differs in significant ways from before the person became ill. Part Three examines how the situation affects him or her. The result can be a return to health, learning to live with incapacity, or preparation for death. Chapter 6 discusses special challenges faced by patients and how to respect the person in this situation. Chapter 7 examines the patient in regards to how his or her intimate and close personal relationships are affected. Ask yourself the following questions as you read about the patient as a person:

- How do my attitudes and conduct convey respect toward a patient?
- What do I need to know about patients to effectively work with them to set reasonable goals consistent with their deepest values?
- How can I best honor and support the patient in the context of his or her intimate and close personal relationships?

CHAPTER

6

Respect for Challenges Facing Patients

CHAPTER OBJECTIVES

The reader will be able to:

- Describe common conditions that create barriers to maintaining wellness
- List the most important changes experienced by persons who become patients in health care institutions and some challenges they face in reckoning with such changes
- Compare challenges facing inpatients, ambulatory care patients, and patients who are treated in their homes
- Identify several types of privileges or accommodations patients may experience
- Describe key characteristics of Molière's Imaginary Invalid that are similar to those of patients today who seem to benefit from remaining ill

---

Ten years ago, if I were setting out to make a film about catastrophic illness and subsequent disability, I would not have cast myself in the lead role. In my prestroke ignorance, I probably would have looked for someone stronger and braver than I—not yet knowing that we are all capable of much more bravery than we think.

—*B.S. Klein*[1]

Most challenges facing patients are related to their transition from everyday routine to the altered role that sick or impaired persons assume in society. The role includes physical, psychological, and spiritual challenges, whether the condition is short or long term. Fortunately, these challenges have received considerable attention in health professions literature and curricula in recent years, so it is likely that you will have one or more courses in which they are discussed. Some common themes are presented here as a basis for your ongoing thought and reflection.

Maintaining Wellness

It is fitting that a chapter on challenges to patients begins with some reflections on maintaining wellness because in recent years there has been much emphasis on maintaining and fostering a healthy lifestyle. Staying healthy seems to be to everyone's advantage—the individual, his or her loved ones, and society. Wellness ensues from maintaining health-supporting habits over a lifetime. As you know, a healthy life ultimately depends on many things including a safe and health-inducing environment. Good nutrition, sleep, exercise, and other health-fostering habits are essential. Freedom from basic want and violence are essential, too. Today thousands of health professionals build practices on the basis of preventative approaches—teaching people some of the essentials of how to remain healthy. A few examples are nutritionists who are involved in school nutrition programs, nurses and nurse practitioners who may work in perinatal or other community education and screening clinics, physicians, and occupational and physical therapists and assistants who focus on safety and health maintenance in the workplace or hold positions in sports or recreational settings. A growing body of literature suggests that the mind and body can develop and grow stronger over an entire lifetime (Figure 6-1).

At the same time, lifelong healthiness is not a goal completely within an individual's own control, even with the help of a safe and health-inducing environment. Almost weekly there are discoveries of new genetic predispositions to illness; scientists have identified scores of environmental toxins, and other health hazards are appearing on the horizon; many people live in conditions of poverty, lacking basic public health and safety conditions, while others suffer unavoidable work-related stress symptoms. Accidents and other misfortunes dash dreams, alter possibilities, and modify relationships.

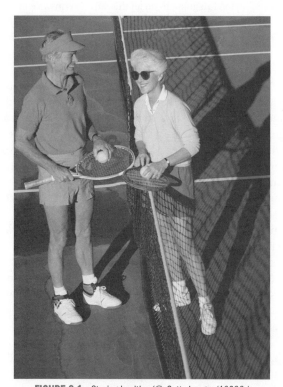

FIGURE 6-1: Staying healthy. *(© Getty Images/10293.)*

Moreover, most of us today have periods of less wellness or more wellness. For example, a person with mild pneumonia or late-onset diabetes or severe atherosclerotic heart disease may function mostly as a healthy person but still may need health care for serious symptoms related to the condition. At best, each of us moves through life on a continuum between maximal health and life-threatening illness or death.

Respect for Patient's Health-Related Changes

The transition from being relatively well to becoming ill or impaired almost inevitably entails change in the form of losses. The loss may take the shape of decreased physical or mental function, as reflected in this excerpt from a young woman who has been working energetically to recover from stroke and then "bottoms out":

> One Saturday morning, you can't bring yourself to get out of bed. Jim [her husband] hears you weeping, comes into the bedroom, and lies down next to you,
>
> "What's wrong?"
>
> "I don't feel like myself. I don't want to get up and face another day in this damaged body. Everything is so hard and I'm just tired of trying to do basic shit, like getting dressed. I just don't think I can live this way. I can't do it."
>
> "Can't do what? Get dressed? Come on, I'll help you."
>
> "No. . . . I don't think I can do all the things that I keep telling everyone I'm going to do. I think I've been saying I'm going to do all this stuff to convince myself. Jim, I can't even put a sock on."
>
> This is not who you are. You feel even worse now because you have unloaded all your fears and insecurities on Jim. All he wants is positive energy from you, and you cannot even give him that. . . .[2]

Persons who lose their sight or other senses, those who lose control of movement or vital body functions, and those who through illness become incapable of making competent judgments may experience a similar sense of loss in some regards, in part due to society's response to various conditions. The loss may also involve a change in physical appearance, such as the person who undergoes an amputation or is scarred after a severe burn.

The significance of these changes for each person is determined by a complex interweaving of several factors such as:
▶ the physical and emotional effects of the pathological process itself,
▶ the alteration in the person's environment or social roles, and
▶ the coping mechanisms the patient has developed throughout his or her life.

Ultimately one cannot predict how a patient will respond. Experience of the significance of the loss is highly personal. Sometimes it is completely understandable to others. The concert pianist who loses an index finger in an accident will experience it as a more profound loss than most of us who might experience a similar trauma. Other times the effect on the patient baffles everyone. Patients will react to you in ways that express their concern about their losses. For example, upon entering a patient's room, the phlebotomist may catch the brunt of the patient's anxiety through comments such as, "Here comes the vampire!" The radiological technologist may be accused of destroying cells with the imaging equipment. Professionals whose diagnostic and treatment procedures require patients to engage in physical or emotional exertion can be accused of sapping a patient's strength. These expressions of anger or fear reflect the challenge a patient is facing in trying to protect his or her body and sense of well-being from further loss.

---

⑨ REFLECTIONS

Reflect on losses you might incur that you think would most threaten your identity and sense of well-being. Name a:

Sensory loss _____

Physical function loss _____

Body part loss _____

Mental capacity loss _____

- Why do you think these specific losses would affect your sense of well-being (and of being "well") more than some other losses you might sustain?
- Do you think your list is similar to that of most people your age? Of persons 20 years older or younger than you? Why or why not?

Loss of Former Self-Image

A natural extension of loss of function or previous physical appearance is the feeling that one's old self is gone. This is especially likely when physical or mental change promises to be prolonged or permanent. Recall the woman described earlier who wept because, "I don't feel like myself. I don't want to get up and face another day in this damaged body." You have probably had the feeling sometimes that you just "weren't yourself" that day or that what you did in a particular situation was not typical of the "real you." For most people, this sense of self-alienation is temporary; however, it may become more long-lasting for a person experiencing significant losses associated with injury or illness.[3]

A patient's feeling of having lost herself or himself may result in part from the conviction that one is largely determined by what one looks like. In other words, one's self-image depends to a large extent on body image (Figure 6-2).

There is a close relationship between appearance, accompanying body image, and sense of self-worth.[4] This is not surprising in a society with a multibillion dollar advertising enterprise stressing appearance above all else, and with it the idea of physical beauty and vitality depicted within narrow norms. Despite the proverb's bidding, most of us still do "judge a book by its cover," and the harshest judgments often are against oneself.

Have you encountered anyone today you thought was exceptionally fit, beautiful, or graceful? Our stereotypes of success and assurance of acceptance often depend on physical appearance. Painful sanctions are imposed on those whose appearance deviates too far from some societally determined standard of normality. A person who encounters illness or impairment must face daily the changes that depart from these stereotypes of success and beauty. The work that accompanies developing a new sense of one's physical self after change in physical bodily appearance brought about by surgery has been explored by one of the authors through poetry:

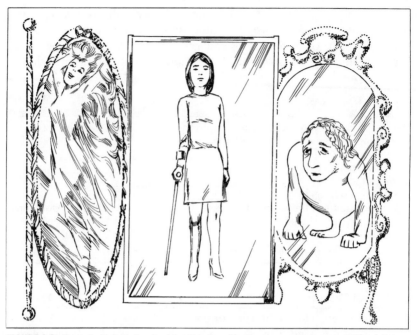

FIGURE 6-2: The patient's fantasies about the distortion of her former appearance may override what she sees in the mirror.

FRENCH WEAVING

I piece together the tattered edges
with illusion net,
laying just the right size squares
over the gaping holes.
Carefully,
arduously
embroider the net to the original.
Trying to match the pattern,
tie up loose ends,
mimic the original curve and detail.
I pick up a thread
of who I once was,
try and attach it,
here,
here,
and here.
My clumsy attempts
only approximate the intricacy of the design.
Yet the untrained eye
cannot see my repair.
Run your fingers over my skin
to feel the flaws.
            —Amy Haddad[5]

⊚ REFLECTIONS

- What is this poet saying? (The title, "French Weaving," is named for an embroidery technique used to repair damaged lace or crochet work. If done by an expert hand, it is hard to see areas of repair, though another expert would always be able to tell.)
- Does this apply to the work patients have to do to help "repair" themselves?
- Name some skills that your health profession has as resources to assist in such repair work.

As you may expect, part of the health professional's success depends on an adeptness at helping the patient either reclaim his or her old image as recovery occurs or, when necessary, discover a realistic and satisfactory new body image. Timing is one important element in your work with patients who are adjusting to changes in body image. There is no preestablished time frame for a man to accept his colostomy or a woman to look at the scar where her breast used to be. Each patient will move in his or her own way and at his or her own pace into this new life territory.

Respect for Necessary Changes in Patients' Values

In addition to being able to identify one's own and others' values, it is imperative to recognize that everyone's values change from time to time. The circumstances that force or enable most people to change their values usually evolve slowly, whereas those that force a patient to do so may appear in a matter of minutes or hours! Illness or injury almost always causes a patient's and their loved ones concern about whether and how the person's values will have to change.

The course of one patient's evolving values is reflected in her response to her condition:

> Daniela Janowski was the star soccer player on her college team at Midtown State College. It came as a terrible surprise when in her mid-20s she began to experience the debilitating symptoms of multiple sclerosis.
>
> It is 6 years later. She is almost totally unable to walk. Her weight has dropped to 90 lb from her previous 125. She suffered one period of deep depression. She says that many people pity her, but she now has come to the happy conclusion that she "has much to live for."

What types of values might Daniela have that would allow her to feel as if there is "much to live for" when so much has radically changed in her life?

The process of reclaiming and replacing values may take weeks, months, or years for any of us. The person who becomes a patient must learn what the illness or injury really means in terms of long-term impairment. Another woman who, like Daniela, had multiple sclerosis told one of the authors that it took her years to stop doing silly things that overstressed her. She said, "It was because I didn't *know* my disease; now I *know* it, like a friend, strange as that may sound. Not knowing was the hardest part … "

As we reiterate in later chapters, the success of adjustment and acceptance to inevitable change is based on the support of family, friends, and those treating him or her in the health professions. One of the greatest gifts you can offer is to be present as a person tries on a new identity with the values that will be fitting for the new situation.

Institutionalized Settings

Although not all people who become ill or injured spend time in hospitals or other health care institutions, the most seriously involved are admitted as inpatients. *Inpatient* is a term applied to those who enter a health care facility to remain there for a period of time.

The necessity of spending time confined in a health care facility may significantly disrupt an individual's personal life, as well as the lives of family, occupational associates, and friends. The challenges associated with the disruption may be primarily social, but it is likely that they will also be economic, owing to loss of work, health care–related expenses, or both. The economic burden is especially acute for a person who is self-supporting or is the breadwinner in a family. A single parent has the burden of finding and paying for suitable caretakers for children. A child, teenager, or other student loses valuable instruction and may fall behind or have to drop out of school. A professional person may have to forego participation in an important project. Whatever the individual's personal responsibilities, he or she is likely to be affected socially and economically.

Psychological stresses compound the social and economic ones. A person often believes that entering an institution for care signals that he or she is not winning the battle of coping with an illness or impairment. This psychological defeat can be as deleterious to his or her welfare as the physical manifestations of the illness itself. In submitting to confinement in an institution, the person finally is admitting openly that the problem is "out of control" and that people professionally qualified to provide certain services are needed on a continuous basis. The patient understandably is anxious about leaving his or her health, and perhaps life, in the hands of strangers but judges that there are no other good alternatives. Sometimes the awareness that the institutionalization took place because of severe stress on family and other caregivers adds to the discouragement.

Challenges Associated with Institutional Life

The disruption of daily and other normal life patterns and coping mechanisms that may accompany patients' admissions is exacerbated by the fact that suddenly they are robbed of both home and important basic privacies. Therefore, having met the initial challenge of admitting to illness or impairment, patients now have to face other changes.

Home

Most people view their home as a safe haven in a complex, fast-paced world. Of course, there are some exceptions, notably people for whom home is a place of loneliness, strife, abuse, or boredom. Occasionally, a person will feign illness to be admitted to—or exaggerate symptoms to remain in—a health care facility just to escape threats to their well-being. These patients require special consideration by health professionals and are discussed later in this chapter.

What makes home so desirable for most people when they are away from it? The answer is that the majority of physical, psychological, and social comforts of home are missing in health care facilities.

Physical comforts take a number of forms. You have undoubtedly walked into someone's room or home where everything is in incredible chaos and disarray. In the midst of the pandemonium, the person or family members appear perfectly at ease; this is their idea of really living! Undoubtedly, you have also entered a home where even the teacups seem to sit primly on shelves, where dust dares not settle, and curtains never ruffle. In the midst of this porcelain perfection, these family members also appear perfectly at ease!

The physical comfort of home may best be described as freedom to extend one-self naturally and completely into one's immediate environment: to do (or not do) what one wishes, when one wishes, and how one wishes. The environment within the home, whether it contains 1 or 40 rooms, has been designed to conform to one's own needs, habits, and desires.

The bed is a good example of how health care facilities often are unable to adequately accommodate the needs and habits of a person. Almost anyone would agree that a good night's rest greatly determines one's outlook on life the next day, and most people acknowledge that their own bed is one of the most important comforts of home. The standard hospital bed is of a given height, width, length, and firmness. Although the hospital personnel stop short of treating patients in the manner of Procrustes, the culprit in Greek mythology who invited his guests to sleep in his guest bed and responded by chopping off the legs of those who were too tall, institutions are usually limited to offering a standard hospital bed.

The obvious difficulties of totally personalizing every patient's health care setting are readily apparent. Hospice is a notable exception, with many hospices giving high priority to encouraging patients to have familiar objects around them. Many nursing homes and long-term care facilities become the final home to residents unable to return to their own dwellings. Many such facilities also are devoting much more attention to providing familiar, comfort-enhancing surroundings. The more that can be done to optimize physical comfort for the patient who is away from home, the more readily he or she will be able to direct energies toward healing, adjusting to dying from a life-threatening illness, or living with impairment.

Psychological and social comforts of familiar surroundings are also sacrificed with institutionalization. A favorite chair for relaxation, a magnifying mirror for applying makeup, a family picture, or a ragged toy may all be symbols of security to the person. The mere arrangement of furniture in a room or the sight of a tree or birdbath in the yard may give a person a sense of well-being. We are told that many patients, upon returning home, burst into tears upon being welcomed by a beloved pet or when noting that a flowerbed has blossomed in his or her absence. All too often these comforts are left behind when the person goes to a health care facility.

Psychological and social comfort may also be experienced in the routine associated with being "at home." It is not at all unusual for a patient who enters a health care facility to become confused about what day of the week it is because important, regularly scheduled events are missing. The person who likes to start the day with a cup of coffee and the morning paper will be unsettled when, in a health care facility, the coffee is served with breakfast and the morning paper arrives just before he or she is scheduled to undergo the first diagnostic test or treatment session of the day. A child who is used to a bedtime story may have great difficulty sleeping without it.

Familiarity is most significantly embodied by people and pets in the home. An older woman may literally live for the companionship of a small granddaughter. A single person may look forward to the weekly visit of a bridge group or housekeeper. Children have the familiarity of family and playmates. The harsh restrictions regarding visiting hours, number of guests, and, most of all, the exclusion of children or pets from the presence of institutionalized patients, may be a source of sorrow in itself.

All of these examples highlight serious but often unstated problems that patients in health care facilities face—to find basic comforts that they have experienced in their homes. In fact, patients do try to retrieve a little bit of home. A remarkable sign is the contents of their rooms and bedside stands. Contents of a stand tell one as much about the patient as the contents of a small boy's pocket does about him (Figure 6-3). Generally, the tabletop is cluttered with greeting cards, photos, or stuffed animals. In the top drawer are stamps, writing paper, religious books or objects, assorted ointments, a Swiss Army knife, a cell phone, and more! One of the authors once found a smoked herring in the back of a drawer after a roommate complained that the patient in the next bed was sneaking fish into his bland diet, and the smell was telling all.

A health care provider who has the opportunity to see into an open drawer will glean much information about the patient's personality and life.

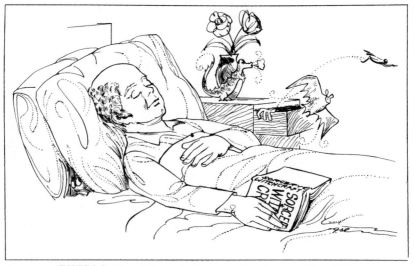

FIGURE 6-3: The bedside stand will reveal untold mysteries about the patient.

You will also learn something about the patient if the room is devoid of personal objects. An empty room may indicate that the patient is not willing to be sick enough to stay too long or is too ill to have even thought about his or her surroundings. Dying patients may want to divest themselves of possessions or get rid of reminders that they will not "get well." Empty rooms may also mean these patients have no one to bring them anything.

Note, however, that a patient understandably may be sensitive about having a caregiver snoop around the room, even if only to read a card attached to a bowl of roses or to linger while hanging up a bathrobe in the closet. Their sensitivity about these seemingly innocent gestures is due to the fact that, in addition to missing the comforts of home, the patient is also robbed of privacy in many ways and may count this additional invasion as inappropriate or annoying.

Privacy

The need for individual privacy may vary from person to person depending on his or her ethnicity, age, other cultural traits, and past experience. Whatever the individual boundaries of comfort, every patient in an institutional setting will experience less control over his or her privacy needs than at home. In many instances inattention by caregivers to this fact is seen by a patient as a glaring sign of disrespect.

◎ REFLECTIONS

Picture this—you are a patient uprooted from your home and placed in a health care facility room. Which of the following do you think will bother you the most?

- You are forced to be in a double room with a stranger as a roommate.
- "Walls" are curtains through which health professionals and others can listen or intrude without warning.
- There is no opportunity to hold a confidential conversation.
- You cannot have a good cry, pray aloud, have an angry outburst, or use the commode without others hearing.
- You cannot lock the door to your room or to the bathroom.
- Love-making with a sexual partner seems out of the question.
- Light switches are out of your reach and can be switched on and off only by persons entering the room.

This scenario illustrates that except in rare circumstances, at least some of your most cherished privacy "props" are removed during institutionalization. For some, privacy is necessary to succeed in certain activities such as sleeping or urinating. If a patient feels that he or she is being watched constantly because of monitors or windows from the hallway, it may be nearly impossible for him or her to conduct the most basic hygienic and other activities of daily living.

Lack of privacy has many cultural nuances that all too often are neglected. In some cultures, the most profound shame would be experienced by a person whose body or bodily functions are exposed to a member of the opposite sex, even a professional caregiver. In some instances a woman would be banned from her community.

Overhearing a conversation of someone else may be a sign of extreme rudeness. Passing gas or belching, vomiting, or crying out in pain may be considered unseemly and cause for great embarrassment. All of those are potential causes for anxiety due to the lack of privacy alone!

The hallmark of the loss of privacy is the hospital gown. Even presidents and kings are not spared the potential indignity of walking down the hall in that garment with the gaping back! You can help patients by making sure they are covered adequately to preserve their modesty.

Whatever the source, the patient robbed of privacy is likely to feel intense discomfort. You can do a great favor to the patient by showing respect through diligence in helping him or her meet the challenge of maintaining personal privacy.

Loss of Independence and Control

Challenges related to the loss of home and privacy are rooted in the far more basic loss of independence or say-so about basic things in a patient's life. The institutional value of efficiency discussed in Chapter 2 allows the facility to be responsive to the many demands of its functioning. At the same time it may create serious problems for the patient who needs time for solitude or religious observance, variety in a schedule, or other resources he or she uses to keep a sense of balance and perspective. Most health facilities impose profound restrictions on independence, many of them unnecessary. For instance, almost every minute of the day is scheduled for patients, their preferences often being unnecessarily compromised in the name of staff efficiency. For others, their choices about how and where they would like to spend their unscheduled time are ignored and are usually significantly limited anyway by policies or institutional practices. Patients are transported or accompanied from place to place for therapy, diagnostic procedures, and other activities, often not knowing where they are headed, how long it will take, or what is going to happen. In many facilities visiting hours are fixed, and the telephone switchboard may prohibit calls from going through after a certain hour at night.

Often the patient's (or other patients') safety and well-being are factors in restricting independence. In Chapter 2 you learned that most health care institutions fall into the category of "partial institutions," meaning that they have freedom to come and go under certain circumstances. However, for many patients it is a challenge to sort out when and how much restriction of their independence is warranted. For example, in some cases, the patient may be on a restricted diet, may not be allowed to have a drink of an alcoholic beverage, may be required to exercise (or to rest) at given intervals, and may not leave the facility. For acutely ill patients, this is a temporary frustration. In the worst case, for chronically ill or permanently institutionalized patients it becomes a way of life. Fortunately, we are in a period when health care institutions are taking a hard look at how respect can be honored more fully while still maintaining a high level of efficiency and patient safety. You will be in a good position to help suggest changes in institutional structures, policies, and functions that will allow its occupants to realize an optimal degree of independence.

Ambulatory Care Settings

More and more procedures are being performed in ambulatory settings. That patient "walks in" for treatment or diagnostic procedures but does not remain. Examples are dentist or doctor's offices, day surgery centers, therapy clinics, and well baby or prenatal clinics. Here institutionalization is brief. In many cases it does not involve an overnight stay.

REFLECTIONS

Have you ever been treated or taken a friend or family member to be treated in an ambulatory care setting such as an outpatient clinic, "Doc in a Box" office in a strip mall, or emergency department?
If so, reflect on the environment of that setting and how it differed from, say, a hospital, nursing home, or a rehabilitation center.
Jot down some notes about it before reading on and then compare your observations with the authors' observations below.

Ambulatory care patients are in the awkward position of sitting on the fence between two worlds. They may appear completely well and therefore not be treated as "sick" or "impaired." However, they are definitely *patients* for the following reasons: physical or mental function is impaired enough to produce discomfort in the person or to result in his or her inability to proceed with some activities formerly taken for granted; symptoms are severe enough to have been openly acknowledged by the person and confirmed by a physician or other health professional; the person has agreed to participate in a treatment or diagnostic regimen that requires regular trips to the health care facility, and the visit takes high enough priority in the patient's life so that other competing activities are sacrificed. For example, ambulatory care patients who receive chemotherapy or renal dialysis must visit the clinic for many weeks, with serious disruptions in their schedules and repeated trips to and from the facility. Each cancellation of an ordinary event and each trip is a shrill reminder of their condition (Figure 6-4).

At first glance, challenges facing such patients may appear almost indistinguishable from those facing inpatients. There are notable differences. For instance, ambulatory care patients may suffer from the loss of self-image even more keenly than inpatients. The person admitted as an inpatient to the health care facility becomes surrounded by others in a similar predicament and is allowed to look and act the part, whereas ambulatory care patients are more like "drop ins" or "visitors" and do not feel as if they have this license; the latter come into the treatment setting for a brief period only and then return to their everyday surroundings where colleagues, families, and others may have no sympathy for what they are facing. The person who is ambulatory also may feel excluded from the "action" that appears to be taking place in the health facility, like a spectator at a game he or she would benefit from knowing how to play but does not. The inpatients know the lingo and can find their way around. The worry about being "out of the know" grows in part from the feeling that institutionalized patients recognize one another, understand the rules, and have a better chance of winning the health caregivers' attention. Ambulatory care patients may feel jealous of those who are in closer contact with the health professionals, assistants, and others they view as being a part of the action.

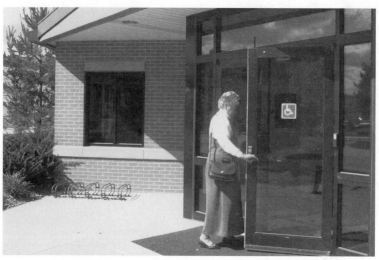

FIGURE 6-4: A patient entering an ambulatory care setting. (© *Corbis.*)

There are other practical challenges for the ambulatory care patient, too. In some instances patients have to fight for time off from work and have difficulty finding—and paying—someone trustworthy to care for children or attend to a homebound spouse or parent. They may lose precious pay or vacation time. The trip to and from the health facility can be so arduous and expensive that the person questions the worth of the visit, especially if when they arrive there is a long wait before being seen.

If you observe that a person receiving ambulatory care is feeling socially isolated, you can help the person overcome this alienation, become acquainted with others, and in other ways help him or her find a sense of belonging in the health care environment. At the same time, you and your colleagues can also help the person see the gains of being able to remain uninstitutionalized rather than having to be admitted as an inpatient to a health care facility.

Home Care Environment

Although home care patients do not have to suffer the trauma of adapting to a strange institutional environment, there are different challenges for persons receiving health care services in their homes (Figure 6-5).

The presence of skilled health professionals and assistants who come to provide sophisticated therapy and professional care is a relatively recent phenomenon. Thus, there is always tension between the true purpose of the home (i.e., a refuge from the outside world) and the home as a site where patients receive technical interventions and care from strangers. Furthermore, homes are not designed to be mini-intensive care units, rehabilitation centers, or long-term care facilities, so they lack equipment, space, and in some cases even electrical outlets or other resources required for equipment that must be brought into the home setting.

The presence of professional caregivers in the home is often met with mixed emotions by patients and families. For patients and their families, on the one hand there

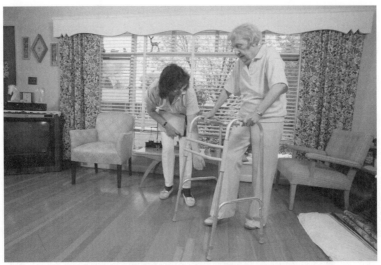

FIGURE 6-5: A home care patient. *(© Corbis.)*

is a sense of relief that assistance with foreign equipment and procedures is at hand and that family caregivers can be relieved temporarily of the burden of continuous care. On the other, professional care in the home inevitably involves an intrusion into personal space, routines, and behaviors. Patients may not know how to treat health care professionals in their homes and thus cannot truly relax or be themselves while the professional care provider is present. Should they treat them as guests and offer them social courtesies such as coffee and cookies? Or should they treat them as hired help, much as one would treat a plumber or electrician who comes to the home to perform a specific task and then departs without an expectation of social pleasantries?

In short, home care is clearly unique in that your services are carried out on the patient's turf, in an environment designed for different purposes than health care. Here the rules and dynamics of a household are the standards for behavior rather than the rules of a bureaucratic organization. It is not surprising, then, that the challenges of maintaining a true level of the comforts that are often lost during institutionalization also face the patient who now must receive care at home.

The Kimura family had been constant companions to their son Noby during his acute recovery and rehabilitation following a train accident that initially left him comatose and then paralyzed. When it was time to take their 20-year-old quadriplegic, ventilator-dependent son home, they wanted him to be a part of the family's life. They and he agreed it would be terrible if he were placed away in a second-story bedroom, so they cleared the dining room of furniture except for the family's small Shinto shrine in the corner to make room for the bed and equipment.

⊚ REFLECTIONS

- What are the strengths of this arrangement for this family?
- What difficulties can you predict for the family because of this arrangement?
- In order to fully assess the challenges for Noby and his family, what else would you like to know about their home? Their family dynamics? Other details?

Let's go to the next step in the Kimura family's adjustment to this dramatic change in their lives:

After 2 months with this arrangement, both Noby and his parents decided this was a poor decision. The family had little privacy when professional caregivers were in attendance. The patient felt like he had no privacy at all. They talked over the situation and came to a new solution: Noby would be moved to the lower-level family room, where he could still be a part of the family life but not the center of all activity. His professional caregivers, as well as his friends, could come and go without coming through the rest of the house. He could invite his parents to watch TV or just sit in the room to talk and he could still enjoy some private time as young men of this age normally need and want.

⊚ REFLECTIONS

1. What new challenges do you predict for the Kimuras in this new arrangement?
2. What family values do you identify in their attempt to be a family again?

Their story illustrates that patients and their families may not appreciate the long-term stress the home care arrangement can cause because initially they are so elated to be together again in their own home environment.

Home care personnel can work with family and patients to plan their schedule and care delivery so that the patient can have enough privacy and the family can develop a sense of appropriate psychological, if not physical, distance between themselves and the caregivers in their home.

Weighing Losses and Privileges

It sounds curious to talk of patients as having privileges, especially in light of the previous sections in which you were introduced to serious challenges that patients face. At the same time, certain accommodations are reserved for anyone who is temporarily struck down by illness or physical or mental impairment. A major feature is that others relieve him or her of certain roles and responsibilities. In Chapter 2 you were introduced to various rights, laws, and social policies that express respect for this accommodation.

Support for a stricken person is an understandable part of the care extended to him or her out of respect for the difficulties that accompany being sick or otherwise

> ⑤ **REFLECTIONS**
>
> • What privileges did you have as a child when you were sick or sustained an injury?
> • What changes did you experience?
> • Which of the following common answers by students also were true of your experience?
>   • Meals were brought to me in bed.
>   • I did not have to go to school.
>   • I had first choice of the toys.
>   • I was exempt from doing the dishes.
>   • I could watch television/listen to the radio/play video games in my room.
>   • I was given a cold washcloth for my forehead.
>   • I got ice cream or chicken soup (or some other special food or home remedy).
>
> Now think about the "negotiation tools" your parents, sitter, or other person in authority used to be sure you were doing all you could to "get well" enough to go back to school, etc.

laid low. However, inherent in the granting of such privileges is a message that these accommodations are also an encouragement to keep up the good fight back to health if that goal is possible. In other words, the privileges are not designed to convey permission for the person to remain in the patient role indefinitely if he or she is capable of recovery. And if recovery is not a reasonable goal, the person is expected to begin to learn the challenge of living well with impairment or preparing for impending death.

The increasing emphasis on the patient's role as an active agent in the process and not just as a passive recipient of professional services is highlighted by the amount of information shared on the Internet, in the daily news, and through other public media sources. Patients today believe that some of the "help" they need is to seek professional intervention, but also that they must have information about their own health that will assist them in the process of healing or adjustment.[6]

It is easy to conclude that a patient who has a lot of information about his or her condition will be better equipped to prepare for whatever lies ahead. This is not necessarily so. A woman who previously had been treated for life-threatening adenocarcinoma of the lung, and who was now undergoing new tests because of a persistent cough, lends insight into how difficult it is to feel confidently in control of one's health or life, especially when there is an underlying threat:

> Bending over the table as a doctor inserted a needle into my back to extract some fluid I started to think about what I would do if a presumably innocent cough turned out to be the sound of the other shoe dropping. I had once had a good reason to listen for that other shoe; I'd had malignant lymph nodes in my mediastinum—the middle of my chest—as well as a tumor in my lung. I had always been amazed at how little time I'd spent listening for it, and what I most disliked about having the needle stuck into my back was that it began to awaken what I'd come to think of as the dragon that sleeps inside anyone who has had cancer. I'd written once that we can never kill this dragon, but we go about the business of our daily lives—giving our children breakfast, putting

more mulch on our gardens—in the hope that it will stay asleep for a while longer. What I hadn't said was what I'd do if the dragon woke up. But, even as I braced myself for the insertion of the needle, it seemed unlikely that lung cancer, a notoriously aggressive disease, would hang around for so long only to reassert itself in the guise of a cough that interfered with my dreams of seeing the Bosporus.[7]

Many patients are resourceful in maintaining hope and participating in their treatment. The arduous preparation for coping with challenges of a prolonged illness or impairment or preparing for death involves more serious losses and understandably fills many with dread. Paul Tillich, a theologian who escaped imprisonment and almost certain death in a Nazi prison camp, wrote a treatise on what happens when all one knows is thrown into disarray. He titled it *The Courage to Be.*[8] This seems an apt way to think about patients.

Choosing to Remain a Patient

We invite you to focus your attention now on the rare situation when a patient who could move beyond the patient role does not choose to do it, or even relishes being in it. Clearly, for the patient, the accommodations received while incapacitated seem better than those granted when he or she is well. One extreme way a person remains in the patient role is to feign symptoms long after they are gone or to fabricate them. Such a patient is engaged in *malingering.*

Sometimes patient problems are so complex or elusive that caregivers mistakenly label the patient a malingerer. The patient may have symptoms of organic illness in the absence of organic pathological signs. This patient is not necessarily a malingerer but may have physical symptoms of a mental illness: He may have a "hysterical symptom" or may have undergone a conversion reaction (i.e., a psychological problem has been converted into an organic, or physical, symptom) that for all practical purposes mimics malingering. Sometimes the organic basis of a condition is difficult to diagnose, and the person may be treated as a malingerer only to later find the cause. Unfortunately, some people are treated as "faking it" for months or years when a serious reason for their symptoms and suffering is diagnosed. Then there are "borderline" cases: *The New Yorker Magazine* profiled a man who woke up after a stint in the hospital, having been hit on the head.[9] When he "came to" he was completely amnesic. However, in the absence of neurological findings substantiating his complete loss of memory, and his apparent contentedness to be taken care of by others while relearning virtually everything, questions surfaced about whether he ever was amnesic. If not, he would qualify as a malingerer, but no one felt certain enough to label him one. A fourth complex situation is the so-called *non-compliant patient,* meaning the patient refuses to follow clear and necessary measures prescribed by the health professionals. Studies of apparent lack of cooperation in following a treatment regimen show that this behavior has many sources, some of which have little or nothing to do with the patient's desire to participate in his or her treatment and healing. Only those who refuse to take necessary measures when able to do so, intentionally undermining treatment attempts, would qualify as a malingerer.

Escape or Financial Gain

You may wonder what patients who malinger gain by their behavior, considering the advantages of a healthy and active life.

Protection from the threatening outside world is one source of motivation. A woman who lives on the streets as a homeless person may find refuge in being in a health care institution, as do many persons in abusive or neglectful home situations. Fear of going back to the front lines of war after an injury or, in the days of the draft, of ever going to the front lines may be cause for malingering. Financial gain may also be a motive. Malingering patients who hate their jobs may fake a work-related injury to draw compensation or, more often, want to remain sufficiently debilitated after an injury to receive sick time or wages while not working. Their situation has resulted in an increasing number of "work-hardening" programs in the workplace that use positive incentives to return persons to work after they have been absent because of illness or injury.

Many of these patients have jobs that are boring or dangerous or offer no opportunity for advancement; therefore, they welcome any means of escape hoping that workers' compensation or some other form of disability insurance will help meet basic needs. In the United States, similar attempts to gain early retirement or to receive extensive disability support are often settled through the court system. The solutions to these issues are complicated and require thoughtful approaches by governments, the health care system, employers, and workers.

Social Gain

Social gain is a third motive. Such patients can manipulate the attention of family, friends, and their professionals when they perceive that this approach is successful. If the results are rewarding enough, an individual may decide that it is not worthwhile to be restored to his or her former symptom-free life.

A perfect example of such a patient is Argan, the malingering patient in Molière's play *The Imaginary Invalid*. He controls everyone in his life by virtue of his "weakened" condition. When his daughter Angélique is old enough to be married, he chooses a physician as her husband. Toinnette, the maid, asks Argan why the physician has been chosen when Angélique is obviously in love with someone else:

> Argan: My reason is that, in view of the feeble and poorly state that I'm in I want to marry my daughter into the medical profession so that I can assure myself of help in my illness and have a supply of the remedies I need within the family and be in a position to have consultations and prescriptions whenever I want them.
>
> Toinnette, boldly: Well that's certainly a reason and it's nice to be discussing it so calmly. But master, with your hand on your heart, now, are you ill?
>
> Argan: What, you jade! Am I ill! You impudent creature! Am I ill?
>
> Toinnette: All right then, you are ill. Don't let's quarrel about that. You are ill. Very ill. I agree with you there. More ill than you think. That's settled. But your daughter should marry to suit herself. She isn't ill so there's no need to give her a doctor.

Argan: It's for my own sake that I'm marrying her to a doctor. A daughter with any proper feeling ought to be only too pleased to marry someone who will be of service to her father's health.[10]

The world thus revolves around Argan's medicines and body functions. His emotional dependency is revealed in his continual tattling to his wife about the annoying Toinnette, who is the only one who confronts him with his hypocrisy. His brother Béralde observes, "One proof that there's nothing wrong with you and that your health is perfectly sound is that in spite of all your efforts you haven't managed to damage your constitution and you've survived all the medicines they've given you to swallow."

Argan quickly counters, "But don't you know, brother, that that's just what's keeping me going. Mr. Purgon [the physician] says that if he left off attending me for three days I shouldn't survive it."[10]

Audiences for 300 years have been laughing at Argan's obvious self-deluding rationalizations. They laugh because they can identify with Argan's reluctance to give up the privileges of the patient's position in society. However, most differ from Argan in that they do not enjoy these privileges enough to create a lifestyle around their symptoms and debilitating disorders.

Respectful Responses to Malingering

You will occasionally meet a person who is malingering and should be prepared to respond constructively and respectfully to him or her. It is understandable that many professional care providers become frustrated when confronted with a patient who apparently does not want to improve but who wants the attention of treatment, often at the price of attention that you and your colleagues judge should be given to other patients. The following case will help you reflect on what you can do:

Marilyn Siegler is a 19-year-old woman who has long had "family problems." Her father is a successful businessman, and her mother is heavily involved in the charitable and social activities of the large city in which they live. From the time she was a child Marilyn has felt that her parents favored her older brother, who now has decided to become a partner in their father's business.

Marilyn has been seen by numerous counselors and psychiatrists since her teen years, when she made a suicide attempt. All agree that her feelings of rejection are the basis for her unhappiness. Several attempts have been made to bring the parents in for family counseling, but they have always been too busy.

Marilyn is a freshman medical student. She went from boarding school to a prestigious private college in a state distant from her home and, upon admission to medical school in this Midwest university, chose to live in a dormitory with other medical school and health professions graduate students. She is friendly and outgoing, though as the year has progressed she has seemed to grow increasingly demanding of those around her. During the past 3 months she has developed a rapidly progressing weakness in her legs and is now confined to a wheelchair. Extensive tests have revealed no physical basis for the disabling symptoms to date. Recently her parents have decided it would be best for Marilyn to return home, where they plan to employ a private tutor for her with the hopes of her being able to complete her first year of medical school.

Jane is living in the dormitory where Marilyn lives. Marilyn has been a patient in the clinic where Jane is currently working as part of her professional on-site preparation. She has observed numerous costly diagnostic procedures being performed on Marilyn to get at the root of her problem and, therefore, knows much more about Marilyn's elusive clinical history than any of the other people in the dorm. She has, of course, never disclosed it to anyone, but it gives Jane a special affection for Marilyn. She does not fully share the feeling of some of her dorm mates who are relieved that Marilyn may be leaving the dorm, saying they are tired of being increasingly called on to assist her.

Last Monday morning the clinic area was unusually full when Marilyn wheeled into the clinic complaining about how exhausted she was. The receptionist took Marilyn to a remote area of some unused private treatment cubicles near the storeroom and an unused bathroom. She asked Marilyn if she could get herself undressed for the test she was about to undergo. Marilyn said she thought she could.

A few minutes later Jane started down the long corridor to check on Marilyn's progress and was astonished to see Marilyn scurrying back from the bathroom to her curtained changing area. Jane could not believe her eyes. Marilyn was walking briskly—and with apparent great ease!

⊚ REFLECTIONS

What should Jane say and do next?
What should the staff supervisors and others do, having this uncomfortable issue to deal with?

Every situation has its own challenges; however, the following principles can guide you when you are a health professional responsible for the care of a patient you suspect is malingering:

▶ Principle 1. Believe the patient until you have legitimately discounted all reasonable evidence that there is a physical basis for the patient's complaint of symptoms. This requires diligence on everyone's part to be thorough in diagnosis. To do less is to stigmatize the patient unfairly, as well as help set a course that may be clinically harmful. In Jane's case even her simple observation needs to be confirmed. For instance, might Marilyn's symptoms be decreased by medication or other clinical factors? This is especially critical because once a person is definitively identified as a malingerer, he or she needs professional counseling. The patient cannot be coerced into wanting to return to society or previous roles and responsibilities until his or her underlying problems are addressed. Health care providers become involved in this problem-solving process by working closely with the psychologist or psychiatrist and by reinforcing conduct that contributes to helping the patient welcome the opportunity to reclaim the degree of healthfulness available to him or her.

▶ Principle 2. Effective teamwork and team respect toward the patient are essential. Employ every team member to assist in the discovery process; if malingering is verified, continue to treat the person respectfully under these unusual circumstances. Respect does not mean that the patient's behavior is acceptable, rather that it warrants the type of care mentioned earlier. Malingering is a stigmatizing label and, once suspected, the attitude of health professionals can turn to neglect or retribution because the patient is "faking it." A common example is seen in the treatment of patients with pain for which no objective basis can be found. If patients are given placebos instead of analgesics to prove that their pain is illusory, they are invariably angry and hurt when they find out about the deception, even though they may have received complete pain relief from the placebo. To avoid the development of an adversarial relationship, the whole team must be prepared to treat the malingering as part of the patient's care package.

▶ Principle 3. Pay attention to comments from family and friends.
Family and friends who have brought concerns about the patient's condition to your attention can be helpful in the discovery process and also should be counted as potential resources for the course that follows. For instance, one of the authors found that a critical conversation had been opened by the wife of a patient when the wife asked whether it was "unusual for daytime wrist pain like her husband's to be so severe that he could not work but it didn't seem to bother him in the evening." When asked what she meant, she said he told her he had been diagnosed with "daytime" pain, but the doctors and others could not find the basis for it. (This last part was true.) It turned out upon further conversation with this wife that the pain disappeared in the evening to the extent that he could spend most nights at the bowling alley using the same arm that kept him from working at a job he had come to despise. That led to additional inquiry of the patient that finally resulted in his being referred for counseling once he was identified as a malingerer, and he eventually went back to work.

▶ Principle 4. As with all sensitive patient issues, confidentiality must be judiciously guarded.
Even in the story of the wife's "disclosure" described in Principle 3, one of the most difficult areas of exploration in this husband-wife situation was to take seriously the information gained from the wife but to use as much skill and caring as possible in getting the patient to raise the bowling issue himself. Even after the patient's malingering had been discovered, the health professionals were bound to honor the patient's right not have the findings of his malingering shared with his wife until and unless he was prepared to do so.

SUMMARY

In this chapter you have had an opportunity to focus squarely on some peculiarities of the patient's challenges during changes that virtually everyone finds unwelcome and difficult in one way or another. Whether the transition involves real or feared losses and adjustments, it involves some degree of a patient's disruption from long-established patterns. Special accommodations the patient receives may be short-lived, especially if he or she seems not to be participating actively in recovery or adjustments that must be made. Some things will be viewed with disdain, distrust, or impatience by persons who make up the fabric of the patient's life.

Malingering is one of the special situations you may encounter, but the principles of good patient care apply to this and other unusual challenges. Your role and skills cannot be divorced from this larger real-life picture that the patient brings to your doorstep. Their challenge then becomes your challenge, too—and one worth meeting well.

REFERENCES

1. Klein BS: *Slow dance: a story of stroke, love, and disability*, Berkeley, CA, 1998, Page Mill Press.
2. Garrison JF, Julia PS: Middleton, MA, 2005, Pinhead Press.
3. Dudzinski D: The diving bell meets the butterfly: identity lost and remembered, *Theory Med Bioeth* 22:33–46, 2000.
4. Wendell S: *The rejected body: feminist philosophical reflections on disability*, New York, 1996, Routledge.
5. Haddad A: *French weaving*, 2001, unpublished (With permission of the author).
6. Purtilo R: Professional-patient relationship: ethical issues. In Reich W, editor: *Encyclopedia of bioethics*, ed 3, Vol. 4, New York, 2004, Macmillan.
7. Trillin AS: Betting your life, *The New Yorker*, Jan 29, 2001.
8. Tillich P: *The courage to be*, New Haven, CT, 1952, Yale University Press.
9. Friend T: Backstory. New man, *The New Yorker*, Feb 27, 2006.
10. Molière JB: *The misanthrope and other plays* London, 1959, Penguin Books. (Translated by J. Wood).

Respect for the Patient's Significant Relationships

A special pattern of communication developed between Robin and Mark (her father) during his hospitalization. Each morning Mark phoned home to tell her about the animal picture on the sugar packet that he had saved from his breakfast tray. One morning Robin explained to Mark that she had a cold, and then, with 3-year-old directness, asked, "What do you have, Daddy?"

After a pause he replied, "I have cancer."

She handed the phone to me and said, "I think Daddy's crying." Though he had never hesitated to discuss his illness with others who asked, he was deeply shaken by the weight of Robin's question and the implications of his answer.

—*S.A. Albertson*[1]

In this excerpt from a book portraying a young family coping with the fatal illness of a dad and husband, we suddenly see a moment when the patient breaks down unexpectedly, touched deeply by the implications of his beloved young daughter's innocent question. The personal life of a patient exists in a web of activities and intimate or close personal relationships that help to provide status, meaning, support, and a sense of belonging to this person. Respect for this fact is immensely important if you are to reach the goal of maintaining the patient's dignity and achieving a truly caring response during your professional interactions with him or her.

Some ways in which patients' intimate and close personal relationships are affected were addressed in the previous chapter including:

▶ loss of the familiar surroundings in which relationships are most easily nurtured,
▶ loss of the patient's capacity to participate fully in the usual fashion, and
▶ sometimes patients cannot meet expectations of others that he or she will return to former roles and functions.

This chapter beams attention on the patient's relationship with family. However, the patient identifies who "family" is. For instance, many people consider their family to include a life partner outside of a marriage relationship, or extended families of cousins, uncles, aunts, and others related by blood and marriage (Figure 7-1). The patient's relationships with close friends, long-time business associates, and others who are important to the patient often are also deeply affected. Special attention in this chapter is devoted to family members or other persons who become caregivers for the patient because their relationship is often dramatically challenged by the new situation. We offer suggestions about how and when you can become a source

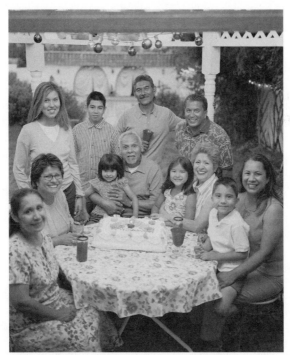

FIGURE 7-1: A patient's relationships with family members and close friends usually are stressed negatively or positively by the situation. *(© Getty Images/AA051759.)*

of support and encouragement to a patient and those close to him or her as they go through stressful and often hard times.

Facing the Fragility of Relationships

Any significant change in a person has the power to alter his or her status and roles in various close relationships. Like a mobile, when one person in a relationship changes, every component necessarily moves, and everyone has to pull together to find a viable new balance point. As patients become aware of changes, they often express concerns of abandonment or fears that they will be unable to contribute to their key relationships in meaningful ways. Whatever else characterizes close relationships during times of illness or injury, one sure thing is that there will be stress. *Stress* usually conjures up only negative feelings, and dictionary definitions support this meaning. But psychologists and others have probed the dynamics of what happens when the stakes are high or the chips are down: Stress is, at its core, a psychological motivator. Stress can have results that are destructive or that enhance individuals and relationships. Rambur and colleagues[2] divide stressful experiences and conditions into negative outcomes of *distress,* and positive ones of *eustress.* In this section we ask you to consider some areas of potential distress with some suggestions for helping all involved to realize eustress opportunities as well.

Among the potential sources of distress during the fragility brought about by change are the patient's concern that others will lose interest in helping to sustain his or her dearest relationships. In some cases the loss of interest is experienced more fully as actual disdain toward the patient. Loved ones and friends who are thrust into the role of caregiving often grapple with similar concerns.

Concern That Others Will Lose Interest

We all hope that our families, friends, and associates will take our problems to heart—fortunately they usually do. However, sometimes patients are unpleasantly surprised by the degree of indifference they feel many people show to the struggle they went—or are going—through. You know from your own experience that this feeling is not limited to persons who become patients. More generally speaking, it can be dismaying to realize that, no matter what momentous event you have been through or are still experiencing, the majority of people in your life do not want to know much about it!

Others' apparent lack of interest may be due to many reasons. For instance, when there is good news to share, some might be jealous of your good fortune or feel that

---

⊚ REFLECTIONS

Almost everyone has experienced the apparent lack of interest in one's good or bad fortune.
- Can you think of an incident in your own life when you were surprised by this?
- How did it make you feel? Describe, if you can, some of the emotions and responses it brought up in you.

their security is threatened by your success; when the news is bad, some may be threatened by that, too, thinking, "There but for the grace of God go I." For that matter, some really do not care much in the first place, even though it was easy and enjoyable to show interest when things were moving along in the usual familiar groove.

In extreme circumstances most people do turn more inward and become self-absorbed, and patients are no exception. Therefore, sometimes a distressed patient becomes extremely boring or demanding, driving others away. Friends and loved ones may assume that the patient no longer really cares about them and lose interest in maintaining the relationship for that reason. As one exhausted young wife exclaimed,

> "I have turned into a service organization! I love Dick but I can't keep this up. He was never demanding like this and I find myself coming to see him less and less because of it! He panics every time I begin to leave, no matter what else I have on my plate. He says he can't sleep if he can't see me. I know he's scared but I am beginning to wonder if he ever really cared about me!"

The truth is that most people expect at least their family and close friends to be there for them when difficult times arise, and it is a shock when that does not happen. One of the authors recounts elsewhere the moment when a 20-year-old patient named David, who had quadriplegia as a result of diving into a shallow pond when he was 19, told her the bad news about his older brother Jim and David's fiancée, Jane. Noticing that something seemed to be troubling David this particular Monday morning, she tried unsuccessfully to encourage the usually loquacious David into conversation. Finally she asked if he had been "on a weekend binge or something."

> "No. But I need a drink."
> "What do you mean, you need a drink?" [long silence] "David! What's the matter?"
> His shoulders sagged lower and I saw the flaps of skin on his chin and belly. . . . Eighty pounds lighter too quickly for his young skin to keep up with his diminishing bulk. He raised his head, barely, and whispered hoarsely from somewhere way back in his throat, or life, "Jane is going to marry Jim."
> For the first time ever, I was without words with David. He looked straight into my eyes, locked in that moment of recognition that we had both lost our footing and were falling.[3]

In your role in the health professions, sometimes you are deeply moved by a terrible event in a patient's life, and, like the therapist in this excerpt, you feel stunned into not knowing what to say or do. She probably did the right thing just then by letting a heartbroken David see that this news was difficult for her to hear because of the enormity she knew it held for him. Later he told her that the tears in her eyes convinced him that she really cared. But as a professional caregiver, one can never be quite sure that the patient will be able to acknowledge support or even feel supported. Over the years the authors have learned never to be surprised when a patient suffers a profound emotional blow due to a breakdown of an important relationship, and to expect that at times the spillover is to distrust anyone to "stay in there" with him or her.

However daunting it may seem, it is always worthwhile to try to offer comfort and hope in such situations. For instance, if you see it coming, you can try to help prepare patients for a disappointment they might encounter if their expectations regarding important relationships seem unrealistic. Just by talking directly to the patient about an obvious absence of someone who previously was present on a regular basis may give the person an opening to discuss his fears or the reality of what is happening. Of course, to pry deeply into the particulars of a patient's intimate or close personal relationships (or the apparent increasing dissolution of one) also can be an unwelcome intrusion into the patient's privacy if the timing is not right. The point is that gentle probing may lead to an opportunity for the patient to talk through and think more expansively about the situation. In fact, sometimes allowing a patient to talk about family, friends, or other social contacts will help him or her start remembering things about the relationships that are treasured and help the patient's focus to turn to strengthening those relationships during this unusual time.

Family members, partners, or friends who become caregivers often go through their own worries about whether others are losing interest in the patient or are becoming indifferent to the negative stresses on the relationship the patient and caregiver(s) are experiencing. Their concerns are founded on their observation that longtime friends and associates are backing off. This seems to be especially true in situations when the one being cared for has undergone a serious and long-standing change in appearance or abilities.

The social functions and activities that partners, families, and friends enjoy with others often dwindle, isolating the patient and caregivers from familiar sources of enjoyment and their feeling of belonging within their larger communities. The loss of a job can further distance them from longtime associates and patterns. For many it is easier to stay away than to face the hard realities with the affected persons. Internal divisions within families also may erupt, often over differing hopes and expectations about who will take responsibility for various aspects of caregiving. The patient may begin to feel as if he or she has caused all the distress and withdraw further from contributing to the vitality of key relationships.

Shunning by Others

Unfortunately, a special burden falls on relationships when the patient has a condition that carries a social stigma of some sort. Loss of a social life may be accompanied by a loss of status. In most such cases what appears to be a loss of interest may be an even deeper disdain and rejection. People who have a diagnosis of AIDS are prime examples of such a group who (by virtue of their illness) may lose their social life or job security. Although great strides have been made in the United States and elsewhere to educate about AIDS, and laws and policies have been put in place to prevent discrimination against the person and family, this disease still has the power to marginalize patients and their loved ones from their communities and important relationships.

Even as we write this book, a 13-year-old boy diagnosed as HIV positive was barred from a private school on the basis that he was a threat to the other 2000 students in spite of his being a responsible adolescent with parents who fully support and are parenting him through this difficult condition. This is putting great strain on not only the boy but also his parents, who have become a target of hate mail and accusations by other parents. Suspicion or confirmation about the source of an HIV infection may be knowledge that some people close to the patient and loved ones cannot accept.

AIDS is by no means the only condition associated with societal attitudes that may be informing why others appear to be losing interest in a patient and those in close relationship with him or her, or worse, shunning him or her. In Christina Lee's excellent book, *Women's Health: Psychological and Social Perspectives,* she points out that depending on their environment, women may be expected to be ashamed of reproductive conditions such as premenstrual syndrome, menopause symptoms, infertility or postpartum depression, obesity, or physically "disfiguring" conditions that lay outside the norms of beauty, and of age-related symptoms.[4] Persons who have undergone abortions or births outside of marriage can be shunned, even by those who were previously close to the person. Sometimes people close to the patient are also expected to feel ashamed for accusations that they had a role in allowing, causing, or worsening a patient's predicament. An example was relayed to us by a colleague who was teaching a 3-week summer course in another city when her husband had a serious heart attack. She recalls the following conversation upon hearing the news that her husband was in the cardiac intensive care unit:

> Cardiologist: Your husband has had a serious heart attack and is in the cardiac care unit.
> Woman: Oh no! What happened?
> Cardiologist: [Explains some medical details.] Was he well when you left?
> Woman: He seemed fine! We have known his heart is bad but we thought it was under control since he has been under your care. [More questions about his condition.]
> Cardiologist: You know he has trouble staying on his diet. Has he been eating correctly?
> Woman (still shaken): I think so! I've been gone for 3 weeks but . . .
> Cardiologist: Oh, yes. Husbands often eat things they shouldn't when their wives are gone.

The woman said that whether or not the doctor was intentionally trying to shame her for not being there when her husband had a heart attack, just by virtue of that conversation she was afraid she would be shunned by his professional caregivers when she returned.

What can you do in your role to help decrease the deleterious effects of others' loss of interest or shunning of the patient or loved one?

Some straightforward suggestions include:

▶ Listen to your own comments with a reflective third ear to think about how they might be coming across to the patient or caregivers. Do they sound off-putting? Blaming?

▶ Facilitate contact with patient and/or family support groups of similarly affected persons.

▶ Be prospective as a resource, suggesting additional supports available at your worksite such as religious counselors, psychologists, or social workers who are skilled in dealing with the negative stresses caused by the situation.

▶ Speak up to counter destructive, shame-inducing attitudes and behaviors in the larger society.

You may think of other ways to decrease the *dis*tress related to both patients and their loved ones who are concerned about real or imagined loss of interest by others, or who are feeling shunned and therefore increasingly isolated.

Weathering the Winds of Change

Patients also justifiably worry about other relationship-related effects of serious illness or impairment from injury. Unfortunately, the change a person undergoes during illness or injury may in some cases cause him or her to become almost a stranger to loved ones.[5] In extreme cases, the established patterns of old relationships becomes unrecognizable in the present situation. For example, a spouse who sustains a traumatic brain injury may become like a child; a long-time business partner who becomes mentally ill may become suspicious or abusive toward family, trusted associates, or clients; or a young man known for his bravado may become fearful of hanging out with the guys after a heart attack, convinced they will see him as a has-been.[6]

However, usually the changes are more subtle, like a chill wind that slices through an otherwise refreshing fall breeze, sending an unexpected shiver of worry across all those in the relationship. One man, a physician named Owen, writes insightfully and sensitively about his increasing sense of disorientation, dread, and fatigue as he watches his wife of almost 30 years, Lezlie, succumb to a fast-growing (and spreading) ovarian cancer—and his inability to "fix it," even though she is in one of the best hospitals in the world where he is a respected physician. He sees the person he knew during their many years together slipping away from him as her symptoms and complications take their toll on this happy family. These sources of suffering are compounded by his guilt when Owen begins fantasizing about a beautiful nurse named Natalie who is one of his wife's professional caregivers:

> So it occurred to me then that this was part of something that had been willed . . . perhaps ordained . . . that Natalie and I would become lovers. There would be this transition as there might be—at least in fictional accounts—when bereaved husbands fall in love with their late wife's caretaker . . .

Natalie accompanies him to a professional presentation he is making in another town. He learns later that their friends and his wife are so worried about his state that they arrange for her to find a reason to go with him. She attends his presentation.

> After the talk, I walked from the conference room with Natalie at my side. I had always been scrupulously faithful to my wife and would remain so. Still, it pleased me to have an attractive woman at my side. Natalie's appearance was striking and there was a seductive quality about her that she was unaware of and that made one think that no one in her life was more important. I craved like an alcoholic in withdrawal. I don't remember what I said to Natalie. . . . It was something to the effect that I, while alone the

previous night, had imagined that she and I had married and that she, too, had become ill. There was a silent moment in which I watched Natalie's face change. She said I had misinterpreted her feelings.

We flew back separately to Boston.[7]

This family member is able to reflect on his situation and regain his bearings so that he can endure the upheaval he, his wife, and their children are living through. He credits their ability to see this through as a couple and family as having been dependent in large part on friends, family, and colleagues who quietly, and sometimes assertively, intervened to provide them support.

⊚ REFLECTIONS

Think about a relationship you hold dear—and would count on the most—if you were to become a patient, like Lezlie, with a serious illness or injury.
- What do you think would be your greatest worry in terms of the changes you knew your condition could impose on your loved one?
- List one or two people you could call on to help you and the other person make it through the hard times of such a change.

Now put yourself in the position of Owen, a family caregiver for your loved one.
- What type of condition that your loved one might incur would be the greatest challenge to your relationship as it now stands? Why (i.e., what values and behaviors have seemed to sustain the "core" of the relationship during other stressors)?

These types of exercises can help you imagine the challenges and concerns patients and their closest resources are facing and sympathetically acknowledge that most people must navigate stresses in their intimate relationships when one person in it is changed by illness or injury. This recognition is extremely important because all too often the health of family or other caregivers has been ignored to the detriment of everyone involved, especially when the new situation requires an intense, long-term (or even lifelong) commitment.

You may ask how important it is for you in your professional caregiver role to gain an understanding of the family or close friend caregiver's situation. The answer is "extremely important." The U.S. Department of Health and Human Services estimates that family and friend (called *informal*) caregiver services will be one of the biggest changes this society will see during your career in the health professions.

Unpaid informal caregivers, primarily family members, neighbors, and friends, currently provide the majority of long-term care services. Informal caregiving will likely continue to be the largest source of direct care as the baby boomer generation retires, with estimates of informal caregivers rising from 20 million in 2000 to 37 million in 2050, an increase of 85%.[8] *

---

* From estimates developed using the National Long-Term Care Summary, Caregivers Supplement and the National Health Interview Survey, Office of Disability, Aging and Long-Term Care Policy; 2002.

Most family caregivers rise to the occasion with remarkable courage, good spirit-edness, and if all else fails, resignation. Still, study after study reveals that the every-day reality of life for most family caregivers begins with the belief that they have an unbounded obligation by virtue of their wedding vows and commitments as parent, spouse/partner, son, or daughter, or "only living relative."[9]

Given these societal assumptions combined with the loving intent of the caregiver, he or she may be faced with:

▶ A frequent occurrence of negative (dis-)stress-related disorders
▶ Serious physical injury from lifting or lack of good judgment because of exhaustion
▶ Social isolation
▶ Depression
▶ Increased risk factor for death (especially among older caregivers).[9]

Family members or other informal caregivers who drop out because they literally cannot take it anymore face acute guilt for abandoning their loved one and often find their action another source of shunning by their already dwindling sources of com-munity support. A burgeoning new industry of counseling and other professional services is popping up everywhere to help take up the slack.

⊚ REFLECTIONS

Pull up the words "caregiver services" on the Internet
What kinds of services are being offered to caregivers?
Are there constraints related to cost or other factors?
How easy does it seem to access the services?
What is missing that you think could help alleviate caregiver distress?

All things considered, persons facing or in caregiving situations often do so with trepidation, and those who through illness or injury have occasioned the need for care have grounds to be anxious about whether they can weather the winds of change. Your efforts can make a great difference.

Enduring the Uncertainties

The issues facing close relationships we have been discussing contain elements of uncertainty. This theme is so fundamental that we now turn to uncertainty to con-sider it directly. At some time in every recovery or adjustment process, a patient's uncertainties loom before him or her (Figure 7-2). Whenever that happens, the reverberations race through intimate and close personal relationships. As a young child put it to one of the authors, "My sickness is like a ghost that hangs around our house. I'm doing OK, then it can creep up on me and 'Pow!' because I can't see it coming. When that happens everybody in my family has to change their plans." His condition was characterized by roller coaster–like exacerbations and remissions, keeping everyone in suspense about what would be possible for all of them from day to day.

One persistent theme is uncertainty about the unsettling effect of it on the patient's close personal relationships. This manifests itself in many ways that professional

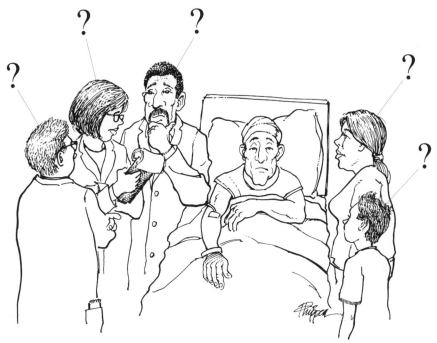

FIGURE 7-2: Varying degrees of uncertainty is a problem patients face during recovery or adjustment, and negative stress reverberates into his or her significant relationships, as well as presenting challenges to professional caregivers.

caregivers must be prepared to interpret and try to respond to respectfully. Behavior changes or comments by the patient will give you clues.

> A young woman is reticent to undergo follow-up tests to check whether or not she remains free of her disease. She may be experiencing uncertainty about what another episode of treatment would mean for her family.
> A man who has believed he was receiving good care in the past suddenly questions your competence when he no longer seems to be improving. His doubts and uncertainty about whether anyone can help him may be prompting the distress.
> An adolescent you have enjoyed working with becomes hostile and aggressive toward you. His anger may be rooted in a growing uncertainty about whether he will be able to participate in an important event in his family's future or hang out with his buddies or go back to playing basketball on his school team.
> An older patient requires constant reassurance. She may be facing uncertainty regarding how to prepare family members or close friends for what she feels is going to happen to her.

Patients who have dark doubts about what lays ahead may be asking a deeper question, although not always directly: "Will you stay with me through this situation, whatever the outcome?" You can respond by assuring the person that you and your colleagues will do everything you can for her or him within your role. Such a question should also be an opportunity for you to gently explore whether this qualm is coming from uncertainty about whether persons important to the patient will be there at some critical juncture or whether they all will be able to make it through their ordeal without your skilled assistance. What can you do then and there to make a sincere effort to decrease their distress? You can:

▶ Make time to provide them with as much certainty about their condition and its future course as your own information and role allow.

▶ Let others who are more qualified to respond to some aspects of the question know.

▶ Exercise restraint by not giving questionable information, instilling false hope around areas of your own uncertainty. The truth will do. The desire to comfort patients by providing false certainty will lead to their feeling of distrust or betrayal in the long run.

Extended family, friends, and other loved ones will also be struggling with uncertainties about the patient's current condition. Responding appropriately to queries from third parties—whether family, friends, or close associates—about the patient's situation should be motivated by your desire to be a positive influence in sustaining their relationships. It is an opportunity to practice your respect for the patient within the context that means the most to him or her. As one wise colleague noted, "You know, when push comes to shove we are just a flash in the pan. It's the family and friends that matter." But if the questions are about the patient's diagnosis, prognosis, or other patient-related matters, you do not have the prerogative to share this information except under certain circumstances, at least in the United States. The Health Insurance Portability and Accountability Act (HIPAA) regulations introduced in Chapter 2 place serious legal constraints on what you may share with anyone other than the competent patient and family members or others he or she designates to receive this information. Health professionals directly involved in the patient's care are also included on a need-to-know basis in order to provide optimum care.

The good intent behind HIPAA regulations is the serious concern that in today's health care system, patient information risks being shared widely, thereby exposing the patient to unwanted or unwarranted invasions of personal privacy. The ethical foundation for keeping this information private is the age-old principle of *confidentiality*. In short, HIPAA constraints and the confidentiality principle affirm the importance of allowing the individual to be the owner of information about his or her health status.

Despite the good intent of these constraints, it can be difficult to know where to draw the line on disclosing patient information so that the higher values cherished by the patient will be respected. These disclosure guidelines can become especially burdensome, threatening the integrity of intimate and close personal relationships. As you learned reading Chapter 3, sometimes communal approaches to decisions are deeply rooted in ethnic or other cultural practices, giving rise to uncertainties on the part of patients, their support groups, and members of the interprofessional health care team if the patient is treated as the sole decision maker. Consider one example:

A 49-year-old Hmong male was dying of liver cancer. The patient had emigrated some years ago from Laos with his wife, four small children, and aging widowed mother to this small Midwestern city and became an influential advocate for the Hmong people living here. As many as 30 visitors occupied the visitor lounges and filled the patient's room to capacity at any given time. When asked if he approved of so many people, the patient said, "Oh yes. They are my brothers and sisters." The patient seemed apprehensive about talking to the physician when the latter tried to get him to talk about his wishes as his disease progressed. He said he could make no decisions without consulting with his family. His wife and teenaged children refused to say anything. Knowing that he would lose the ability to make decisions at some point in the near future, the interprofessional team watched intently to try to figure out who the key decision maker, or decision makers, should be. He slipped into unconsciousness and in a few days became short of breath. Someone needed to be consulted about a decision as to whether the patient should be resuscitated if he stopped breathing or his heart stopped. Because they had no way to determine a designated spokesperson, they chose two of the older men whom the team recognized as being at the patient's bedside every day. But as soon as the discussion began, the room became crowded as the other visitors pushed closer. Murmurs arose every time the interpreter conveyed to the two what the physician had said. The two old men wore their suspicion and confusion in their deeply creased faces.

After a long group consultation one of them stepped forward and said they did not understand many things, but they wanted to be present when the patient died. At this point, the physician decided to make the patient a "no code," meaning that the patient would not be resuscitated. As he lay dying the extended family began chanting, lit candles, and performed various rituals around him. Their activity continued for some time after he died.

The interprofessional team involved in the patient's care talked about this situation for a long time afterwards. They were convinced that neither the patient nor the old men had sufficient certainty about what they were expected to do in this strange environment, leaving them with uncertainty, too.

⊚ REFLECTIONS

- If you were a member of this team, what would you like to know about the patient and these members of the Hmong people that might help you in caring for this patient and honoring his intimate or close personal relationships?
- Make a list of your areas of uncertainty in one column on a sheet of paper. In a second column next to each one, indicate how you might go about getting information.
- What resources should your workplace offer health care providers to decrease the distress of uncertainty about how to respond well in this kind of situation?

Recall the discussion in Chapter 3 on cultural humility that requires your ongoing self-reflection and critique as lifelong learners. Willingness to continue to reflect on what we need to know in order to provide patient-centered care better equips us to provide more certainty to a patient regarding his desire to honor his cultural practices and those of his loved ones whether or not all such differences can be honored within the health care context.

A second occasion for high uncertainty can arise around longstanding habits of who makes decisions between a couple or among family members. This case is an apt example.

Oscar works in a chemical processing plant, his occupation since he was a teenager. He did not get the chance to finish high school because his dad died in a plant accident and he had to become the breadwinner for his mom and three siblings. He says that one of his biggest accomplishments, which "woulda made my dad proud!" was to get his GED in the evening school offered through the plant. His youngest brother, Walter, lives with him and has since their mom died about 20 years ago. Walter was let go from school after the sixth grade on the basis that he was "slow," though Oscar always doubted this "diagnosis." Oscar thought a better explanation is that when Walter lost his baby teeth, his adult teeth never came in. When he tried to talk, the other kids laughed and made fun of him, calling him "grandpa" because so many of the old people in this impoverished town were without teeth or dentures. Walter was in his middle teens by the time anyone mentioned the possibility of dentures to Oscar. A social worker at the local community clinic helped to get the dentures for Walter, but to this day, his childhood experiences have left scars on his personality and self-esteem. Whenever he makes even a small mistake, he suffers, calling himself a "dumbbell." Fortunately, since receiving dentures his pronunciation, nutrition, and appearance have improved.

Oscar was able to get Walter on at the plant, and Walter has done well there. Over the years the other guys have grown used to his self-effacing personality, have come to appreciate his hard work and big heart, and know that there is more to him than may meet the eye initially. Oscar watches out for him, too, menacingly confronting anyone who treats Walter disrespectfully.

Over the past several months, Walter has been wheezing. Oscar notes that he is going to bed earlier and earlier, always with some lame excuse. Some of the guys ask Oscar if Walter is OK because he seems so short of breath and is sweating so much. Oscar finally convinces Walter to go to the company clinic. The nurse practitioner who sees Walter and Oscar allows Oscar to stay with Walter while he undergoes tests. However, when the tests come back, the physician asks Oscar to leave the room and shares the bad news with Walter that he has emphysema. He explains that it is in its early stages and the physicians think that he may benefit from entering a clinical trial of a medication that they hope will help relieve the progressive deleterious symptoms of the condition. Walter is paralyzed by this news, saying that Oscar will have to make that decision and insists that the doctor tell Oscar everything he has just said. The doctor gently tells Walter that it is best if the caregivers be able to talk with him directly about these decisions.

But Walter grows stony cold and looks distrustful. Once included, Oscar listens authoritatively, saying he will take responsibility for making the decisions about what will happen next and declines the offer of a social worker who would be willing to talk with the brothers. He refuses the literature about the study. They both just laugh when the young physician asks if they would like to talk with a chaplain about this. But later, while Walter is filling out some paperwork, Oscar confides to the nurse practitioner who had seen them together on their initial visit that he knows the physician disagrees with his making the decisions, and he is frightened he might make the wrong one.

Again, when they discuss it among themselves the health care providers are uncertain about what to do, understandably reluctant to turn over the decision-making authority to Oscar for a decision that is so important to Walter's life and well-being. To them, ethically and legally Walter is a competent, middle-aged adult and should be making his own decisions even though both he and his brother seem to assume that Oscar will do so.

⊚ REFLECTIONS

- If you were one of the caregivers in this situation, can you think of ways you might bring more certainty into these brothers' understanding of why the professionals are hesitant to accept the decision-making arrangement?
- What, if any, additional information about their relationship would you need to help decrease your team's uncertainty about how to proceed?

The dynamic between Walter and Oscar sometimes can be observed among older patients in marriage relationships. Their conviction that the husband "is the boss" and makes the decisions is all that some couples can fathom. For a husband suddenly to be left out of the information loop and lose his decision-making authority role may be extremely disorienting to both parties, adding a new level of uncertainty to an already difficult period in their life together. The actual dynamic of a relationship is not always easy to unravel. For instance, some caregivers of elderly parents may appear to have overridden the patient's self-confidence sufficiently for them to become beholden to the other; a suspected prostitute and pimp relationship parading as a common law marriage can be hard to detect, and other abusive relationships can be extremely challenging to disentangle.

What can professional caregivers do to decrease the negative stress of their own uncertainties as much as possible when the issue is who will speak for the patient?

▶ Family meetings approved by the patient can become an avenue of fact finding and clarification for all involved;

▶ Ethics committees or ethics consultants are a mechanism to help navigate situations that the professional caregivers find unethical or illegal and therefore cannot accept;

▶ Documenting such patient requests in the patient's clinical record signals to other members of the health care team why you are relying on someone other than the competent patient in decisions about his or her health care regimen;

▶ The help of professionals qualified to detect unhealthful relational dynamics should be sought for the benefit of all involved; and

▶ Reminding each other on the team often that the goal of any such discussion and discernment is not ultimately to decrease your own distress but to do so only when the patient's distress has been fully addressed.

Having reviewed some important uncertainties patients and their loved ones face, as well as the ripple effect of uncertainties you face in such situations, we turn in the next section to economic challenges and how these challenges affect the patient's intimate and important personal relationships.

Close Relationships and Health Care Costs

In today's health care arena, at least in the United States, many patients' most significant relationships will be dramatically impacted by costs associated with health care–related expenses.

The authors of *Uninsured in America: Life and Death in the Land of Opportunity* paint a sobering and well-documented profile of the many ways that illness (physical and mental), injury, and necessary caregiving by loved ones act as portals into what the authors call the "death spiral." The death spiral is their metaphor for "the deep changes taking place in American society as the demarcation between rich and poor . . . hardens into a static barrier between the caste of the healthy and the caste of those who are fated to become and remain sick."[10] Their conclusion is that, except for the wealthiest today, persons in relationships touched by serious illness or injury are forever more vulnerable to severe financial duress. This may come about by the cost of the initial health care episode, the necessary changes in employment made by the person or family caregiver, or the decreased likelihood of being able to find health insurance coverage for future conditions and ongoing maintenance. An adult's values may include that of being a good provider for those dependent on him or her, but the loss of opportunity to earn money for a time (or permanently) may be compounded by the high cost of medical and other health care bills. The patient who decides to make a highly desirable change in life direction or lifestyle with a loved one may feel prohibited from doing so by the reality of the desperate financial distress the illness or injury has caused.

Their distress may express itself in depression or cause patients to make health care choices you do not understand. It is well known that many instances of so-called "noncompliance" on the part of patients are occasioned by the cost of medications, treatments, devices, or services. Patients need to weigh those goods against that same money being spent for food, housing, or other necessities for themselves and their children or others dependent on those resources.

As a professional caregiver, you are in a good position to be an advocate on behalf of patients and their family or other caregivers. Fortunately many health care educational programs include courses designed to help you understand the financial mechanisms supporting or constraining what you can offer in the way of services and assurances. This can give you some certainty about how, and if, to talk realistically about what is available. Beyond that, what does advocacy entail in such a situation?

1. Inform patients and their caregivers of available institutional resources (e.g., social workers) who can help them maneuver through the often confusing web of bureaucratic procedures they must traverse in order to receive essential services.
2. Be attuned to community services that patients, families, and others in caregiver relationships with the patient may be able to access.
3. Educate yourself regarding the basic language and concepts of health care financing and how it operates in your area of expertise so that you can contribute to discussions and strategies about it in areas relevant to your role. Attend educational conferences or in-service sessions addressing these areas of your professional practice.
4. Document instances in which you are forced by inadequate or unjust policies to say "no" to interventions or services you know will strengthen the relationships most critical to the patient's quality of life. For example, in the United States, Medicaid, Medicare, or private insurance reimbursement practices often control the number of days the patient is eligible for treatment, placing both professional and family caregivers in an untenable position.
5. Judiciously gather empirical data regarding treatment effectiveness and patient outcomes to assist policy makers in creating cost-effective approaches to care.
6. Work directly with your colleagues and professional organizations to influence legislation or other policy in your institution, state or province, and nationally.
7. Implement innovations in your workplace to address the strengths and weaknesses of cost-containment policies.

In short, although many of the family's financial burdens will remain outside of your sphere of responsibility or influence, these steps can be taken for you to be a positive force for them and for all coming down the road in similar situations.

Re-valuing Significant Relationships

Bookstores brim with titles like *Ten (or a Hundred) Places to Visit before You Die*. On the scale of opportunities for deep human flourishing, an even more compelling book should be *Ten People to Spend More Time with Whether or Not You Are Dying*. Having reviewed some questions and problems patients and their loved ones face, this final section of the chapter ends on a positive note, turning to the enrichment that can be realized in relationships touched by adversity (Figure 7-3). Most of this chapter understandably has dealt with the negative effects of stress, resulting in distress, and your role in helping to ameliorate it. There are, gratefully, some positive aspects that the stressor of illness or injury can sometimes motivate, leading to what Rambur and colleagues[2] call "eustress." "Eu" is a Greek prefix meaning "good" or "positive" or "beauty."

A stressor can shock one into putting priorities in order and focus on what is really important. One of the authors received an e-mail from a niece this morning that illustrates this point:

"Today I am telling special people in my life how much I love them and appreciate them. I lost a dear friend to a heart attack today. He was only 42 years old. Too

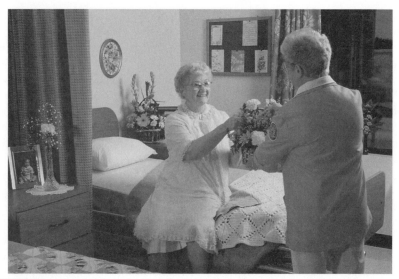

FIGURE 7-3: Often adversity can lead to renewed energy for and commitment to significant personal relationships. *(© Corbis.)*

young!!! He left behind a wife and little girl. I feel so bad for them . . . I got the news this morning just before work and began thinking of different memories of the past and wishing I had spent more time with them. I love you."

Many people faced with illness or injury discover that it prods them to reflect on the value of significant relationships, past and present. You will sometimes be brought into the patient's thoughts or plans as the person reflects about things done and left undone in regard to his or her relationships.

⊚ REFLECTIONS

- Although it is difficult to place yourself in a future situation, try to reflect on the following:
- If you learned that you had a serious medical condition that would likely lead to your death in, say, the next year or so, do you think there are relationships you would like to mend or enrich?
- Can you name a particular relative or close friend whom you would probably spend more time with?
- Are there things you would like to say to someone dear to you?
- Are there relationships you would now feel free to shed?
- Are there old friends, relatives, or others you would want to call or go to visit?

This reflection may give you a glimpse of the urgency with which you might invoke the help of professional caregivers if you thought they were a resource for fulfilling one or more of your relationship-related goals.

Longstanding breaches with a friend or loved ones are the biggest challenge for most patients. We have noted that sometimes a patient is surprised to feel a stirring to make amends. Of course sometimes a past trauma weighs so heavily on a patient or family member that he or she never fully recovers from it, and their relationship remains mired in anger or grief. At other times, the illness or injury highlights a deeper burden of estrangement the person has been carrying. Fortunately, there is hope that today our increasing understanding of depression and of profound delayed responses to serious earlier trauma (post-traumatic stress syndrome) will provide an escape for many more people who in the past have been locked into these burdens.

The good news, too, is that most people do recover or adjust sufficiently to take stock of what is really important in their lives. A young couple may decide their differences are not that important after all and try to make a new life together. A man who felt he was too busy for golfing may decide to take the opportunity to resume regular golf games with his long-time buddies and the camaraderie that they enjoy. An older woman may decide to move out of a secure but harsh job environment to find a new position where she believes she will find more support and her impairment will be more accepted.

Religious beliefs and images can help provide meaning to the patient's experience and aid in healing or adjustment of intimate and close personal relationships, too. The following is one example. You may be familiar with the words in Psalm 23 found in the Hebrew-Christian scriptures. There is a portion that reads, "He [God] makes me lie down in green pastures. He leads me beside still waters; He restores my soul." Herman, a middle-aged man with colon cancer, said that this was God's way of getting him to "lie down" so that his soul would be restored enough for him to get his relationship with his children back on course. Although many people would have a hard time thinking of colon cancer as a "restoring moment," the professional caregiver was wise enough to use this man's religious image to support him through trying periods. Later she heard the man laughing with a son who was saying he hoped he would not have to be knocked off his feet in order to take care of what was important!

The stories of a difficult situation becoming the springboard to a new release into life are legion.

Sometimes patients will ask your advice or even intervention, and at times you may feel you are faced with a dilemma about what to say or how much to get involved. A good general rule of thumb is to be mindful of the nature of respectful health care provider and patient relationships. You have been gaining some ideas about that as you have read and reflected on the chapters in this book. Some helpful guidelines for maintaining appropriate professional boundaries are discussed in more depth in Part Five. However, any written guidelines also assume you recognize that whatever you can reasonably do will mean a lot to that patient. The result is that often you will have the satisfaction of watching patients or former patients use their conditions, however unwelcome they were initially, as opportunities to think things over and start afresh, in the process rejuvenating or bringing new perspectives to their close relationships.

SUMMARY

The personal life of the patient involves a web of activities and relationships that help to provide status, meaning, support, and a sense of belonging to this person. The most immediate intimate relationship for most people is their family; therefore, showing respect for the patient and assessing the stressors facing the patient means thinking about how his or her predicament affects the family and vice versa. The fragility of relationships in general is often increased by the fears and realities facing patients, their loved ones, and other supporters. Sometimes they see interest and support falling away; they may suffer from the changes that are taking place and from the uncertainties that lay ahead. Financial burdens are almost always an added stress. In all instances, the patient's responses are influenced by those closest to him or her. In turn, those near the patient become enmeshed in the concerns, new responsibilities, and changes. Those who become family or other "informal" caregivers represent a growing group of persons who can be at risk for injuries, burnout, and other debilitating conditions and require the professional caregiver's respect and considered attention to help them all nurture their most treasured relationships. The good news is that illness or injury may also become an opportunity for relationships to draw on their past strengths and find renewed vitality and vision. One of the most critical and ultimately satisfying contributions you can make in your professional capacity is to engage in behaviors that express genuine care for everyone in the patient's circle of key relationships.

REFERENCES

1. Albertson SA: *Endings and beginnings: a young family's experience with death and renewal,* New York, 1980, Random House.
2. Rambur B, Vallett C, Cohen JA, Tarule J: The moral cascade: distress, eustress and the virtuous organization, *J Organiz Moral Psychol* 1(1):41–54, 2010.
3. Purtilo R: The story of David. In Haddad AM, Brown KH, editors: *The arduous touch: women's voices in health care,* West Lafayette, IN, 1999, NotaBell Books/Purdue University Press.
4. Lee C: *Women's health: psychological and social perspectives,* London, 1998, Sage Publications.
5. Zuckerman C: 'Til death do us part: family caregiving at the end of life. In Levine C, editor: *Always on call: when illness turns family into caregivers,* New York, 2000, United Hospital Fund of New York.
6. Akin C: *The long road called goodbye: tracing the course of Alzheimer's,* Omaha, NE, 2000, Creighton University Press.
7. Surman OS: *After Eden: a love story,* New York, 2005, iUniverse.
8. Dept. of Health and Human Services Committee: The future of long-term care in relation to the aging baby boom generation, Report to Congress, May 2003, p. 38 (report online) *http://aspe.hhs.gov/daltcp/reports/ltcwork.htm.* Accessed September 25, 2012.
9. Purtilo R: Social marginalization of persons with disability. In Purtilo R, editor: *Have HAMJ ten: Ethical foundations of palliative care for Alzheimer disease,* Baltimore, 2004, Johns Hopkins University Press.
10. Sered SS, Fernandopulle R: *Uninsured in America: life and death in the land of opportunity,* Berkeley, 2005, University of California Press.

PART THREE

Questions for Thought and Discussion

1. Name some technologies and procedures that your profession uses to evaluate or treat patients. If you have seen them used, how do they seem to you to have a possible negative effect on a patient's dignity? For those that might have demeaning aspects, what can you do to help maintain respect toward the patient during the application of these procedures?

2. A patient asks you if she can bring her friend to treatment with her. You know that this patient has been asking a lot of questions and seems to be anxious. When the friend comes, she starts asking you some of the same questions that the patient asked you previously. Some are what you would take as private matters. You want to honor the patient's privacy and so are hesitant to respond. The friend states, "You know how anxious she gets. I just want to be able to reassure her, and I can't do that without knowing what is going on."

   You ask the patient what she would like you to share, and she just shrugs her shoulders. You really cannot tell whether the shrug is a passive resignation or what! Not feeling completely comfortable with your answer, you say to them that you are not free to share information with anyone unless the patient is more positive that it is OK. At that she shrugs her shoulders again.

   What steps can you take to show this patient and her friend respect in spite of your concerns about the patient's privacy?

3. A single woman in her 60s comes to you with symptoms you know are related to the stress of her position as the primary family caregiver for her elderly father who has Alzheimer's disease. You know the best thing for her is to have some respite from the situation. You first ask her about other family members who might share her responsibility, but she claims to have none who are willing or able to help share her burden. Her situation seems perilous to you, and you begin to think of a perfect society where she would not be stuck in this seemingly endless and intense situation. List all the things you can think of to design an environment for her and her father so that both can realize the respect they deserve.

PART FOUR

Respect through Communication

Just as history does not exist in nature, but is created in the telling, so, too, autobiography and the patient's case history emerge out of interactions, which mean that they are at the same time both less and more than the "facts" of the case.[1] Chapter 8 focuses on how we understand our patients by examining the ways the patients' stories are created. Illness and injury are milestones in patients' lives. The clinical record is one place where the experience of the patient is set into words by individuals other than the patient, words that are shared with the whole health care team. The format, syntax, perspective, and language we use to tell the patient's story deserve your attention as much as the content. It becomes apparent that it is not enough to merely describe the chronology of events that bring patients to us.

You will want to understand why things happened the way they did, what meaning the patient gives to the experience, and what the patient expects from you.

To come closer to understanding the meaning your patients give to their experience, you will depend on your ability to communicate. The most immediate "tool" you have available to you for respectful interaction is your own communication, whether that tool is used verbally or nonverbally. What you say, how and when you say it, and how you communicate nonverbally through gestures and other types of physical messages will set the tone for everything else that happens in the relationship.

Chapter 9 focuses on components of respectful interaction in verbal and nonverbal aspects of communication. As you read and reflect on all the types of messages you give and receive, think back to Part One, especially to the parts of those chapters addressing values and culture. It is almost certain that you will work with colleagues and patients from countries and backgrounds different from your own. These differences are evident as we attend to patients and listen to what they choose to include in their stories and what is left unsaid. Consider how the challenge of communicating both verbally and nonverbally, face-to-face or from a distance, is enhanced and influenced by these factors.

REFERENCE

1. Greenhalgh T, Hurwitz B, Why study narrative? In: Greenhalgh T, Hurwirtz B, editors: *Narrative based medicine: dialogue and discourse in clinical practice*, BMJ Books, London, 1998.

The Patient's Story

When you have mouth sores you think very carefully before even trying to take a bite of food; even something as innocuous as a yogurt smoothie is like swallowing a handful of nettles. This also happened to be the time when my hair truly fell out. Because I couldn't eat my weight had dropped alarmingly. I happen to be one of those people who look a wreck when I have a mere head cold; I look horrible out of all proportion to my symptoms. This time when I looked in the mirror I was truly alarmed. This was not a case that the Look Good–Feel Better people could solve.

—J. Hooper[1]

For many decades, most health professionals believed that if they carefully observed a patient and listened to the patient's responses to the numerous questions they posed, then they could arrive at an accurate clinical diagnosis and treatment plan. However, this approach to understanding the patient's experience or story in order to offer effective interventions is not sufficient for several reasons. First, asking an established list of questions to arrive at a diagnosis of any type shapes the story along health care lines, not the "lived" experience of the patient.

Second, the patient's role is passive in this traditional model of interviewing and ignores the fact that a "new" story of what is wrong, what needs to be fixed or needs attention, is being unilaterally created by the health profession. This chapter offers a different way of viewing what happens during interactions between health professionals and patients, as well as an understanding of the roles both play in creating the patient's story.

Human beings experience illness, injury, pain, suffering, and loss within a narrative, or story, which shapes and gives meaning to what they are feeling moment to moment.[2] One may say that our whole lives are "enacted narratives." Another way to understand this is to think about life as an unfolding story. Narration is the forward movement of the description of actions and events that makes it possible to later look back on what happened. And it is through that backward action that we are able to engage in self-reflection and self-understanding.[3] Illness and injury are milestones in a person's life story. "The practice of medicine is lived in stories: 'I was well until …' 'It all started when I was doing …' are common openings of the medical encounter."[4] Think about an illness or injury "story" from your own life. How does your story begin? Is your story a tragedy or a comedy? Who has a starring role? Who has a supporting role? All of these elements of an illness or injury story tell us a lot about who you are as a person, how you see the world, and what is important to you. The same is also true of the patients you encounter in clinical practice.

Much of this book has emphasized that health professionals are called into a particular relationship with patients because of the importance of the illness experience or serious injury. The medium of that relationship is the patient's story. This chapter will help you grasp the importance of paying attention to the unique and personal story of a particular patient's life beyond the more general suggestions we have offered so far. Because the final focus of all of our efforts in health care is the patient, the insights that arise from viewing the patient's account of what is meaningful about an illness or injury experience are essential to delivering high-quality care. Furthermore, narrative analysis or narrative theory can offer ways for health professionals to understand the stories that patients tell from a variety of perspectives. We highlight how different voices offer different stories of the patient's predicament. We briefly explore some of the basics of narrative theory and apply it to health care communications, such as textbooks, scientific journal articles, and the medical record. We go beyond professional, scholarly literature to the humanities to include some examples of literature such as poetry and short stories to give you an opportunity to read and think in different terms about patients' and health professionals' experiences.

Who's Telling the Story?

When a patient enters the health care system, regardless of the place of entry, an exchange of stories begins. It might be hard for you to consider the patient's "history" portion of a traditional history and physical examination to be a kind of story, but it is. So are the entries in a medical record and the scientific explanation of a particular pathological condition in a textbook. Even within the health record, for example, many individuals who are members of the health care team contribute their voices and perspectives to the single entity of the patient's health record.

Montgomery has convincingly argued that all knowledge is narrative in structure.[5] Although her work focuses on the physician and patient encounter as a story, her insights apply to all health professional and patient encounters. In these encounters, the patient tells the story of an illness or injury, which she notes is an interpretive act in that the patient chooses certain words and not others and reports some incidents and not others. The physician [health professional] then interprets the story and translates it into a list of possible diagnoses. Frank suggests that the physician's story is guided by the notion of "getting it right." "Diagnostic stories are about getting patients to the appropriate treatment as quickly as possible."[6] From the patient's perspective, however, getting it right may or may not be what is important. For example, a patient who has a chronic illness such as multiple sclerosis might have a story that is guided by figuring out how to cope with the unpredictable nature of the disease, or a dying patient might want to address challenges to his or her faith. Getting to a correct diagnosis does not seem like the appropriate response to either of these patients' stories. The act of interpretation begins by really listening to what the patient is trying to say.

Narrative theory helps us understand what patients are experiencing and to appreciate or adopt others' perspectives.[7-9] Narratives pull elements together such as events, characters, and setting in a meaningful way. If we think about a novel as one type of narrative, the preceding explanation makes sense in that we expect that every novel will include events, characters, and setting arranged in some manner. The novel will also include a plot, point of view, and motivation so that we can understand why the characters act the way they do. It is only when we apply these components of *narrative theory* to written communication within the health care setting that things get confusing because the genres are so different. One way to help clarify the application of *narrative theory* to clinical practice is to begin with the narrator or the person who tells the story. You will see that when the narrator shifts, so does the content of the story.

From the Patient's Perspective

One way to highlight the different ways that the same story can be viewed is to look at it from various perspectives. For example, how is a cerebral vascular accident (CVA) seen from the perspective of the patient, written about in the medical record, and described in a medical textbook? Before we look at these different "stories" about a CVA, consider the most basic differences in language here regarding what we call the neurovascular injury in question, a *cerebral vascular accident,* or, in common language, a *stroke.* Think of all the metaphoric meanings of the word "stroke" that are stripped away by the use of the clinically sterile term: cerebral vascular accident. Even this technical term uses a word that leaves room for interpretation because an accident connotes a variety of meanings. An accident is unintended, not foreseen. Think about how we would view this diagnosis if the term were *cerebral vascular event* rather than *accident.* What is the difference between an event and an accident? Next consider how health professionals distance themselves even further from the patient's experience by replacing "cerebral vascular accident" with the acronym "CVA." We will now return to the patient's perspective with a personal account of a man who had a stroke. He recounts his experience in the past tense. This is common because most patient stories are recollections.[10]

The following is an excerpt from a much longer account of the stroke that changed this person's life:

> On May 23rd, 2004, I was reading a Hopalong Cassidy novel by Clarence Mulford, the best western author ever, late at night when an artery on the right side of my brain burst and began bleeding into my skull. I suddenly experienced the mother of all headaches. Headaches for me were rare. I'd had fewer than five in my entire life. As I read, the words on the page broke apart into individual letters that started crawling off the page like ants off a paper plate. It was a hallucination, and it wouldn't be my last. I walked to the bathroom to get some aspirin, the only pain reliever on hand. I felt "removed," very "spacey." I looked in the mirror as I passed by and was shocked by what I saw. My mouth drooped on the left side. Suddenly my bowels knotted up and my stomach did a flip. My face looked like melted wax. I suspected I was having a stroke because of the droop. I remember seeing Kirk Douglas after his stroke. Following a short bout of diarrhea, I vomited. This worried me because I'd seen many animals let go from both ends when they were fatally injured. My left leg wouldn't work, and my left arm felt like it was made of wood. Walking was impossible. I fell more than a dozen times while returning the thirty plus feet to my bed. Each time I got up, only to fall again. I refused to just lay there. My thinking was confused and clouded, but I vaguely knew I was in trouble.[11]

The description is written in the first-person voice. *Voice* is the personality of the writer coming through the words on the page. Voice can give the reader an indication of the uniqueness of the person who is speaking in the text. When a writer uses the first-person voice, it feels as if the writer is talking directly to the reader. The story begins with what could appear to be an unnecessary detail in that the patient tells us what he was reading and his opinion of the author's work. Although we do not need to know which western novel he was reading or even if he was reading at all, this information gives us some insight into how the patient marked the moment the stroke began and a bit about his values and tastes.

⊚ REFLECTIONS

- What did you notice first about the patient's story? What does the patient's choice of words (e.g., "artery," "hallucination," "vomited") tell you about him?
- What sorts of emotional reaction, if any, did you have to the patient's story?

This is probably not the first time the patient told the story of his stroke, although it could be the first time that he actually wrote about his experience. In the telling and retelling of landmark experiences such as the trauma associated with a stroke, "the narrative provides meaning, context, and perspective for the patient's predicament. It defines how, why, and in what way he or she is ill. It offers, in short, a possibility of understanding which cannot be arrived at by any other means."[12] When a patient begins to tell you the story of his or her illness, you might be able to discern whether this is a familiar, often told story or if the patient is still trying to figure out what happened and make sense of the experience. Clearly, only in retrospect could the patient know that "an artery on the right side of my brain burst." He includes this information in his written account to help make sense out of what happened, but he could have easily left that clinical explanation out of his story and just provided the facts of what progressed that night.

Health Record

Beginning with the patient's direct experience of the trauma that he has undergone, let us move forward in time to a different setting and interpretation of the story of his CVA and what is happening to him. The patient reports that he was eventually discovered by his brother and taken to an emergency department at a local hospital. In a hospital, one of the vehicles for communication between health professionals who care for a specific patient is the health record. The health record might be handwritten but is today more commonly electronic health records (EHRs). How might the patient's story continue in the EHR? Here are three typical entries, the first from the nurses' notes, the second from the medical progress notes, and the third from physical therapy. Assume that they were written 3 days after the patient was admitted to the hospital.

Nurses' Notes–7/18/20__ Impaired physical mobility; impaired verbal communication R/T aphasia; unilateral neglect; fear and anxiety

9:00 A.M.

AM Assessment Notes: Pt. irritable and tearful. Repeatedly asked for "book" but no books found in bedside stand. Pt. then pointed to photo of his wife on over-bed stand. Pt. calmed down when reassured wife would visit soon. Pt. ignores L arm when moving in bed. Pt. needed assistance with breakfast. Poor appetite.

Plan: Continue to support pt.; consult with speech, occupational, and physical therapy as needed; use every encounter to support communication; obtain picture board; remind pt. to attend to L arm and leg affected by sensory alteration.

Physician's Progress Notes–7/18/20__ Dx: R hemisphere hemorrhagic infarct.; Pt. stable; echo, CXR, repeat MRI; contact speech/OT/PT for rehabilitation assessment.

Physical Therapy Notes – 7/18/20__:

S: Pt. teary. No c/o pain.

O: Alert, oriented to place and person. Cooperative with therapist but is impulsive. Range of motion is within normal limits. Flaccid paresis in left upper limb. Left lower limb strength is zero. Poor hip extension, hip adduction and knee extension. Minimal spasticity in left lower limb extensor mm. Pt. demonstrates denial of left upper and lower limb. Could not assess sensation due to emotional labiality. Pt. needs maximal assist to roll in bed and supine to sit. Sitting balance is poor. Did not stand patient.

A: Left hemiparesis. Dependent in mobility and basic activities of daily living. Good rehabilitation candidate with goal to achieve ability to perform bed mobility and transfers with minimal assist and ability to locomote via walking with assist.

P: Recommend for inpatient stroke rehabilitation when medically stable.

> ### ⊙ REFLECTIONS
>
> • What do you notice first about these versions of the patient's story?
> • Do you understand all of the terms and language?
> • Do these more objective, clinical renderings of the patient's illness give you different insights into what you can do to help the patient?

Clearly, there is a difference in how the patient and health professionals describe what is going on. In Chapter 9 we discuss the use of jargon in health care and how it serves a useful purpose of facilitating communication between health professionals but also works to distance patients from caregivers. The jargon in these sample entries from a fictitious medical record almost becomes impenetrable to a novice in the official language of health care. Did you understand all of the terms and abbreviations? What is "flaccid paresis?" Did you know that "R/T" means "related to," that "echo" is shorthand for "echocardiogram," and that "CXR" is an acronym for "chest x-ray?"

Although the patient describes his experience of having a stroke in the first-person voice, the EHR refers to him in the third person. He is now "Pt.," which is shorthand for "Patient." In the assessment notes from the physical therapist, the patient is almost completely invisible in the account. We will discuss point of view in more detail later in this chapter. It is sufficient here to note the type of voice used in writing and the implications of using a particular voice. Third-person voice distances us from what is going on in the narrative. The EHR may even move further away from these textual accounts to drop boxes that merely require a check or click to categorize the diagnosis or problem and the plan of care. One final comment about all health records, whether written or electronic—they are essentially monologues with each member of the health care team entering information and offer little to no opportunity for interaction.

Consider one more version of the patient's story, this one even further removed from the personal experience of a CVA. In a current medical diagnosis textbook, the clinical signs and symptoms of an intracerebral hemorrhage (ICH) are described as follows:

> Although not particularly associated with exertion, ICHs almost always occur while the patient is awake and sometimes when stressed. The hemorrhage generally presents as the abrupt onset of focal neurologic deficit. Seizures are uncommon. The focal deficit typically worsens steadily over 30 to 90 minutes and is associated with a diminishing level of consciousness and signs of increased ICP such as headache and vomiting.
>
> The putamen is the most common site for hypertensive hemorrhage, and the adjacent internal capsule is usually damaged. Contralateral hemiparesis is therefore the sentinel sign. When mild, the face sags on one side over 5 to 30 minutes, speech becomes slurred, the arm and leg gradually weaken, and the eyes deviate away from the side of the hemiparesis. The paralysis may worsen until the affected limbs become flaccid or extend rigidly. When hemorrhages are large, drowsiness gives way to stupor as signs of upper brainstem compression appear. Coma ensues, accompanied by deep, irregular,

or intermittent respiration, a dilated and fixed ipsilateral pupil, and decerebrate rigidity. In milder cases, edema in adjacent brain tissue may cause progressive deterioration over 12 to 72 hours.[13]

What does this final version of the patient's story tell you? How does this technical version mesh with the patient's account? The authors of the medical text are not concerned with a specific patient who has an intracerebral hemorrhage. The description is general, one written for health professionals, hence the use of highly technical terms, and one that can be applied to all patients who suffer a stroke. The symptoms are described as a matter of clinical, scientific fact, not of personal experience. You might be thinking, "Perhaps this is not all bad. A general description helps a health professional learn what to expect when a patient has had a cerebral hemorrhage." The danger lies in accepting the textbook description as "fact" or the truth as opposed to just one more interpretation of what a CVA is and means to individual patients. To assist you in scrutinizing the narratives you encounter in clinical practice, turn now to some basic concepts from narrative theory.

Awareness of Literary Form in Your Communication

When you see a poem on a page, even if you do not know anything about poetry, you recognize it as a poem because of its form and structure (i.e., the way it looks on the page). Because it is a poem, you also know that the particular words the poet chose are important. In poetry, every word matters. It is unlikely that you look at the writing in your textbooks, even this one, in the same way. Yet any type of written communication (whether on paper or digital) has a form and structure, subtle or obvious. By paying attention to these aspects of the various types of written communication you encounter in clinical practice, you can develop an appreciation for how language is used and its impact on your thinking and behavior. Two assumptions from narrative theory applicable to narratives encountered in health care are that (1) language is not transparent and (2) language does not reflect the whole reality of what is going on.

Language Is Not Transparent

The language of narrative does not function like a clear glass that lets messages flow between sender and receiver. In other words, it is not transparent.[14] No language is neutral or "colorless." This is true of any narrative whether it is a story, a case study, or an article in a scholarly, professional journal. Scientific writing (this includes the writing in a patient's health record) does not call attention to itself the way language does in a poem, play, or novel. As you saw in the sample entries in the medical record of the patient who had the CVA, there were no metaphors, similes, or figures of speech. The nurse did not write, "I walked into the room and found the patient sobbing his heart out." The physical therapist didn't note, "The patient is as helpless as a newborn kitten." Yet if the nurse and therapist used this type of language we would understand what they meant regarding the patient's grief and vulnerability. Professional writing in health care is devoid of these kinds of richer descriptions, but it is based on and created in a particular context for a particular purpose. The closest we get to an emotion in the nurses' notes is in the phrase "Pt. found tearful," but there is no mention of grief, loss, or the depth of his sadness, just an observation. However, the decision of the nurse to mention the tears in her note indicates that the emotional state of the patient is as important as his physical condition.

In Chapter 9 you will discover that one skill you must learn in your professional preparation is to write in this technical, objective manner to communicate with other professionals. Robert Coles describes an interaction with one of his teachers when he was in medical school. Although it involves physicians in training, it is applicable to all health professions. "He remarked that first-year medical students often obtain textured and subtle autobiographical accounts from patients and offer them to others with enthusiasm and pleasure, whereas fourth-year medical students or house officers are apt to present cryptic, dryly condensed, and, yes, all too 'structured' presentations, full of abbreviations, not to mention medical or psychiatric jargon. No question: The farther one climbs the ladder of medical education, the less time one has for relaxed, storytelling reflection."[15] How and what one writes about the patient's story of illness or injury is a choice and should be a conscious one. Although you need to learn enough jargon to know what colleagues are saying, you do not have to be limited by it. Rita Charon, a general internist trained in literary theory, does not begin patient interactions with a battery of questions. Instead, she begins her interactions this way (Figure 8-1):

> I find that I have changed my routines on meeting with new patients. I simply say, "I'm going to be your doctor. I need to know a lot about your body and your health and your life. Please tell me what you think I should know about your situation." And patients do exactly that—in extensive monologues, during which I sit on my hands so as not to write or reflexively call up their medical record on the computer. I sit and pay attention to what they say and how they say it: the forms, the metaphors, the gaps and silences. Where will be the beginning? How will symptoms intercalate with life events?[16]

⊚ REFLECTIONS

- Why do you think Charon states she has to "sit on her hands" while the patient is telling his or her story?
- What is the hardest part of listening to a patient's story for you?

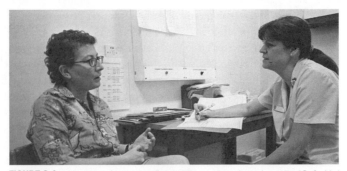

FIGURE 8-1: A health professional listening while a patient shares her story. *(© Corbis.)*

Language Creates Reality

Rather than reflecting reality, language creates reality.[14] For example, without thinking much about it, most health professionals would say that a patient's history in a medical record states the case as it is. In other words, the history is simply recorded observation. Yet the language used actually creates the reality of the case insofar as it frames the kinds of questions we ask about it, how we seek answers, and how we interpret what we find. It also sets limits on what we observe or even consider. Refer to the structure of the physical therapist's notes. Did you know what the letters S, O, A, and P that preceded the physical therapist's entries meant? The SOAP charting method is one way to record information in clinical records. The words being abbreviated by SOAP are *subjective* (usually a direct quotation from the patient), *objective* (the health professional's observations or description of the situation), *assessment* (the health professional's interpretation of the situation), and *plan* (actions to be taken to solve the problem presented).[17] The opening step in SOAP charting, subjective, involves interpretation on the part of the health professional because a choice is made about which quote to include among the many things a patient might say. The quote is an important choice because it is a springboard for the rest of the entry. Furthermore, the whole structure of SOAP charting requires one to think of patients as individuals with problems that need professional resolution, which shapes our thinking about the patient and what we attend to in our interactions.

Language can also be used to exclude others. A clinical ethicist noted this manipulation of language on medical rounds:

> As I began to watch this process more carefully, it became apparent that the physicians spoke a language which was quite understandable when they thought the ethical issues were fairly clear and where there would probably be some consensus but resorted to high code when they felt uncomfortable with the decision(s) before them or when there was dissent in the group.[18]

So when things were easy and comfortable, everyone spoke the same language. When things got tough, the physicians switched to a technical language that allowed them to distance themselves from the discussion and enabled them to dominate it as well.

The use of extremely technical language, or "high code," creates an atmosphere that prevents lay people from participating in the conversation. In addition, scientific language and information are more highly valued than what the patient has to say, as poet and physician Jack Coulehan notes:

> Witness the time devoted on rounds to discussing serum magnesium levels as compared to the time spent discussing the patient's experiences. When the patient's narrative (variously called "subjective," "qualitative," or "soft" data) conflicts with laboratory or radiographic findings (considered "objective," "quantitative," "hard" data), the narrative is usually given the lesser weight; it might well be ignored or minimized and the patient attacked for being a "poor historian."[19]

Although the language may vary from profession to profession, generally speaking the health professional's language will prevail over that of the patient.

Contributions of Literature to Respectful Interaction

Health care practice is a rich metaphor for so many archetypal human dramas, featuring such riveting themes as life and death, loss and hope, and love and hate. All play out in different scripts, some meaningful and others trivial, each experience providing its own opportunity for wonder at the infinite capacity for human invention. There is an increasing emphasis on the use of literature, a specific type of narrative, in health professional education. The premise is that studying literature about illness, death, or caregiving will help you, the student, relate more personally to patients, hear patients' stories more clearly, and make decisions that reflect a humane appreciation of patients' situations.[20] Reading novels, stories, plays, and poetry is a means of participating imaginatively in other lives; it encourages you to construct your own stories in relation to the ones you are reading. Consequently, you will come to know yourself better, too.

Literary Tools

Narrative literature, and by this we mean language used in an intensified, artistic manner, can be used to offer a fresh way for you to understand the encounter between health professional and patient. You can use some simple literary tools such as point of view, characterization, plot, and motivation to examine *narrative literature* and, as you have seen, the usual types of narrative writing in health care communication, such as the patient's medical record.

Point of View

This is a good place to begin because it gives you an immediate sense of who is speaking to you through the poem or story. As you think about point of view, here is a simple question to get you started: Who is the narrator of the piece? In a health record, the point of view is always third person. Health professionals talk about the patient in the third person, even avoiding pronouns whenever possible; that is, the patient is referred to as "Pt." not as "him" or "her." In the excerpt from *Harrison's Principles of Internal Medicine, 18e* that described a CVA earlier in this chapter, the point of view is that of an omniscient, authoritative narrator, but one who is almost invisible. The personal voice is deeply hidden in scientific and professional writing, yet it is there.

Characterization

Also in good narrative, characters bring their whole intricate selves to the story. For instance, if the character in a story or a drama is a physical therapist, you will also learn that he is a son, maybe a husband and father, a friend, and a softball coach. You may also learn that he smokes and has tried to quit many times, cheats at cards, and loves pizza. As the narrative unfolds, you appreciate how multiple, often conflicting, interests and identities figure in the twists and turns of his motivations and decisions. You follow along, getting the feel of his prejudices, fears, passions, and pains. Then, if you are lucky, the magic of transference will take you on a journey into the story and eventually into the byways of your own life, but from some new and different angle. The lived quality of narrative is what makes it plausible. "I could be him," feels the reader. "I've been there, too." On the other hand, some characterizations can cause discomfort, which can teach us about our "unspoken, unacknowledged, and often unknown fears, biases and prejudices."[21] Learning about what makes you uncomfortable is equally valuable as the characters or principles that you identify with when reading a novel, short story, or play. All of this knowledge has implications for your interactions with patients who may be similar to you or very different from you.

Plot and Motivation

Narratives of clinical interest tend toward plot in their structure rather than the more basic narrative of a simple story. In his oft-cited work, *Aspects of the Novel*, E. M. Forster explains the difference between a simple story and a plot: "in a story we say 'and then—and then …' in a plot we say 'why?'"[22] Why do the people in a particular clinical narrative make certain choices and act in specific ways? You can examine the motives of the individuals in clinical narratives in the same way that you can those of characters in a short story or novel. Once again, you may have to try harder to find motivation in clinical narratives because so much work goes into hiding the feelings or emotional reactions of health professionals. Even emotional outbursts by patients are written to appear objective and "clinical." Consider the "plan" portion of the nurse's note presented earlier in the chapter: "Continue to support pt.; consult with speech, occupational, and physical therapy as needed; use every encounter to support communication; obtain picture board; remind pt. to attend to L arm and leg affected by sensory alteration."

⊚ REFLECTIONS

* What are the motives of the writer, in this case the nurse?
* Is there any indication of the feelings or emotional reactions of the nurse?

Poetry

Literature written from the patient's perspective is particularly helpful to health professionals to gain insights into the experience. Poetry is one form of literature that deliberately calls attention to the specific words in the poem, as well as how the words are placed on the page. There are many definitions of poetry, but the following description of poetry perhaps captures it best: "Poetry gives pleasure first, then truth, and its language is charged, intensified, concentrated."[23] The following poem explores the poet's experiences as a patient with a colostomy. We suggest that you read the poem at least twice before reading the questions to help you appreciate it.

A RARE AND STILL SCANDALOUS SUBJECT

From Susan Sontag's *Illness As Metaphor*

The title of my confession
is "Colostomy." The word,
cured and salted,
sizzles on my tongue.

This is shame:
standing naked at the sink,
unsnapping the adhesive flange
from my abdomen.

I couldn't have imagined
the stoma, the opening,
red glistening intestine.
Peristalsis moves it like a caterpillar, hatched
from a visceral cocoon.

My life depends on the stoma,
which insists on gratitude,
gurgling, "Listen to me,"
but I place my hand over it,
even now when I am alone.
—R. Solly[24]

After you have read through the poem, you should be able to recognize who is speaking, what his situation is, and to whom he is speaking.

These are just a few questions to help you begin to understand the poem and find meaning to take away to help you in clinical practice.

---

⑨ REFLECTIONS

- Before reading on, take each stanza in turn. What mood is the author trying to convey?
- Refer to the poem's title, "A Rare and Still Scandalous Subject." The title is taken from a book by Susan Sontag. What is the "subject" in the title the poet is talking about?
- What is it like for the narrator of the poem to live with a colostomy?
- Why is the poem a "confession"?

Short Stories

A short story should be complete, which means it should have a beginning, a middle, and an ending. Stories should also have proportion (i.e., the parts of the story should be in proportion to one another). Generally, more time is devoted to the beginning than the ending. Finally, a story should be compact. Every incident in a story must point to a solution, favorable or unfavorable, to the problem introduced at the beginning of the story.[25] The same literary tools that apply to poetry also apply to fiction. It is important to understand that the narrator in both poetry and fiction is not necessarily the author. Authors can create narrators who are more or less involved in the story. Consider the following short story about a nurse and long-time patient in an intensive care unit.

Morning Visitors

Mr. Johnson doesn't look so good today. I noticed it as soon as I walked into the room this morning. As I go through his chart, all the numbers are the same. His vital signs and his labs are all rock stable. He's been here a long time, not looking very good, but today he looks a little greener or bluer or whiter, or something. Perhaps the smell in the room has changed, or the ventilator sounds a little more high-pitched. I can't put my finger on what it is, but something is different. . . . His immobile features give me no clues for what's giving me this sense of deterioration.

Even in a coma he seems to be maintaining a dignified expression. I imagine him saying, "Don't worry, dear, I'm fine," but I feel uneasy as I go about his familiar morning care and medications. He looks like such a nice man, and he would no doubt be mortified by the spectacle of his stuffing coming out, as he leaks onto the bed like a sawdust doll.

Mrs. Johnson, the wife, is very gracious and soft-spoken. Her clothes are elegant and her hair is always beauty-parlor perfect. Her face is wrinkled but still beautiful, and her eyes are clear blue. She comes in every day and asks the same questions. Things don't change much. She stands quietly by his bed, always refusing to sit down, and squeezes his hand.

I recognize the even sound of her heels before she enters the room. I've fixed him up to look nice for her visit, but he still looks below par. She enters, scans the room, and then looks as though she smells smoke. We discuss his lungs, his vital signs, the plan of the day, the usual things. There is no concrete change to offer her, as we look at each other's worried faces.

"I don't know why, but he doesn't look as good today," I finally say.

"No, he doesn't. He looks sadder today," she says positively.

She goes to take her place by the bed, and I take my cue to leave the room for awhile. She always leaves at the same time, before the next round of medications and treatments. She wouldn't dream of being a bother.

I imagine the two of them going out for dinner, probably to a nice place where they know the owners and order the same dishes each time. They eat slowly, drink slowly, talk quietly, enjoy each other's company. . . . He squeezes her hand under the table.

The consciousness in Mr. Johnson's brain is like an eel languidly S-ing through smooth dark weeds. A few rays of light from the water's surface make little spotlights on the sea bottom, but mostly the eel S-es along in dull monotonous ecstasy.

A cluster of neurons in the frontal lobe simultaneously galvanize themselves for the struggle to be Mr. Johnson. "I am not an eel!" they cry. Mr. Johnson floats to the surface. One lidless eye just manages to break the surface tension of the water and take in the upper world. A spaghetti of plastic tubing threaded through a bank of blinking pumps is above his head, and the tubing snakes toward his head and chest. His chest is being mechanically inflated with bigger whooshes of air than feels comfortable.

Mr. Johnson gasps like a fish beached on a merry-go-round. The ventilator shrieks in outrage at having its cycle thrown out of phase. His vital signs climb upward on the monitor until the alarms are all going off.

Mr. Johnson's bedside is usually a harmonious humming of happy machines, but right now all the alarms are going off. I scurry over to see what's going on and I'm happy to see that his vital signs have gone up instead of down. I walk closer to his bed and see one eye is barely open and darting around like a sardine. His body tenses up and one arm stirs, just a little. The hand on the awakened arm starts groping around.

I take and squeeze his hand, partly to keep it from grabbing any of the equipment, and speak directly into his good ear.

"Mr. Johnson, you're in the intensive care unit." His eye darts toward me and stays, but looks unfocused.

"You've been here about a month. Your heart is healing. You're doing okay. Your wife comes every day to be with you. She just left."

These are the most encouraging things I can say without lying.

"Mr. Johnson, can you squeeze my hand?"

He squeezes my hand spasmodically, and then he suddenly looks gray and exhausted. His hand and arm go limp, his eye closes, and his vital signs sink back down to their usual numbers.

Mr. Eel Johnson sinks back to the seabottom. He thrashes around a moment and then goes back to S-ing through the smooth dark weeds.[26]

◎ REFLECTIONS

- From this short story, what do you know about the narrator of the story?
- Did he or she treat Mr. Johnson with respect? Why or why not?
- What emotions and reactions is the author trying to evoke in you, and how is this accomplished?
- The author uses strong imagery in the story, the ocean floor and sea creatures, to contrast with the clinical images of intensive care. What insights do these images provoke?
- The machines in the intensive care unit react with emotion. Why would the author use such a device? What does it tell you about the use of technology in cases like Mr. Johnson's?

The story form of narrative expands beyond the basic facts of most health care interactions into the experience of the event creating an opportunity for reflection on your reaction to challenging patients.

Illness Stories/Pathographies

A third type of literary narrative is the *pathography,* a form of autobiography or biography that describes personal experiences of illness, treatment, and sometimes death. "What it is like to have prostate cancer," or "How I live with multiple sclerosis," or "What it means to have AIDS" are examples of the typical subjects of *pathography* that help us understand the experience of illness and endow it with meaning.[27] Some pathographies have developed on the Internet on discussion forums or blogs.

The "Leukemia" narrative is one example of an electronic narrative in a discussion group format that evolved from an introductory post in 1991 from Phil Catalfo, the father of a 7-year-old son, Gabe, who was diagnosed with leukemia. The discussion group on the WELL (Whole Earth 'Lectronic Link) conference site allowed for an ongoing discussion between Phil Catalfo and numerous respondents who added to the story as it continued through the course of Gabe's illness and eventual death in 1998. The whole discussion is archived on the WELL site.[28] The Internet allows for, and perhaps encourages, this type of interactive and public form of a pathography.

Refer to the quote that opened this chapter by Judith Hooper. Hers is not the usual description of a patient's experience with chemotherapy after breast cancer surgery. Hooper's pathography from which this quote is taken would probably be character- ized as an "angry pathography," even though it is laced with sarcastic humor. In angry pathographies, the author expresses frustrations and disappointments with the health care system in general and with particular programs or health professionals. The cartoon by Miriam Engelberg is another form of a pathography in which she uses humor to address the often taboo subjects of cancer (Figure 8-2).

She is satirizing the most common form of pathography, the testimonial type, in which the author offers uplifting advice and guidance to others who are faced with

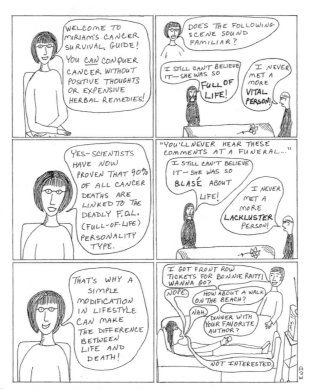

FIGURE 8-2: The F.O.L. Gene. *(From Engelberg M: Cancer made me a shallower person: a memoir in com- ics, New York, 2006, Harper Paperbacks.)*

the same disorder or problem.[29] Pathographies offer you yet another type of narrative to help you understand your patients and their struggles.

Where Stories Intersect

After exploring all the various ways a story can be told, you might wonder: "What is the true story?" The health professional must listen carefully to the patient's story but also understand that the patient does not know the "whole truth" either; the patient is not always accurate. There are clearly differences between the patient's experience and the health care professional's explanation of the experience. So how do we get coherence, if not the true story? The first step to a coherent, richer account could be to recognize the dialogical nature of narrative as Frank affirms:

> We tell stories that sound like our own, but we do not make up or tell our stories by ourselves; they are always co-constructions. Stories we call our own draw variously on cultural narratives and on other people's stories; these stories are then reshaped through multiple retellings. The responses to these retellings further mold the story until its shape is a history of the relationships in which it has been told.[6]

The kind of exchange described by Frank among a patient, health professionals, and family members produces a fuller interpretation of the patient's story than any one person could produce including the richest account a patient could offer.[30-32] Perhaps viewing the interview process as "building" a history rather than "taking" a history from a patient would be a step in the right direction. Building suggests collaboration and the positive outcome of mutual work rather than taking something from the patient and making it your own.[33]

SUMMARY

Literary explorations of the subjective and interpersonal responses of patients, family members, and health professionals to the tensions encountered in health care settings can engage you in your own personal questions and reflections about your response to similar situations in your clinical practice. Narrative, in all of its forms, offers a way of seeing the deeper, subtle nuances involved in your interactions with patients, families, and peers, thereby improving the chances that the opportunities for showing them due respect are not missed or behaviors misguided.

Your role in your patients' stories will vary from assisting them to recover to witnessing their deaths. Whatever roles you take, recall that you also bring your own unfolding story to the relationship. You will build a story with each patient you encounter that becomes another part of the unfolding narrative of both of your lives.

REFERENCES

1. Hooper J: Beauty tips for the dead. In Foster P, editor: *Minding the body: women writers on body and soul*, New York, 1994, Anchor Books.
2. Donald A: The words we live in. In Greenhalgh T, Hurwirtz B, editors: *Narrative based medicine: dialogue and discourse in clinical practice*, London, 1998, BMJ Books.

3. Churchill LR, Churchill SW: Storytelling in the medical arenas: the art of self-determination, *Lit Med* 1:73–79, 1982.

4. Hatem D, Rider EA: Sharing stories: narrative medicine in an evidence-based world, *Patient Educ Couns* 54:251–253, 2004.

5. Hunter KM: *Doctors' stories: the narrative structure of medical knowledge*, Princeton, NJ, 1991, Princeton University Press.

6. Frank AW: From suspicion to dialogue: relations of storytelling in clinical encounters, *Med Humanit Rev* 14(1):24–34, 2000.

7. Bruner J: *Acts of meaning*, Cambridge, MA, 1990, Harvard University Press.

8. Sharf BF, Vanderford ML: Illness narratives and the social construction of health. In Thompson T, Dorsey A, Miller K, Parrott R, editors: *Handbook of health communication*, Mahwah, NJ, 2003, Lawrence Erlbaum, pp 9–34.

9. Charon R: *Narrative medicine: honoring stories of illness*, New York, 2006, Oxford University Press.

10. Robinson JA, Hawpe L: Narrative thinking as a heuristic process. In Sarbin TR, editor: *Narrative psychology: the storied nature of human conduct*, New York, 1986, Praeger.

11. Little ME: *Stranger in the mirror*, Bloomington, IN, 2006, Author House, pp 24–25.

12. Greenhalgh T, Hurwitz B: Why study narrative? In Greenhalgh T, Hurwirtz B, editors: *Narrative based medicine: dialogue and discourse in clinical practice*, London, 1998, BMJ Books.

13. Smith WS, English JD, Johnston SC: *Chapter 370. Cerebralvascular diseases*. In: Longo DL, Fauci AS, Kasper DL, Hauser SL, Jameson JL, Loscalzo J, editors: *Harrison's principles of internal medicine*, ed 8. Retrieved December 19, 2011 from http://www.accessmedicine.com/content.aspx?aID=9145753.

14. Donley C: Whose story is it anyway? The roles of narratives in health care, *Trends Health Care Law Ethics* 10(4):27–31, 1995. 39–40.

15. Coles R: *The call of stories: teaching and the moral imagination*, Boston, 1989, Houghton Mifflin.

16. Charon R: Narrative medicine: attention, representation, affiliation, *Narrative* 13:261–270, 2005.

17. Weed LL: Medical records that guide and teach, *N Engl J Med* 278:593–600, 1998. 652–657.

18. Rogers J: Being skeptical about medical humanities, *J Med Humanit* 16(4):265–277, 1995.

19. Coulehan J: Pearls, pith, and provocation: teaching the patient's story, *Qual Health Res* 2(3):358–366, 1992.

20. Davis C: Poetry about patients: hearing the nurse's voice, *J Med Humanit* 18(2):111–125, 1997.

21. Wear D, Aultman JM: The limits of narrative: medical student resistance to confronting inequality and oppression in literature and beyond, *Med Educ* 39:1056–1065, 2005.

22. Forster EM: *Aspects of the novel*, New York, 1927, Harcourt, Brace.

23. Drury J: *Creating poetry*, Cincinnati, 1991, Writers' Digest Books.

24. Solly R: A rare and still scandalous subject. (Unpublished. Reprinted with permission of the author.)

25. Mueller L, Reynolds JD: *Creative writing: forms and techniques*, Lincolnwood, IL, 1992, National Textbook.

26. Shay E: Morning visitors in Cortney Davis and Judy Schaefer. *Between the heartbeats: poetry and prose by nurses*, Iowa City, 1995, University of Iowa Press, pp 169–171.

27. Hawkins AH: *Reconstructing illness: studies in pathography*, West Lafayette, IN, 1993, Purdue University Press.

28. Catalfo P: *Leukemia, introductory posting (16 January 1991), topic originally numbered 453, health conference, the WELL (Whole Earth 'Lectronic Link)*. Retrieved December 19, 2011 from http://www.well.com.

29. Engelberg M: *Cancer made me a shallower person: a memoir in comics*, New York, 2006, Harper Collins.

30. Poirier S, Rosenblum L, Ayres L, et al: Charting the chart—an exercise in interpretation(s), *Lit Med* 11(1):1–22, 1992.
31. Brody H: "My story is broken, can you help me fix it?" Medical ethics and the joint construction of narrative, *Literature Med* 13(Spring):85–87, 1994.
32. Manoogian MM, Harter LM, Denham SA: The storied nature of health legacies in the familial experience of type 2 diabetes, *J Fam Communic* (10):40–56, 2010.
33. Haidet P, Paterniti DA: "Building" a history rather than "taking" one: a perspective on information sharing during the medical interview, *Arch Intern Med* 163:1134–1140, 2003.

CHAPTER
9

Respectful Communication in an Information Age

CHAPTER OBJECTIVES

The reader will be able to:

- Compare and contrast models of communication
- Describe basic differences between one-to-one and group communication
- Identify four important factors in achieving successful verbal communication
- Assess three problems that can arise from miscommunication
- Discuss two voice qualities that influence the meaning of spoken words
- Identify two types of nonverbal communication, and describe the importance of each
- Describe how attitudes and emotions such as fear, grief, or humor affect communication
- Give some examples of ways in which time and space awareness differ from culture to culture
- Discuss ways to show respect through effective distance communication
- Identify seven levels of listening and describe their relevance to the health professional and patient interaction

After surgery last May, my first memory upon awakening in the ICU was a feeling as if I were choking on the ventilator, and of desperately wanting someone to help me. I could hear the nurse behind the curtain. I lifted my hand to summon her, only to realize I was in restraints, immobilized. I felt as if I were being buried alive. Lacking an alternative, I decided to kick my legs until someone came. This worked. The nurse came and suctioned me briefly, then disappeared behind the curtain. Still afraid and still feeling as if I needed more suctioning and the presence of another near me, I kicked again. She returned, this time to lecture me on how I mustn't kick my legs.

And then she left.

—*S.G. Jaquette*[1]

Talking Together

Patients rely on verbal communication to try to explain what is wrong or seek comfort or encouragement from health professionals. Yet they may have difficulty with

159

the language itself, with finding the right words, or they may literally be unable to speak and have to resort to gestures, such as the patient in the opening scenario of this chapter. Unable to use words to convey her needs, she spoke the only way she could—she kicked her legs.

The greater responsibility for respectful communication between you and a patient lies with you, although both must assume responsibility. By examining interdependent components of effective communication, you will gain insight into this critical area of human interaction. Health professionals rely on verbal, nonverbal, written, and electronic forms of communication to share information, plan care, and collaborate with others on the health care team.

In your work as a health professional you will be required to communicate verbally with a patient to (1) establish rapport, (2) obtain information concerning his or her condition and progress, (3) confirm understanding (your own and the person with whom you are communicating), (4) relay pertinent information to other health professionals and support personnel, and (5) educate the patient and his or her family. Periodically, you are expected to offer encouragement and support, give rewards as incentives for further effort, convey bad news, report technical data to a patient or colleague, interpret information, and act as consultant. Naturally, you will be more comfortable with some activities than with others, according to your own specific abilities and experiences. Nevertheless, all health professionals should be prepared to perform the entire gamut of communication activities.

Verbal communication is instrumental in creating better understanding between you and a patient. However, this is not always the result. You will often be able to trace the cause of a misunderstanding to something you said; it was probably the wrong thing to say, or it was said in the wrong way or at the wrong time. The way words travel back and forth between individuals has been the subject of a great deal of study in the communication field. Several models have been proposed to graphically describe what happens when two people exchange the simplest of words.

Models of Communication

Although the following quotation focuses on the exchange of information between the physician and patient, the same can be said of all health professionals as they communicate with patients. As you read the quote, recall the differences between how a patient tells his or her story that was elaborated in Chapter 8 and the traditional model of questioning to arrive at a diagnosis described here.

> It is revealing to examine how this flow back and forth between physician and patient is shaped, what is revealed or requested, when, by whom, at whose request or command, and whether there is reciprocal revelation of reasons, doubts, and anxieties. When we look at the medical context, instead of a free exchange of speech acts we find a highly structured discourse situation in which the physician is very much in control. Some patients perceive this sharply. Others more vaguely sense time constraints and a sequence structured by physician questions and terminated by signals of closure, such as writing prescriptions.[2]

Communication understood in this way involves the transfer of information from the patient to the health professional so that a diagnosis or plan for treatment can be made. The focus is on the "facts" and generally begins with a question about what brought the patient to the health professional. However, once the initial complaint is stated, there appears to be little time or attention devoted to other patient-centered concerns.[3]

Think of some reasons this is problematic. For example, the first complaint that a patient mentions may not be the most significant. More important, the patient may take a health professional's hurried rush through a discussion as an overt sign of disinterest and disrespect. Most interactions with patients take the form of "interviews" rather than a conversation or dialogue. Health profession students take great pains to learn this interview technique designed to reveal, by the process of data gathering and elimination, the patient's health problem. The interview becomes a means to an end, the end being a diagnosis, problem identification, and treatment plan. As was noted in Chapter 8, this end may not be the one the patient is seeking. Furthermore, by strictly following the interview model of communication, the health professional effectively controls the introduction and progression of topics. This pattern of communication involves the use of power and authority but remains largely hidden from awareness. Patients may literally be unable to get a word in edgewise during the time they have to speak with health professionals.

Imagine yourself changing your view of communication to one of a dialogue or conversation so that you can focus your attention on different aspects of the process such as minimizing the disparities in power and creating opportunities for true understanding between you and the patient. Even including questions and prompts like, "Tell me more about that," or "What have you tried that helps?" offers greater opportunity for communication than mere "yes" and "no" types of questions. Also, keeping quiet and letting a patient tell his or her story is especially effective to build trust and gain a sense of what is most important to the patient. Figure 9-1 conceptualizes communication,

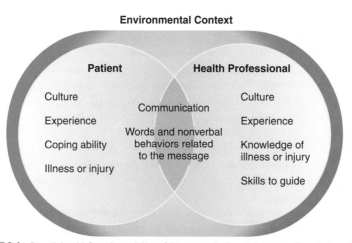

FIGURE 9-1: Essential and influencing variables of the communication environment. *(From Keltner NL, Bostrom CE, McGuinness T: Psychiatric nursing, ed 6, Philadelphia, 2010, Elsevier.)*

both verbal and nonverbal, as the bridge between you and a patient. The model also includes some of the primary and secondary cultural characteristics introduced in Chapter 3 that influence what each party brings to the dialogue. All of these factors (and others not listed in the figure) have an impact on the interaction.

The Context of Communication

Figure 9-1 places the two parties who are communicating within an environmental context. Where, with whom, and under what circumstances the dialogue or conversation takes place can have a profound influence on the process and outcomes of the interaction. Clinical encounters between you and your patients are, according to Arthur Frank, a particular form of dialogue: "Most of the particularities generate tensions: stakes are often high for both parties, time is often limited, intimate matters are being broached between comparative strangers, power differentials intrude, and—not last but enough—both parties often have idealized expectations for what should take place."[4]

Thus, the internal context of this exchange between you and the patient sets it apart from everyday conversations. The external environment also has an impact on the process and outcome of your dialogue. Because of technology, you may find yourself communicating with the same patient in a variety of contexts (e.g., face-to-face in a clinical setting, talking on the telephone, corresponding via e-mail).

Face-to-Face or Distant

If someone is standing or sitting right in front of you, the type of interaction is different from what occurs on the telephone or through an e-mail message, text, discussion board, or chat room. What varies most between face-to-face interactions and those that occur across distances is proximity and the degree of relative anonymity. When we are in direct personal contact with another person, there are fewer places to hide our fears and discomforts. In fact, knowing this, some health professionals specifically choose areas of practice in which they will have little direct contact with patients.

When you have the opportunity to meet face-to-face with a patient, all of the possible ways of communicating can be engaged. Each sense can be a source of information about the other. This explains, in part, why the exchange is that much richer and, to some, more frightening than those that take place from a distance.

We will discuss various forms of "distant" communication tools later in this chapter. During your career there is a good chance you will use all sorts of devices to communicate with patients. Perhaps at some time in the future, a holographic, computer-generated version of yourself and the patient will virtually "interact" with each other. Face-to-face interactions with health professionals will continue but will be more and more supplemented by other forms of communication technology (Figure 9-2).

For example, surveys show that patients want to be able to e-mail their clinicians to get test results and ask questions.[5] Online communication with patients has many positive attributes such as the verbatim record of the transaction between patient and health professional. However, e-mail is not well suited to urgent problems nor

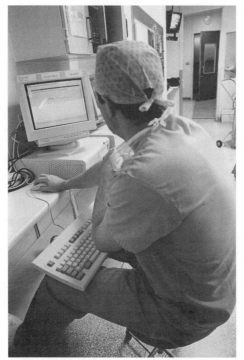

FIGURE 9-2: Online communication with patients has both its advantages and its drawbacks. *(© Corbis.)*

does it contain the nonverbal components of communication that are crucial to understanding.

One-to-One or Group

Before you begin any type of interaction with a patient, you should make sure the patient knows who you are and what you do. This sounds so basic that it hardly seems worth mentioning. However, some health professionals are so focused on getting on with the diagnostic examination or asking questions that they forget the introductions. Of course this is not necessary if you are seeing a patient often. If you have met before, but there has been some time between your interactions, it does not hurt to reintroduce yourself and explain your role. In addition, always wear your name tag with your name and professional role clearly displayed.

If you are meeting a patient for the first time, be sure to use his or her full name. Do not presume to address a patient, unless the patient is a child, by his or her first name until the patient gives you explicit permission. Ask the patient how to pronounce his or her name if there is any doubt about the correct pronunciation. The 6-year-old niece of one of the authors was highly insulted when her pediatrician continually mispronounced her first name after being corrected. The child said, "How would she like it if I kept saying her name the wrong way?" So even children noticed a lapse in respect.

After you introduce yourself, tell the patient what you do in a few sentences. It is helpful to practice this explanation with a sympathetic audience such as relatives or friends who will tell you if you are being too technical or confusing. Having established this initial rapport, you can now devote your attention to the patient before you and vice versa. We will address matters such as facial expression, gestures, and touch later in this chapter. All of these nonverbal forms of communication may override verbal messages, and this is especially obvious in a face-to-face interaction.

Working with an individual patient is far different from working with a group of patients. You will have the opportunity to interact with groups of patients or patients and their families or friends in addition to individual patients. Thus, it is important to become knowledgeable about group functioning because much of what you plan for and deliver may be accomplished through a group process. To have a constructive effect in a group setting you must be familiar with how a group influences individual behavior and the forces that operate in any group. The groups you interact with as a health professional may be spontaneously formed for a short period of time, such as a group of diabetic patients currently on the unit who come together for instruction about their diet, or they may be groups that will interact for longer periods of time, such as a support or therapy group in a rehabilitation setting. You will also work with interdisciplinary groups or peer groups in clinical practice. We focus here on the behavior that occurs when any group interacts and how you can improve the functioning of a group process whether you are the facilitator or a group member.

Groups that remain together over a period of time appear to go through various stages of development, and the behaviors during each can help you understand group process. The first stage is one of orientation or "groping." Members try to figure out what the purpose of the group is at this initial stage. If you are working with a group of patients, it is important to identify the specific goal of the group or what is to be accomplished in a specific time frame. When you are in the leadership or facilitator role, you can do a lot to increase the effectiveness and decrease the anxiety and confusion of the group by clearly providing structure. The second stage of group process for groups who continue to work together is the "griping" stage. Members of the group express, either openly or covertly, frustration and anger with the group process. This phenomenon seems to symbolize the group members' struggles to maintain their own identity and still be part of the group process. Stage 3 is the "grouping" stage where members figure out how to work together for a common purpose. Finally in stage 4 the group moves to the "grinding" stage, where they cooperate and focus on the task at hand.

Of course, not all groups move through these stages in a straightforward manner. Group composition can change, disrupting the growth process. Also, in the frantic pace of contemporary health care, groups come and go quickly; therefore, many times, little cohesion can be achieved. In other words, you may find yourself constantly working in the "groping" stage of group development, with your role remaining one of providing guidance and structure.

Institution or Home

In Chapter 2 we discussed a variety of environments in which patients receive care today. Whatever the environment in which you encounter patients, for social, psychological, and financial reasons, there is a strong tendency to medicalize the setting. So even in settings such as a skilled nursing facility or the patient's home, medical props and devices shape the atmosphere.

It is evident to health professionals who work in patients' homes that they are viewed as guests, at best, or intrusive strangers, at worst. Home care places the health professional on the patient's turf. Communication in the home care setting is shaped by that environment. Health professionals are more deferential, more attuned to asking before doing. Other health care environments, such as intensive care units or emergency departments, do not even pretend to be "homelike" or welcoming to patients. The sights, sounds, smells, and urgency of these high-tech environments have a profound impact on patients, particularly because this environment is often foreign and threatening. Consider this excerpt from a poem involving a mother who gets her first glimpse of her child in a critical care unit in a hospital.

INTENSIVE CARE

… I am called.
But nothing prepares me for what I see, my child

in her body of pain, hooked to machines. Grief
comes up like floodwater. Her body floats on a sea

of air that is her bed, a force field of sorrow
that pulls me to her side. I touch pain I know

I have never felt, move into a new land
of nightmare. She is so still. Only one hand

moves, fingers oscillate like water plants risking
the air. Machines line the desks,

the floor, the walls, confirm the deep pink
of her skin in rapidly ascending numbers. One eye blinks. . . .
    —L.C. Getsi[6]

Sensitive communication depends on an appreciation of the effect of the environment on what transpires between you and the patient.

Choosing the Right Words

The success of verbal communication depends on several important factors: (1) the way material is presented (i.e., the vocabulary used, the clarity of voice, and organization; and (2) the tone and volume of the voice.

Vocabulary and Jargon

As we note in Chapter 8, the descriptive vocabulary of the health professional is a two-edged sword. A student must learn to offer precise, accurate descriptions and must be able to communicate to other professionals in that mode.

Technical language is one of the bonds shared by health professionals among themselves. In contrast, highly technical professional jargon is almost never appropriate in direct conversation with the patient. It cuts off communication with the patient. It is imperative that you learn to translate technical jargon into terms understandable to patients when discussing their condition or conversing with their families. Only in the rarest instances are patients schooled in the technical language of health care sufficiently to understand its jargon, even in today's world of the Internet, television, podcasts, and other health care–related media resources. Even when the patient happens to be a health professional, it is important to use easily understandable language when talking about what is happening with him or her. Do not assume that the therapist or nurse who is your patient is conversant in all areas of health care. The safest approach in working with another health professional who is your patient is to take a cue from the patient and use only the technical language that he or she introduces.

Another common area for miscommunication is when the health professional and patient literally speak different languages. As was mentioned in Chapter 3, the world is often literally at our doorsteps because of the influx of a variety of refugees and immigrants into the United States. It is a rare health professional who does not routinely encounter language barriers with patients.

Numerous options exist for bridging these language barriers including interpreters, bilingual health professionals, and untrained volunteers. There are several reasons to avoid the use of family members and other untrained volunteers as medical interpreters such as:

▶ Interpreters close to the patient may not be able to disregard their views regarding the situation, which can bias the information that is shared.[7]
▶ Family interpreters, in particular, often speak as themselves rather than merely providing accurate information between parties.[8]
▶ Untrained interpreters often lack knowledge of medical terms, which can lead to miscommunication and misdiagnosis.
▶ Untrained interpreters may be emotionally harmed because of the stress of performing an essential activity for which they are not prepared.[9]

This is not to say that formally trained interpreters are the only or best recourse. Limited data indicate that the use of nonverbal supplementation to verbal communication can help lead to sufficient understanding between health professional and patient.[10] Also, patients may not trust formally trained interpreters for a variety of social and cultural reasons, so again it is best to take your lead from the patient. If possible, a combination of the languages involved and nonverbal signs might be the best alternative when a patient refuses a trained interpreter. The main goal is to find a neutral and accurate means of communicating across language barriers. [9]

Choosing the right words is a special challenge when working with patients with changes in mental capacity such as patients with Alzheimer's disease. In a study of caregivers who worked with patients with Alzheimer's disease, a "yes/no" or forced choice type of question (e.g., "Do you want to go outside?") rather than an open-ended question (e.g., "What would you like to do?") resulted in more successful communication.[11] Family caregivers of patients with Alzheimer's disease also found that using simple sentences was more effective than other communication strategies, such as slow speech.[12]

Thus, as always, the general rule has exceptions, and you will have to assess what types of questions work best with each patient. Of course, the way to respectful communication is to try as much as possible to talk to patients as equals (because that is what the majority of patients want) while remaining flexible in your style to meet individual patients' needs.

Problems from Miscommunication

Several problems arise when miscommunication occurs because the health professional is unable to communicate with the patient in terms understandable to him or her.

Desired Results Are Lost

The health professional attempts to understand the patient's complaints. Often the descriptions are too vague or too difficult to classify. Rather than continue to work to understand the symptoms and their significance for the patient, the health professional immediately turns to the more objective criteria of laboratory and other diagnostic findings and bases treatment programs on experience described in the literature or derived from a large number of other patients. This "miss" in communication all too often inhibits the results the health professional wished to achieve and could have achieved, had effective communication with the patient been established.[13] Once again, when the health professional viewed the interaction with the patient as merely the transfer of information, the opportunity for true discourse was lost.

Meanings Are Confused

Another common area for miscommunication is when the health professional and patient are both using the same word but ascribe different meanings to it. In a qualitative study of diabetic patients and their physicians, it was found that different conceptions of the term "control" affected the ability of patients and their physicians to communicate effectively.[14] Although the physicians in the study acknowledged the numerous physical, psychological, and social obstacles to treatment, they did not focus on these aspects of the disease when they interacted with patients. Rather, they focused almost entirely on managing blood glucose numbers. This led to a great degree of frustration on the part of the patients.

Doubt Arises about the Health Professional's Interest

Another problem that can result from using technical language is that the person to whom you are speaking will not be convinced that you really want to know how he or she feels. In addition, your choice of words can unintentionally hurt the patient. For example, after her first prenatal visit to the doctor, a pregnant teenager reported to her friends, "The doctor wanted to know about my 'menstrual history.' I didn't know what that was. Finally, I figured out she was talking about my periods. Why didn't she just say that? I felt so stupid."

When the health professional persists in using "big words" or technical language, the patient may interpret this as a sign that his or her problems are not important. The complexity and impersonality of a health facility will undoubtedly be communicated to the patient if health professionals are unwilling to explain carefully to the patient, in understandable terms, his or her condition and its treatment. The amount that is accomplished within any allotted period of time, rather than the actual amount of time spent, will convince the patient that the health professional really cares. If the patient cannot understand what is being said, little will be accomplished.

The mastery of appropriate vocabulary, then, includes being able to communicate with your colleagues but at the same time being willing to converse with patients in words they can understand. You will, in essence, need to become "bilingual," translating from professional terms to common everyday language. When this is accomplished, it is more likely that the patient will be able to do what is requested, will respond accurately to your questions, and will be convinced that you care about him or her.

Clarity

In addition to using words that are too technical for the patient to understand, a health professional may not speak with sufficient clarity to free the patient from uncertainty, doubt, or confusion about what is being said. What is the difference between the two? Lack of clarity can result if you launch into a lengthy, rambling description of treatment options (e.g., not realizing that the patient was lost at the outset). Even a highly organized, technically correct, and objectively meaningful sentence can be unclear if it is poorly articulated or spoken too softly or hurriedly. Lack of clarity can result when patients become preoccupied with one particular facet of what you are saying and consequently interpret everything else in light of that preoccupation.

It is surprising to some students that patients may be too embarrassed to ask them to repeat something, and so patients rely on what they think they heard. Patients are sometimes hesitant because they are a bit awed by you as the health professional and so try to act sophisticated instead of asking you to repeat what you said. Patients may be awed primarily because they realize that health professionals have skills that can determine their future welfare and that, regardless of their influence in the business or social world, they are at your mercy in this situation. Some ways to help enhance the clarity of your communication follow.

Explanation of the Purpose and Process

Clarity begins with helping the patient understand why you are there and what you plan to do. As we mentioned earlier in this chapter, you first establish the purpose of your interaction when you introduce yourself and explain your role. This general introduction should be followed by a statement of the purpose of this particular encounter (i.e., what is going to take place at this time and why). Thus, you and the patient know what the goal of the interaction is from the start. Because the patient may be tired or uncomfortable, it is also helpful to state at the outset how long the interaction will take and what the patient will likely experience (e.g., "The head of this instrument may be a little cold at first when it touches your skin," "When you get up on the table we will ask you to roll onto your right side," and "Push this call button if you want to get out of bed."). Questions the patient asks will then help you decide what more you need to say.

Organization of Ideas

Think ahead about how you are going to present your information. You can quickly confuse a patient by jumping from one topic to the next, inserting last-minute ideas, and then failing to summarize or to ask the patient to do so. Failure to systematically progress from one step to the next toward a logical conclusion is usually caused by (1) your own lack of understanding of the subject or of the steps in the procedure or (2) ironically, a too-thorough knowledge of the subject or procedure. The former causes the patient to have to figure out the relevant facts, whereas the latter causes the speaker to leave out points that are obvious to him or her but not to the listener. In either case, it is advisable to organize the description of a procedure or test into its component parts and then to practice describing it to a friend who is not familiar with the procedure. That person will be able to identify any obvious steps that have been omitted. Complicated information should be broken down into manageable chunks so that the patient is not overwhelmed by everything that follows. This is especially true when the information involves bad news.

Augment Verbal Communication

Verbal information and instructions alone are not always adequate to ensure clarity. Written notes or instructions, diagrams, videotapes, and nonverbal demonstrations are highly desirable adjuncts to the spoken word because they may help the person organize the ideas and information more fully.

Tone and Volume

Paralinguistics is the study of all cues in verbal speech other than the content of the words spoken. Although paralinguistics is considered part of the realm of nonverbal communication, we will discuss tone and volume here because they are so closely connected to the content of speech. Sometimes a person's voice or volume belies his or her words. Any vocalized sound a person makes could be interpreted as verbal communication, so besides your words you will communicate "volumes" with the tone, inflection, speed, and loudness of the words you use.

Tone

Each of us tries to communicate more than the literal content of our messages by using different tones of voice of the same spoken message. An expression as short as "oh" can be used to express anger, pity, disappointment, teasing, pleasure, gratitude, exuberance, terror, superiority, disbelief, uncertainty, compassion, insult, awe, and many more. Try this exercise with "no," "yes," and other simple words or phrases to fully grasp the rich variety of meanings a word can convey when you vary the tone and inflection.

Tone is a voice quality that can actually reverse the meaning of the spoken word. When the patient's response is puzzling to the health professional, the latter should be alert to the tone in which the patient communicated a message or reacted to a statement. For example, if the patient asks, "Am I going to get better?" the health professional can inadvertently confirm the patient's worst fears by hesitating then answering in a not-too-convincing tone, "Why, of *course* you will."

⦾ REFLECTIONS

Give several meanings to the simple question, "What are you doing?" by varying the tone in which it can be spoken. Try to mimic the tones of the following people: (1) a man telephoning his wife at midday; (2) the man's wife, who has just caught their 2-year-old son writing on the living room wall with a purple crayon; and (3) the 2-year-old son trying to make up to the mother after being scolded.

Volume

Tone and volume are closely related voice qualities. An angry person may not only spit out the words indignantly but may also alter the volume of the message. For instance, it is possible to communicate anger either by whispering words through gritted teeth or by shouting them.

Voice volume controls interaction in subtle ways. For instance, if one person stands close to another and speaks in an inordinately loud voice, the listener invariably backs away. On the other hand, a soft whisper automatically causes the listener to move closer. Thus, literally and symbolically, the volume of the voice does control distance between people.

Whatever you say, you must make certain that the patient can hear you. An easy way to assess if you are speaking loudly enough is to ask the patient to repeat instructions rather than just solicit "yes" or "no" responses. Make sure the patient can see your face when you speak because some patients need the physical cues of your expression and the movement of your lips to understand what is being said.

Choosing the Way to Say It

Your educational experience will provide you with the right words, but you will send many other messages to patients in addition to the spoken word. The most basic of nonverbal forms of communication is the manner in which you think, feel, or act—your attitude. We will begin our discussion of attitudes by presuming the inherent good in one another. We presume an attitude of mutual trust and respect. Most health professionals maintain a caring attitude toward patients, and their way of speaking to them helps to communicate this genuine concern. On rare occasions, however, you may feel anger or disdain for a patient. In Chapter 13 we address some types of patients who present a challenge in this regard.

Attitudes and Emotions

One variable that is frequently overlooked and has considerable impact on the exchange of information is the patient's emotional and mental state and attitudes. Examples are anger or fear that complicate communication and the management of his or her condition. If you want to effectively communicate with a patient, you must be knowledgeable about his or her mental state. You do not have to perform an exhaustive mental status examination to determine a patient's ability to comprehend, his or her orientation to the task at hand, or his or her ability to follow directions. You can obtain this information as you interact with the patient. If there is any doubt as to the patient's general cognitive ability, you can use one of the many screening tools available to assess general mental functions such as the Mini-Mental State Examination developed by Folstein and colleagues[15] or the shorter, and thus more easily administered, Short Portable Mental Status Questionnaire.[16]

The attitude or feeling that a health professional has toward the patient will help to determine the effectiveness of spoken interaction, too. Attitudes and emotions that are commonly encountered among health professionals are fear, grief, and a sense of humor.

Fear

Patients are often afraid for many reasons. Fear may present itself as stony silence, clenched fists, profuse sweating, or an angry outburst. Patients may not recognize the emotion that they are experiencing as fear, so you must be watchful for the signs of fear and do your best to help reassure the patient.

The specific situations in which health professionals' fears arise are just as numerous as those for patients. How will your fear manifest itself during spoken communication? Fear can arise when the health professional is inexperienced or the patient is threatening in some way. In the following exchange from Samuel Shem's satire "Mount Misery," a new psychiatric resident interviews just such a patient:

> "So, Dr. Dickhead, tell me about yourself," Thorny said.
>
> Uh-oh. Surely this was backward—*I* was supposed to be asking about *him.* "I'm the new resident." I felt a sharp pain in my palm. I was clutching my key ring so hard the keys were biting into my flesh. "You?"
>
> "Got here a month ago from New Orleans. My daddy's rich, made a fortune burnin' trash down Cancer Alley. Calls himself the Burn King of the Bayous. I did okay till I was eighteen, 'n' got sent north to Princeton. Lasted about three months. You look kinda tentative, Doc. Scareda me?"
>
> I was, but I wasn't going to let *him* know it. "Nope."[17]

The patient, Thorny, began this exchange by putting the physician on the defensive. No one likes to be called an obscene, derogatory name. Furthermore, the patient took control of the interview process from the inexperienced physician. Finally, the patient brought direct attention to the fact that the physician was scared. Here was an opportunity for the physician to be honest with the patient and acknowledge his fear. By denying his fear, he amplified its presence, and it remained a roadblock to future, candid communication. Of course, it is not prudent to announce to all patients when you are fearful. Patients count on the confidence and courage of health professionals. So as with all things, you must consider your relationship with the patient and the circumstances that would suggest disclosure of fear and other emotions.

Grief

Patients have a variety of ways of dealing with grief, but it is likely that you will see people at the worst times of their lives and come to witness many different reactions to profound loss. It is important to prepare yourself to comfort patients and family members dealing with grief and also to deal with your own feelings. Sharing your sorrow or tears with a patient or family member is often deemed "unprofessional." However, letting a patient know how deeply you feel about their situation is not always inappropriate. If you remain too stoic, patients may think you do not care. Striking the right balance between some distance and sharing grief are evident in the following account of a struggle by a neurosurgical resident when she has to tell a patient he has a terminal brain tumor:

> I sat down and delivered the news. I hinted at the ultimate implications of his diagnosis, but I didn't want to hit this too hard too soon. I wanted to give him some time to digest the shock of the unexpected. I looked at his wife, his infant daughter, and at him. He nodded his head, slowly, calmly. I wanted to provide them with some hope so I started, reflexively, to enumerate all the treatments he could receive that would give him the best possible chance. I reassured him that he was young and healthy, which would put him in a more favorable category.
>
> I felt I had done enough talking at that point, so I stopped and sat in silence, a natural invitation for questions. I looked at the three of them. His wife was starting to cry, silently.
>
> Then, without warning, I started to cry, too, then sob, interrupting the silence. My usual calm professional demeanor had broken down. I was struck by a harsh paradox: the vision of this young vibrant family sitting with me in the present, clashing with my knowledge of biology and how this tumor was about to change their lives. I could see the future too clearly.
>
> The patient continued to look at me, stoically, nodding his head. He exhaled audibly and then thanked me. I didn't deserve much thanks, though. I worried that my unbridled outpouring of grief had wiped out any shred of hope. Chances are that if the surgeon is bawling, the prognosis is dismal. I calmed down, hugged his wife, and left the room, passing his friends in the hallway and looking downward to shield my face. I walked straight out to the hospital garage and drove right home.[18]

> ### ⊙ REFLECTIONS
>
> - Because the prognosis was bleak, the message that the neurosurgeon related was accurate but was it appropriate?
> - Would the patient necessarily lose all hope as the surgeon feared?
> - What might be another outcome of the neurosurgeon's expression of grief?

Humor

A subtler, often effective way of dealing with a problem or hiding fear is through the use of humor. Health care settings can be full of banter, laughter, and jokes, some of which serve useful purposes, whereas others are destructive. Humor can be used wisely to help patients cope with stress related to their illness and accompanying problems.

In communication between the patient and the health professional, joking and teasing can be used constructively to (1) allow the person to express hostility and anxiety, (2) permit exploration of the humor and irony of the condition in which he or she is placed by illness or injury, and (3) reduce tension. Shared humor and a good laugh can often defuse anxiety in tense situations and open up connections between you and the patient. The following story by a psychiatrist highlights the mutual benefits of humor:

> I had one patient in therapy for a year who was completely bogged down in inappropriate guilt, always ready to take the blame for anything that happened to anybody anywhere in the world. She was, as usual, castigating herself, when I interrupted with, "You know, I don't mind the things you have done to the economy. I don't even mind the fact that you're responsible for high inflation. I don't even mind the taxes you cause me to pay. But I'm just madder than hell at you for causing it to rain the past three days."
>
> There had been a sharp intake of breath when I started. Her worst fears had been realized: *I* blamed her too! The seconds ticked by. First there was a small smile—just a twitch of the lips, really—then a grin, followed soon by a giggle, then a guffaw—which I joined. We literally laughed until we cried.[19]

In the preceding situation, the psychiatrist was an experienced health professional and knew the patient well. Both of the components, experience and familiarity or a bond with the patient, and good timing need to be present for humor to be therapeutic and not destructive. The same psychiatrist compared humor to nitroglycerin: In the proper hands it serves a useful purpose, but in the wrong hands it can cause great harm.

The inexperienced health professional and the layperson are often shocked by the openness with which patients joke about themselves. For instance, patients whose legs are paralyzed often joke about rubber crutches and icy surfaces, both of which are real threats in their present situations. Persons with disfiguring injuries call themselves "freaks." Their joking helps to alleviate their anxiety about these problems. Patients with temporary or permanent sexual impotence also may joke a lot about sex. It is helpful to recognize their joking as one means of expressing difficult thoughts and emotions.

The use to which humor is put will determine whether it fosters respectful inter-action or is a poor substitute for direct confrontation. "When used appropriately, humor can have positive psychological, communication, and social benefits, as well as positive physiological effects."[20] When used inappropriately, such as making fun of patients who are challenging or are perceived to be responsible for their own health problems, humor can be hurtful and disrespectful. Although you may witness derogatory jokes about certain groups of patients, you should not join in, and you should remember that this is unacceptable behavior.

Communicating Beyond Words

In this section we turn our attention beyond vocal utterances designed to engage us in dialogue and conversation to consider all the additional (or substitute) ways we enter into communication with patients and others. Collectively these means are often referred to as *nonverbal communication*. The majority of communication is nonverbal with estimates of 7% of the message being verbal and the other 93% being nonverbal communication.[21] In a systematic review of the literature from 1975-2000 of studies of office interactions of patients and physicians, the following nonverbal behaviors were positively associated with health outcomes: head nodding, leaning forward, direct body orientation, and uncrossed legs and arms.[22] All of these non-verbal behaviors and others that follow are easy to adopt so that they become second nature when you interact with patients.

Facial Expression

Earlier in this chapter, you were asked to consider the variety of messages conveyed by altering the tone and volume of the spoken word "oh." It is possible to omit the word altogether and, with only a facial message, convey a variety of emotions.

Eye contact generally communicates a positive message. There is a powerful, immediate effect when we gaze directly at another person. If two people genuinely like each other, they will position themselves so that they look into each other's eyes. The distance between them as they face each other further communicates how they feel about each other. Distance as a form of nonverbal communication is discussed later in this chapter.

Even without eye contact, the rest of the face reveals many things. The presence or absence of a smile and the genuineness of a smile are all clues to a person's emotional state. Grimaces from pain, the vacant stare of a child with a fever, and the bland affect of a depressed patient provide important information that speaks volumes without the use of any words. Your own facial expression need not be somber but should be friendly and open. This is preferable to an overly cheerful demeanor that does not permit a patient to express his or her true feelings.

Gestures and Body Language

Gestures involving the extremities, even one finger, can suggest the meanings of a message. Consider the mother who folds her arms when a child begins to sputter an excuse for coming home late, the man who clenches his fist, or the adolescent girl twisting a lock of her hair. What unspoken messages are they sending? Refer to the patient scenario that opened this chapter. She would be considered a "non-vocal" patient because she was intubated. Because the patient had no other way of communicating her fears and her need for the presence of the nurse, she kicked her legs. Gestures like this are often used by patients who cannot communicate verbally, and they are often misunderstood as anxiety. The patient may indeed be anxious but is often trying to convey a message. "The nurse may administer a sedative and/or apply restraints when the more appropriate management would be to identify and implement communication strategies that meet the particular needs of the patient to communicate effectively."[23]

Unlike the nurse in the opening scenario, many health professionals develop the skill of truly reading the meaning of the gestures and behaviors of patients. In more than one study, staff members in nursing home settings have demonstrated the predictive value of certain changes in nonverbal behavior in patients and the development of acute illness. One study found that the nursing assistants' documentation of signs of illness preceded chart documentation of acute illness by an average of 5 days.[24] Another study noted that the highest positive predictor values were for lethargy, weakness, and decreased appetite, each of which correctly predicted acute illness.[25] Understanding subtle and obvious gestures is an important component of learning respectful communication.

Physical Appearance

Stereotypes are formed from outward appearances. In some instances, a person tries to adopt a stereotyped manner of dressing or speaking in the hope of being identified with a particular group.

Some health professionals adopt a stereotyped manner of dress (the uniform) to be identified easily within the world of health care. The "uniform" may include clothing, a patch, a pin, a lab coat, or a name tag or badge. Certain instruments also identify the person: the nurse's stethoscope dangling from the neck or the laboratory technologist's tray.

⊚ REFLECTIONS

What are the implications of wearing a white coat, scrubs, stethoscope, and other readily identifiable professional attire while engaging a patient in the admission process?

Touch

In all societies, individuals come into physical contact with each other all the time, but the context is crucial (i.e., they tend not to put their hands on each other except in well-defined social and cultural rituals). However, upon entering a health facility, regardless if they like or dislike physical contact, people may have to allow themselves to be palpated, punctured with needles, squeezed, rubbed, cut, examined, manipulated, and lifted.

These unusual touching privileges are granted to health professionals by society. Licensing of health professionals is primarily a protection against the charge of unconsented touching *(battery)*. In Chapter 11 you will learn about the boundaries, including physical ones, that must be maintained, even when legitimate touching is recognizable as part of the therapeutic encounter.

Fortunately, the comforting touch is usually regarded as legitimate, and you have in it a powerful tool for communicating caring (Figure 9-3). The positive effects of a caring touch are sometimes observable in the patient. For example, you may observe one or more of the following: a lowering of the patient's voice, a slowing and deepening of the patient's breathing, or a spontaneous verbal response like a sigh or "I feel relaxed." A physician who was seriously ill commented on how much rubbing his back meant to him: "The nurse giving a back rub was so incredibly important to me. It was profoundly human—an act of caring. Even with painkillers, there's suffering and pain. Those back rubs were ... somebody affirm[ing] that I mattered."[26]

People pick up signals conveyed by your manner of touching. This is often related to your appearance, the speed and ease with which you move, and the quality of your touch. The sensation received by the patient when his or her arm is lifted by the health professional's cold, clammy hand sends quite a different message from the gentle support of a warm, dry hand. The reassuring hand resting on a patient's shoulder sometimes speaks more loudly than the kindest words. Patients should be

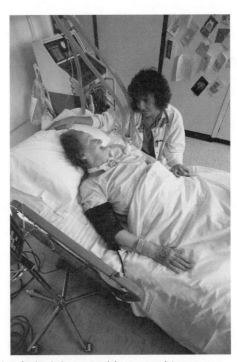

FIGURE 9-3: A health professional who uses touch in an appropriate manner communicates caring to his or the patient. *(© Corbis.)*

touched with respect for the person who lives inside the body being manipulated. Even if our touch is less than perfect, perhaps a bit clumsy, patients are generally deeply grateful for being handled with care by another.

Patients will be much more aware of this touching than the health professional, who has become used to touching patients. The experienced health professional probably has so firm a concept of his or her good intentions that the question of inappropriateness or improper familiarity never arises. However, touch, as one form of nonverbal communication, does involve risk. It may be a threat because it invades an otherwise private space or it may be misunderstood. So, an explanation before touching a patient is always in order.

Proxemics

Proxemics is the study of how space is used in human interactions. For example, authority can be communicated by the height from which one person interacts with another. If one stands while the other sits or lies down, the person standing has placed himself or herself in a position of authority (Figure 9-4).

Height is sometimes an unwitting message to a patient when the person is confined to a bed, a treatment table, or a wheelchair. In many instances, the relationship would be improved if the health professional would move down to the patient's level. An important rule for respectful interaction whenever you are talking to a patient is to sit down. This signals to the patient your willingness to listen and gives the impression, even if this is not true, that you are not going to rush through your time together.

Another aspect of proxemics is the distance maintained between people when they are communicating. In his now classic *The Hidden Dimension,* an intriguing book that explains the difference in distance awareness among many different cultural groups, anthropologist Edward T. Hall defines four distance zones maintained by healthy, adult, middle-class Americans.[27] In examining these zones, you may also be better able to understand how they differ from those of other cultural and socioeconomic groups. Dr. Hall stresses that "how people are feeling toward each other at the time is a decisive factor in the distance used." The four distance zones are as follows:

1. Intimate distance, involving direct contact, such as that of lovemaking, comforting, protecting, and playing football or wrestling.
2. Personal distance, ranging from 1 to 4 feet. At arm's length, subjects of personal interest can be discussed while physical contact, such as holding hands or hitting the other person in the nose, is still possible.
3. Social distance, ranging from 4 to 12 feet. At this distance, more formal business and social discourse takes place.
4. Public distance, ranging from 12 to 25 feet or more. No physical contact and very little direct eye contact are possible. Shopping centers, airports, and city sidewalks are designed to maintain this type of distance.[27]

Health professionals perform many diagnostic or treatment procedures within the personal and intimate distance zones. You may have to invade the patient's culturally derived boundaries of interaction, sometimes with little warning. Consider, for instance, the weak or debilitated patient who comes for treatment and must be

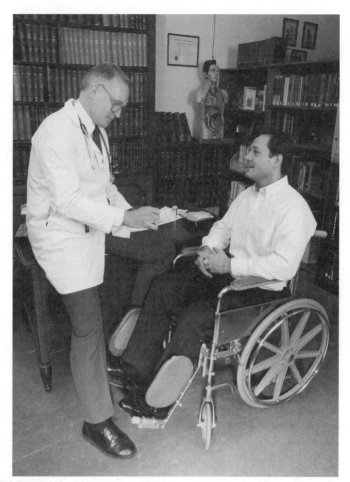

FIGURE 9-4: Standing over a patient in a wheelchair is inappropriate nonverbal behavior. *(© Getty Images/18164.)*

helped to a treatment table. To get the patient on the treatment table, you might have to "embrace" the patient and, in some cases, actually lift the patient to the table, deeply invading his or her intimate zone.

When you work with an ethnic or cultural subgroup outside of your own experience or travel to other parts of the world, culturally defined uses of space are readily apparent. In addition, you may become aware of some things that you did not expect to be part of the interaction. For instance, body odors become more apparent when you are working at close range. In mainstream American society in which a man or woman is supposed to smell like a deodorant, a mouthwash, a hair spray, or a cologne, but not a body, it is not surprising that some health professionals find the patient's body odor offensive, sometimes nauseous; some admit that it so repulses them that they try to hurry through the test or treatment.

Patients will respond to the health professional's odors, too. An x-ray technologist confided to one of the authors that one of her biggest shocks while working in a mission hospital in India came when her assistant reluctantly admitted that patients were failing to keep their appointments because she "smelled funny," making them sick. The "funny" smell turned out to be that of the popular American soap she was using for her bath.

Bad breath is a problem. What constitutes "bad breath?" It is not necessarily the smell of garlic, onion, tobacco, or alcohol. Its definition depends on who is asked the question. The health professional who is unwilling to try to go beyond his or her own culturally derived bias of distance awareness (with its accompanying distance zones for interaction) will have difficulty in communicating with many patients. While working at close range, your reaction to body and breath odors will affect interaction. Most patients are far too ill or preoccupied with their problems to have sweet-smelling breath, and others are not aware that they are being hustled out quickly because of the salami sandwich they had at noon.

Adhering to a patient's need to maintain an appropriate distance reinforces the patient's ability to feel secure in the strange new world of health care institutions. By handling distance needs respectfully, you are helping the patient to find himself or herself in the sometimes frightening vastness of the unknown health care environment into which he or she has been cast.

Differing Concepts of Time

A culturally derived difference that affects nonverbal communication is how people interpret time. The right time and the correct amount of time are relative, depending on one's cultural perspective. One aspect of the time dimension that directly affects the patient and health professional interaction is the scheduling and maintaining of appointments with patients. Most health professionals are punctual and expect their patients to be the same. In fact, the health facility operates each day on a schedule. Harrison points out that "punctuality communicates respect while tardiness is an insult." However, "in some other cultures to arrive exactly on time is an insult (it says, 'You are such an unimportant fellow that you can arrange your affairs easily; you really have nothing else to do.'). Rather, an appropriate amount of tardiness is expected."[28] You may find that a patient is scheduled to arrive at "10 o'clock health-professional time" but arrives instead at "10 o'clock patient time," feeling no need at all to explain or apologize.

The amount of time spent in rendering professional service may also vary from one culture to another. How should a given amount of time be spent so that the patient benefits most? By middle-class American standards, you should greet the patient briefly and begin treatment or a test without delay. If you rush in setting up equipment, the patient may interpret it to mean you care enough to hurry. When the treatment is over, the patient usually leaves immediately.

However, in some cultures, if the treatment does not begin as soon as the patient arrives, it does not matter as long as it will eventually be done. Rather than rush into the procedure itself, you should first inquire about the weather, the family, and other things that may be important to the patient, sometimes spending several minutes in this way.

During the actual treatment or test, you may hurry, but good-byes must not be short and rushed. One of the authors worked in an African village where she was expected to slowly enter the room, then greet the patient for a few minutes. The treatment or test could begin immediately after that, but at no time could she rush around the room. To rush while the patient remained seated was an unspeakable insult that could only mean that the health professional believed herself more important than the patient.

These examples give you an idea of the rich variety of ways in which time may have to be organized within different cultural contexts to convey respect toward the patient and others.

Ways of operating within and indicating time, then, are highly relative. The few examples presented only skim the surface of differences in time awareness among different cultures. As mentioned in Chapter 3, you should always take possible differences into consideration when working with people whose cultural backgrounds are different from your own, recognizing that both distance and time awareness are deep seated and culturally derived. A person is usually not consciously aware of how he or she interprets time and distance, and so neither factor is easily identified as the cause of misunderstanding. Clearly, culture influences the interpretation of verbal and nonverbal communication in terms of time or distance.

Communicating across Distances

Much of the literature regarding communication between the patient and health professional has taken for granted that the two parties are within close proximity of each other. In many cases today, because of the mobility of society and technological developments, health professionals and patients can communicate across great distances. In addition, you may work with colleagues on the same complex patient problem and yet geographically be in two different cities. All of the techniques to enhance communication in general apply to communication across distances, but they must be adapted to the special demands created by miles between a patient and health professional instead of inches.

Written Tools

Written communication includes information about diagnostic tests and evaluation observations, progress notes about patients, instructions to patients to perform activities, informed consent documents, and quality assurance surveys to obtain information from patients about services rendered. Whatever the reason for the written communication, there are distinct advantages to its use over verbal communication. Written communication has the advantage of visual cues. The reader has control over the pace of absorbing the information and can reread the information any number of times. However, written communication demands a high degree of accuracy. All written communication should clearly state and define the reason it is being sent. The content should be well organized. Clarity and brevity are also hallmarks of good written communication.

The vocabulary must be fitting for the recipient. Although Institutional Review Boards that make judgments about research involving human participants are supposed to guarantee that consent forms are readable and understandable, study after study demonstrates that they are too long and complex. A recent review of the literature on consent forms for human participants in research reveals that consent forms are getting longer and that there is greater consistency in the description of risk.[29] The length of consent forms is certainly a problem because the more information that is given to people, the less likely it is for them to understand what is being proposed. Clear, concise written messages will be more easily understood and problems prevented if both verbal and written forms of communication can be used.

Voice and Electronic Tools

Since the telephone has become so much a part of our lives, you may not even notice how much you use it to communicate with patients. In an ambulatory setting, the phone may be your only contact with a patient between visits. It is best not to rely solely on this communication modality. It is especially important not to give bad news over the phone or try to explain a complicated evaluation finding or treatment plan. However, exchanging information or data such as blood glucose levels or electrocardiogram printouts electronically is an effective and efficient adjunct to other forms of communication.

Telephones can also be used to triage patient care.

Telephone triage is the process by which a health care provider communicates with a client via the telephone and, thereby, assesses the presenting concerns, develops a working diagnosis, and determines a suitable plan of management. Determination of the seriousness of the situation will dictate whether the client can be cared for at a distance or whether a more comprehensive in-person evaluation is in order.[30]

Of course, as we noted earlier, use of the telephone to render care must be done cautiously, particularly when you determine what follow-up is necessary.

Voice mail should be used with care. When you order a sweater from a catalogue over the phone or check your savings account balance, you generally do so with automated voice mail. But person-to-person communication that is so necessary to respectful care is missing when a computerized voice is on the other end of the telephone. However, a benefit of voice mail is the opportunity for a patient to leave a detailed message about a question or problem and avoid playing "phone tag" with health professionals.

E-mail is another form of electronic communication that is becoming more and more a part of health care practice. Although e-mail will not replace face-to-face visits, it can augment the health professional and patient relationship by providing a way to seek advice and follow up on tests or changes in prescriptions or a plan of care. Another advantage is that there is a written record of the exchange that both parties can refer to in the future.

Although e-mail may assist in communication, its use depends on the availability of a personal computer and a knowledgeable user on both ends. Needless to say, not everyone has access to a computer but access is slowly but steadily increasing even in developing countries. In some cases, advanced communication technology may be the best solution to providing health care to people who would otherwise not be able to travel to places with the latest innovations in health care. The World

Health Organization (WHO) views *telemedicine* as one of the most promising methods of health delivery to the developing world where the need for quality health care vastly outstrips the ability to deliver it. WHO defines telemedicine as, "The delivery of health care services, where distance is a critical factor, by all health care professionals using information and communication technologies for the exchange of valid information for diagnosis, treatment and prevention of disease and injuries, research and evaluation, and for the continuing education of health care providers, all in the interests of advancing the health of individuals and their communities."[31] As you will note, this use of information and communication technologies includes all members of the health care team, not just physicians, and for broader purposes than health delivery to patients who are at a distance. Of course, there are numerous barriers to the implementation of telemedicine systems such as high costs and lack of technical expertise, but the potential benefits appear to outweigh these negative factors.

Effective Listening

A considerable portion of a health professional's day is spent listening to patients and colleagues in person or over the telephone. Elizabeth Smith describes the following levels of listening and suggests that health professionals are usually involved in the more complex levels, cited first:
1. Analytical listening for specific kinds of information and arranging them into categories
2. Directed listening to answer specific questions
3. Attentive listening for general information to get the overall picture
4. Exploratory listening because of one's own interest in the subject being discussed
5. Appreciative listening for aesthetic pleasure, such as listening to music
6. Courteous listening because one feels obligated to listen
7. Passive listening, as in overhearing something; not attentive to the matter being discussed[32]

Most people lack the skills to listen effectively. If you are one of them, two goals for your further development are (1) to improve listening acuity so that you hear the patient accurately and (2) to ascertain how accurately a patient has heard you. The first step to achieving these goals is to examine the reasons messages get distorted. Besides the often-overlooked but important possibility of a hearing deficit, there are at least three reasons a health professional or patient distorts a verbal communication.

Distorted Meaning

First, a mind-set or frame of mind may distort meaning. It is the result of past experience. In this case, a person fails to listen to the spoken words or to note subtle individual differences because he or she is sure of what the other person will say. A poignant example of people talking at and across each other and not really communicating in the health care environment is the following dialogue poem between members of the health care team and the mother of an infant in the neonatal intensive care unit. The mother speaks in stanzas 1, 4, and 7.

PATIENT CARE CONFERENCE

"I just want them to show some respect for me ... to understand that I'm her mother."

"What she has to understand is these doctors are busy; they can't stand around waiting for her to come and besides, she doesn't always understand anyway."

"I'm leaving here and I'm glad of it. I've never been anywhere they let the nurses talk back like they do here. In Alabama, the attending is the only one allowed to talk to the family and he does, so it's all coordinated. This group of nurses sides with the family and sets us up to be the bad guys."

"I don't leave often. If I go to the store, the nurses know when I'll be back. Don't they have some legal thing that requires my permission before they do things to her?"

"What you have to understand is we have talked to her. I heard Dr. Smith on the phone with her just the other night. He went over each of the possible outcomes. We can't help it if she forgets. Maybe she should call us to see what's going on. That might fit her schedule better. I'm sure whoever is on call could deal with her."

"Well, so the pulmonary guys said the lung was blown. We didn't ask that. Why are we always blamed for not telling her? She didn't ask the right service."

"He said changing her trach wasn't considered a procedure. OK. So what should I call those things I don't want them doing to her without me here?"

"What she has to understand is ..."[33]

⊚ REFLECTIONS

- Beneath the misunderstandings conveyed in the poem, what other communication issues are going on in the patient care conference?
- What are the attitudes of the health professionals described in the poem?
- What do you read "between the lines" in the poem about listening?

The patient's mother becomes just another mother in the neonatal intensive care unit, not a unique person with her own concerns and needs. Because the listeners, the health professionals, have made up their minds about what they will and will not hear, the mother's voice gets lost.

Search for Familiarity

In addition to the risk that meaning becomes distorted, distortion can occur because most people tend to force an idea into a familiar context so that they can understand it quickly and ignore aspects of it that do not fit this context. This tendency is, of course, related to their mind-set but is also a defense against possible change. It may be that a person's inability to accept new concepts is a result of a basic lack of self-understanding. Thus, the weaker or more ill-defined a person's self-image, the greater the need to resist ideas that are more complex or ambiguous.

Need to Process Information at One's Own Rate

The rate at which incoming information can be processed varies significantly. This is partially, but not entirely, due to differences in innate ability. Overconfidence or too little confidence in predicting what will be said also determines whether a person will cease to process incoming information. If a person is overconfident, boredom settles in. If a person has too little confidence, he or she tends to become overly anxious and tune out the message. Active listening also requires undivided attention. If a person is distracted by too much sensory input, he or she will not be able to listen.

The rate and level of understanding at which you direct communication will alter the listener's ability to process the information. Thus, it is important that you have some knowledge of the patient's basic intelligence and past experience with a subject. The listener's set, the need to defend existing precepts, and the listener's innate intelligence both determine how accurately he or she will hear a message. Sometimes you will be the poor listener, and at other times the patient will be.

Taking all these factors into account, you cannot completely control how effectively a patient listens, but you can become a more effective listener. By simply restating what the patient has said, you can confirm part of a message before proceeding to the next portion of it. In addition, the following are some simple steps to more effective listening:

1. Be selective in what you listen to.
2. Concentrate on central themes rather than isolated statements. Listen in "paragraphs."
3. Judge content rather than style or delivery.
4. Listen with an open mind rather than focus on emotionally charged words.
5. Summarize in your own mind what you hear before speaking again.
6. Clarify before proceeding. Do not let vague or incomplete ideas go unattended.

The underlying theme in most discussions about listening is that it is a deliberate act. You must make a conscious decision to be fully present and engaged in the patient encounter in order to really understand what a patient is trying to tell you.[34]

SUMMARY

The purpose of this chapter was to give you an overview of numerous components of respectful communication. You will communicate in many ways with your patients: in person and across the miles, verbally and in writing. It may seem impossible to pay attention to the context of communication, the words you choose, your attitude, and the nonverbal messages you send all at the same time. However, good communication is like any skill: It takes practice. If you are willing to truly listen to your patients, they will assist you in refining and improving your communication skills throughout your career in health care.

REFERENCES

1. Jaquette SG: The octopus and me: the nursing insight gleaned from a battle with cancer, *Am J Nurs* 100(4):24, 2000.
2. Smith JF: Communicative ethics in medicine: the physician-patient relationship. In Wolf S, editor: *Feminism and bioethics: beyond reproduction*, New York, 1996, Oxford University Press.

3. Byrne PS, Long BE: *Doctors talking to patients*, London, 1976, Her Majesty's Stationery Office.

4. Frank A: From suspicion to dialogue: relations of storytelling in clinical encounters, *Med Humanit Rev* 14(1):24–34, 2000.

5. Grover F Jr, Wu HD, Blanford C, et al: Computer-using patients want Internet services from family physicians, *J Fam Pract* 51(6):570–572, 2002.

6. Getsi LC: Intensive care. In Getsi LC, editor: *Intensive care—poems by Lucia Cordell Getsi*, Minneapolis, 1992, New Rivers Press.

7. Phelan M, Parkman S: How to work with an interpreter, *Br Med J* 311:555–557, 1995.

8. Schapira L, Vargas E, Hidalgo R, et al: Lost in translation: integrating medical interpreters into the multidisciplinary team, *Oncologist* 13:586–592, 2008.

9. Seidelman RD, Bachner YG: *That* I won't translate! Experiences of a family medical interpreter in a multicultural environment, *Mt Sinai J Med* 77:389–393, 2010.

10. Watermeyer J: "She will hear me": how a flexible interpreting style enables patients to manage the inclusion of interpreters in mediated pharmacy interactions, *Health Communic* 26(1):71–81, 2011.

11. Ripich DN, et al: Training Alzheimer's disease caregivers for successful communication, *Clin Gerontol* 21(1):37–56, 1999.

12. Small JA, et al: Effectiveness of communication strategies used by caregivers of persons with Alzheimer's disease during activities of daily living, *J Speech Lang Hear Res* 46(2):353–367, 2003.

13. Bergsma J, Thomasma DC: *Health care: its psychosocial dimension*, Pittsburgh, 1982, Duquesne University Press.

14. Freeman J, Loewe R: Barriers to communication about diabetes mellitus: patients' and physicians' different view of the disease, *J Fam Pract* 49(6):513–542, 2000.

15. Folstein MF, Folstein S, McHugh PR: Mini-mental state: a practical method for grading the cognitive state of patients for the clinician, *J Psychiatr Res* 12:189–198, 1975.

16. Pfeiffer E: A short portable mental status questionnaire for the assessment of organic brain deficit in elderly patients, *J Am Geriatr Soc* 23:433–441, 1975.

17. Shem S: *Mount misery*, New York, 1997, Ballantine Publishing Group.

18. Firlik K: *Another day in the frontal lobe: a brain surgeon exposes life on the inside*, New York, 2006, Random House.

19. Chance S: *A voice of my own: a verbal box of chocolates*, Cleveland, SC, 1993, Bonne Chance Press.

20. Buxman K: Humor in critical care: no joke, *AACN Clin Issues Adv Pract Acute Crit Care* 11(1):120–127, 2000.

21. Argyle M: *Bodily communication*, ed 2, London, 1988, Routledge.

22. Beck RS, Daughtridge R, Sloane PD: Physician-patient communication in the primary care office: a systematic review, *J Am Board Fam Pract* 15:25–38, 2002.

23. Grossbach I, Stranberg S, Chlan L: Promoting effective communication for patients receiving mechanical ventilation, *Crit Care Nurse* 31(2):46–61, 2011.

24. Boockvar KS, Brodie HD, Lachs MS: Nursing assistants detect behavior changes in nursing home residents that precede acute illness: development and validation of an illness warning instrument, *J Am Geriatr Soc* 48(9):1086–1091, 2000.

25. Boockvar KS, Lachs MS: Predictive value of nonspecific symptoms for acute illness in nursing home residents, *J Am Geriatr Soc* 51:1111–1115, 2003.

26. Klitzman R: Improving education on doctor-patient relationships and communication: lessons from doctors who become patients, *Acad Med* 81(5):447–453, 2006.

27. Hall ET: *The hidden dimension*, New York, 1966, Doubleday.

28. Harrison R: Nonverbal communications: explorations into time, space, action and object. In Campbell JH, Hepler HW, editors: *Dimensions in communications: readings*, ed 2, Belmont, CA, 1970, Wadsworth.

29. Albala I, Doyle M, Appelbaum PS: The evolution of consent forms for research: a quarter century of changes, *IRB: Ethics Human Res* 7–11, 2010, (May-June).
30. DeVore NE: Telephone triage: a challenge for practicing midwives, *J Midwifery* 44(5):471–479, 1999. 425–429.
31. World Health Organization: *Telemedicine: opportunities and developments in members states, report on the second global survey on eHealth (Global Observatory for eHealth Series, 2)*, Geneva, Switzerland, 2009, WHO Press.
32. Smith E: Improving listening effectiveness, *Tex Med* 71:98–100, 1975.
33. Ogborn S: Patient care conference. In Haddad A, Brown K, editors: *The arduous touch: women's voices in health care*, West Lafayette, IN, 1999, Purdue University Press.
34. Shipley SD: Listening: a concept analysis, *Nursing Forum* 45(2):125–134, 2010.

PART FOUR

Questions for Thought and Discussion

1. In groups of three, have one student act as a patient with an injury, such as a fall off a ladder; have the second act as the interviewer trying to find out how the client was injured; and have the third student critique the interview process. Change roles three times so that all get to play each part. What works well, and what does not?

2. Write out instructions for a simple procedure such as using a cane or giving a subcutaneous injection that a patient might carry out at home. Share the instructions with a classmate, and see if he or she is unclear about any of the written instructions. What other modes of communication would make the instructions clearer? Work together to improve clarity.

3. Dennis is a 24-year-old man who has had surgery to control his epilepsy. Unfortunately, postoperatively he remains somewhat confused and apprehensive about health care settings. His wife brings him to your department, and you can see his anxiety. You must perform some tests on him that will not hurt him but will require his cooperation.

   a. What parts of this setting may be causing his anxiety?

   b. What aspects of your appearance may be causing his anxiety?

   c. What steps will you take to establish communication with him?

   d. How may his wife be helpful in facilitating effective "dialogue" between you and Dennis?

4. You verbally instruct an intelligent young businesswoman in the use of a home-treatment device and ask her if she understands what you want her to do. She assures you that she does. The next week when she returns, you discover that she has done exactly the opposite! You are dumbfounded.

   a. How will you react, and what will you say when your patient glowingly reports that she did exactly what you said and you realize that she did exactly the opposite of what you said?

   b. List the possible communication reasons your patient failed to do what you asked of her.

5. Find a standard "case study" in a professional journal. Rewrite it from the patient's perspective.

PART FIVE

Components of Respectful Interaction

In Part Five you have an opportunity to integrate many of the concepts you have encountered in this book so far. In Part One you were introduced to the centrality of the idea of respect in the health professions. You also were encouraged to reflect on your personal values and key institutional and societal forces that make up the larger value system in which health professionals work. In Parts Two and Three you focused on the parties who make health care a personal phenomenon—you and the patient surrounded by his or her loved ones and the health care team. Part Four provided you with an opportunity to learn how challenging it is to communicate with patients and others in a way that allows the deeper meanings of their situation and the health professional's role to emerge. In this part you will need to use everything you have learned from this book so far as the focus turns squarely on the particulars of the health professional and patient in their relationship.

Sometimes it does not appear so on the surface, but the relationship between you and a patient is significantly different from a friendship. When the similarities and differentiating characteristics are carefully defined and understood, you will enjoy the satisfaction of knowing that you, too, have achieved a habit of respectfully exercising the privileges of your role.

Chapter 10 describes some strong conceptual beams in the bridge that allow you and the patient to connect with each other in ways that allow you to meet the appropriate goals of your relationship: trust and trustworthiness, the importance of reassurance, attention to transference, a commitment to courtesy as a gateway to caring, skillful handling of dependencies in the relationship, and the desire to empower the patient toward his or her own goals. Chapter 11 discusses how establishing and maintaining respectful boundaries helps achieve the goal of comfortable closeness in your relationships with patients, distinguishing it from a friendship. Together these chapters outline the type of relationship in which respect is bountifully expressed.

Professional Relatedness Built on Respect

The reader will be able to:

- Describe how trust and trustworthiness give shape to the idea of respect between patient and health professional
- Assess the roles of competence and reassurance in strengthening the necessary connections between you and the patient
- Explain the phenomena of transference and countertransference in the health professional and patient relationship
- Contrast courteous behaviors with casualness and how each is perceived by the patient to bridge the gap of estrangement between you when you first meet and as the relationship develops
- Give some examples of what it means to focus on caring behaviors
- Distinguish contractual characteristics of the health professional and patient relationship from covenantal characteristics and evaluate the role of each

Of course the questions had to do only with illness. By the time he was through, this young man would know all about her years in the sanatorium, about her hysterectomy, and about her damaged lungs—and that is all he would know. Laura was amazed to discover that she was struggling to make a connection on another level. In a hospital one is reduced to being a body, one's history is the body's history, and perhaps that is why something deep inside a person reaches out, a little like a spider trying desperately to find a corner on which to begin to hang a web, the web of personal relation.

—M. Sarton[1]

In this chapter you have an opportunity to take the insights you have gained from the book so far and put them together in the context of your relationship with patients. The authors have encouraged you to think about how you would respond to some relational challenges, but now you have the background to focus directly on the relationship. Your situation is like a bridge that needs strong supports because you and the patient always remain individuals, but your mutual goal is to be able to "bridge the gap" between you in ways that meet those goals (Figure 10-1).

Some characteristics described in this chapter are essential for any relationship to thrive. For example, trust and reassurance are fundamental. A psychological

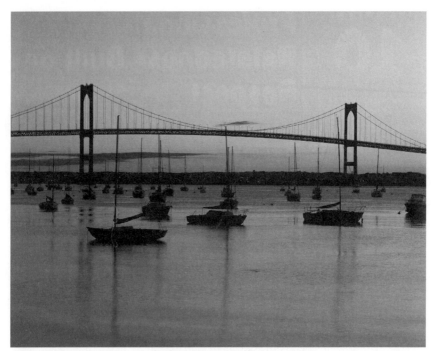

FIGURE 10-1: The health professional and the patient always remain individuals, but their mutual goal is to be able to "bridge the gap." *(© Getty Images/16032.)*

phenomenon called *transference* can always be a factor in how you view and respond to another person, and they to you. At the end of the chapter we come back to the idea of professional caring, emphasizing everyday behaviors that express it.

Build Trust by Being Trustworthy

Trust connects the patient's ability to feel that he or she is being respected by you with your intent to provide your professional services. In the traditional physician-patient relationship, trust was thought to mean having blind faith in the physician. This type of *trustworthiness* was just about all that health care providers had to offer because until the beginning of the 20th century, a patient had less than a 50% chance of benefiting medically from an encounter with a physician. This total reliance on trust as the support beam allowing the two individuals to "meet" meant that the doctor should be benevolent and protective toward patients.

Modern insights regarding the role of trust in human relationships are molding the understanding of the health professional and patient interaction today. In the view of developmental psychologists, trust plays a central role in a person's developmental task of figuring out when to depend on others and when to be cautious. Therefore, a professional is worthy of trust when patients feel secure to exercise their decisional capacity appropriately. But what, exactly, does such trustworthiness look like in the day-to-day health professional and patient relationship? In an article entitled "Engendering Trust in a Pluralistic Society," Secundy and Jackson make the following observation:

> When a patient speaks of trust in a health care setting, he or she is essentially speaking about a comfort level, a feeling of safety, a belief that he or she can rely on people with power not to hurt or exploit him or her . . . Such positive feelings can ensure appropriate cooperation and compliance during the course of an illness. When such feelings are absent or ambivalent, the patient's behavior can influence outcomes negatively. There are several areas in which trust is relevant: The patient can trust or distrust the system of health care itself, the specific institution or setting in which health care services are being delivered, and the person or persons providing service or care.[2]

For each area of trust experienced by the patient, the health professional has done his or her part by being trustworthy.

Competence and Trust

Competence is:

▶ knowing what you know and are skilled to do,
▶ a commitment to diligently stay current on the research and management of conditions within your scope of practice,
▶ being aware of your professional and personal shortcomings, and
▶ applying the communication skills discussed in the previous section of this book.

You have learned that a patient's request for your services is usually generated by the presence of a sign or symptom that manifests itself in the form of pain, lack of ability to function, or some other discomfort. The patient counts on you and your colleagues, all strangers to the patient, to learn his or her diagnosis, what it means for his or her everyday life, and what he or she needs to do to initiate and follow a treatment process. People also seek your counsel about how to stay healthy and prevent health-related difficulties.

In each instance patients come to you having to decide whether or not to trust that your professional training prepares you to competently address pertinent health-related needs and questions. Your role in the relationship is to be trust*worthy* through actions that demonstrate you are there to meet their reasonable expectations in ways you are professionally prepared to do. Their trust grows as you interact with them. At the same time, for genuine trust to take root in the relationship the patient also must be convinced that he or she is viewed as something more than a symptom or an interesting medical case or a body part (Figure 10-2). Unfortunately, health professionals and institutions are sometimes insensitive to the messages they are conveying in this regard. For example, the "bone clinic," the "allergy clinic," the "heart specialist," and the "obstetrics nurse" all convey images of body parts or symptoms rather than living, breathing human beings. Some have called this phenomenon "thinging." In it the patient is made to feel more valued for the "interesting thing" that he or she is bringing to the health professions setting than because of being a person with a human need.

Common sense suggests that patients should not trust you if you seem more interested in their diagnosis or symptom than in what these mean to their well-being as persons. To the extent that you recognize the mistake of "thinging," you will have

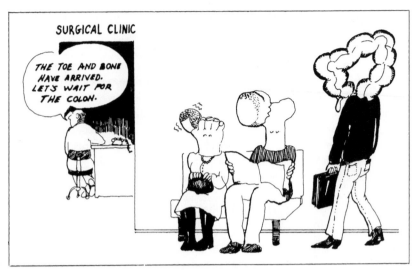

FIGURE 10-2: Professionals' view of patients. *(From the Swedish translation of Health Professional and Patient Interaction: Vård, Vårdare, Vårdad.)*

taken a giant step in engendering a genuine bond of trust as the bond between you and the patient.

Sometimes being judged as trustworthy by patients is not completely in your control no matter how well intentioned you are. You are a part of a system. For example, government or institutional policies determining your course of intervention may shortchange a patient or discriminate against a group, resulting in their understandable lack of trust in the system or in you personally. This does not relieve you of responsibility. Being trustworthy requires that, as you learned in Chapter 2, you participate in the change of deleterious or unjust policies whenever possible.[3] Rogers and Ballantyne found in their study of women patients that when they felt themselves to be among the safe, privileged variety (e.g., white, economically well off, younger) they may develop a distorted trust in the health professional to make policies work on their behalf when that is not the case. The result can be care that is no more suited to this patient than to the one in a socially disadvantaged position.[4]

In most cases you are also one member of an interprofessional health care team, and this, too can have an impact on whether the patient will believe you are trustworthy to deliver competent care. Being trustworthy requires some things you can do, such as:

▶ be an alert and active participant in team decisions appropriate to your expertise,
▶ communicate throughout your relationship with what you judge the challenges are in the patient's situation and what you are doing to address them, and
▶ let the patient know when you are going to tap the expertise of others more expert than you.

Occasionally, health professionals find themselves in awkward situations knowing that the patient's trust might be based on unreasonable expectations. For example, consider the case of Mrs. Gleason, her family, and the team:

Mrs. Gleason, a 70-year-old homemaker, has had amyotrophic lateral sclerosis (ALS) for just over a year. Mrs. Gleason and her family have gone on the Internet and learned that ALS, also known as *Lou Gehrig's disease,* is a progressive neurological disease affecting all voluntary muscles of her body. Most patients become weaker and weaker until they die, usually of respiratory arrest. Mrs. Gleason has only a small amount of movement left in her legs but can get around in a wheelchair. She is in the hospital for treatment of pneumonia that is probably due to weakness of her swallowing muscles, allowing aspiration of her mouth contents into her lungs. Her weakness has accelerated since hospitalization, even though her pneumonia is responding to antibiotics. She is discouraged, knowing that the aspiration will continue and that in her present state it is unlikely she will go home. Her family realizes she is probably past the point of her ability to live independently. They feel unable to care for her in any of their own homes but are afraid of the terrible effect it will have on her when she learns this news. They ask the physician, Jaime Sills, to do anything she can to reassure their mother that she will be OK.

Jaime decides to request a reevaluation by speech therapy and occupational therapy with the goal of determining the maximum swallowing function she has necessary for eating and any possible way she might be able to function well enough in her activities of daily living to manage in her own home with home health care assistance and the family's periodic help. Both therapists are extremely guarded in their conclusions, believing that her potential for a return home is minimal.

Jaime Sills calls a family meeting with Mrs. Gleason, the children, the nurses primarily responsible for her care, and the therapists. As the family feared, Mrs. Gleason is devastated, saying that she trusted them to help her and now they have let her down. The family, too, becomes assertive, telling the team that increasing her therapy at least would have given her some chance of a longer stay at home. No amount of reasoning about other alternatives open to all of them seems acceptable at this moment in time. Jaime Sills tells them that a social worker will be glad to work with them to further explore their options.

This situation was uncomfortable for the health professionals who felt they had Mrs. Gleason's interests at heart but could not meet her and the family's expectations. In the end all you can do in such situations is to continue to search for ways to give the patient and family a basis for exploring new options open to them.

Honesty, Reassurance, and Trust

To be "assured" is to have a feeling of confidence and certainty. Reassurance helps restore that feeling when it is lost. No matter what their differences in other regards, all patients trust you to offer honest reassurance about what they can reasonably expect from their encounter. *Reality testing* is a term often used in the health professions to denote that the care provider keeps the patient on track from setting unattainable goals. Although as noted in Chapters 3 and 8, not all cultures treat your direct communication with a patient as the appropriate means of dealing with a diagnosis, prognosis, or treatment decision, the appropriate spokesperson on behalf of the patient expects honest reassurance. Even then a more general expression of reassurance must be directed to the patient. For example, you may be able to offer reassurance about ways to cope with a changing body or about resources available to help him or her adjust to the new situation.

Chapter 6 recounts some major ways that life's "slings and arrows" can shake one's confidence in the way the world will respond and one's certainty about what is reasonable to expect in the future. *Reassurance* is a powerful bridge-building beam, giving the patient confidence to rely on your word and think differently about his or her situation. The act of reassuring requires offering information that you can stand behind with certainty yourself, however minimal an effect you believe it will have on the patient. Reassurance may also take the form of your willingness to respond to difficult questions about areas that are causing anxiety for patients or their families.

◎ REFLECTIONS

Think of a time in your life when someone tried to reassure you.
- What did the other person say or do that worked?
- Can you recount an example of when someone tried to reassure you but it didn't work?
- Why did their attempts fail?
- Finally, have you ever been falsely reassured, only to find out later that the false or misplaced reassurance shook your trust in that person?

You can use these personal experiences with confidence they will help guide you when you are faced with patients' or family's worries. When your attempts at reassurance are unsuccessful, use your own experience of when others' attempts to reassure you failed. That can help you become aware of what might be going on in the mind of the patient. Further gentle probing may help to uncover the patient's cause for concern and give guidance to the direction your reassuring words or gestures should take. At the very least your reassurance that you are trying your best to work on their behalf in this difficult time for them is always appropriate. Your creativity about how to retain or regain their confidence in themselves and the relationship must be an intentional part of your work plan. Overall, in your practice you will find that the time and activities you devote to reassurance will be as varied as patients themselves, but it will always be worth your effort to express your respect in this manner.

Integrity in Words and Conduct

Integrity comes from the root integritas, meaning "wholeness." The cultivation of integrity is the commitment you make to yourself to temper your attitudes and conduct so that patients can experience a high level of consistency between what you say and what you do. They can observe fittingness between their needs and your demeanor and actions, providing the evidence they need for them to confidently place their trust in you.[5]

That attitudes and actions must be consistent with your reassuring words for professional closeness to develop is illustrated in the novel *I Never Promised You a Rose Garden:* The ward administrator tells Deborah, "It [the cold pack] doesn't hurt— don't worry." Those words sound like words meant to generate reassuring comfort and Deborah's willingness to cooperate with the health professional's plan. However, Deborah, who is undergoing treatments in a psychiatric hospital and is frightened of what has already been done to her in the name of treatment, has exactly the opposite response. She thinks, "Watch out for those words . . . they are the same words. What comes after that is deceit."[6] Her situation illustrates that the words meant to be reassuring did not have the intended effect of engendering her confidence in the health professionals, because in the past, their conduct was not consistent with their words.

Integrity is not a character trait that only patients with long-term relationships with health professionals count on. Alice Trillin, the author of the quote at the beginning of this chapter, was on high alert from the moment Dr. Kris began his examination. He won her confidence in a one-time interaction.

The patient's reliance on the professional's integrity also extends to his or her experience with teams. Teams were first designed to help coordinate care so that the patient could experience a kind of collective integrity across the system. However, today sometimes the patient's encounter with multiple members of a team breaks down confidence that there is "a plan" shared across units and among team members, and the patient experiences a fragmentation of services. The good news is that "[t]he culture of team care is a culture of interprofessional communication, with constant heads-ups and inquiries about what ought to be done with patients. In that sense, the culture of team care approximates the best that ethics seeks when it joins the team to help create the most humane and encompassing solutions(s) to the problems(s) at hand."[7] The potential for professional closeness is knitted into the fabric of teams, but in the end each individual on the team must strive to be sure that his or her own and the team's integrity is at work to help ensure that the patient's confidence is well placed.

Tease Out Transference Issues

The psychotherapeutic notion of *transference* can help you understand certain kinds of behavior some people might exhibit toward you when you enter into a professional relationship with them. Transference has its root in the theories advanced by Sigmund Freud and further developed by other psychologists who employ this term to convey the process of shifting your feeling about a person in your past to another person.[8] A young man, angry that his father "ruled with an iron hand," might conclude, "Here it comes again!" and respond aggressively to the health professional as soon as he is reminded of his father. One of the authors knows a male nursing student who prepared extensively and carefully to provide care to his first obstetrics-gynecology patient. A part of the clinical evaluation was to conduct a personal exam on her. Upon entering the patient's room he said, "Good morning. I'm a student who is going to be your nurse today and I will be examining you." The patient took one look at this bearded, 6-foot-plus student and said, "Oh, no you're not! You look too much like my son, honey!" His supervisor, who had just stepped into the room, caught this woman's reaction and judged that to disregard the patient's discomfort would be a sign of disrespect. Instead she used the occasion as a teaching moment with the student, explaining that this type of transference sometimes happens. Everyone was relieved that this patient was reassigned to another student nurse.

Transference can be negative or positive. A negative transference interferes with trusting the support beams necessary for venturing confidently into a relationship. Examples are the aggressiveness of the young man and discomfort stimulated by the similarity of the student to the woman's son. For reasons patients sometimes cannot identify or express, their comfort level is low and guard is up. At the other end of the spectrum, positive transference, the good feelings a patient transfers to the health professional, can promote a well-working relationship.

It is not always easy to tell whether the transference will create a problem. A young nurse caught a new male patient staring at her. Finally, he shook his head and said, "Man, I could have sworn my first wife walked in when you came into the room. The resemblance is startling!" Of course, this raised some questions—and the woman responded by saying, "Well, is that a good or bad thing?" He said, "Both!" So she was still in the woods on this one. She felt she had no choice in this case but to continue with the patient, watching for further signs that this man's association seemed to be affecting his responses and their relationship. (There were none, and the matter never came up again.)

The patient is not the only party in the relationship who experiences transference. *Countertransference,* the tendency to respond to a patient with associations of others in one's life, takes place every bit as often. A health professional may transfer feelings to the patient on the basis of name, physical appearance, voice, age, or gestures. Any one of these can increase the chance of countertransference. It is up to you to be self-aware about such associations and adapt your behavior to correct for any negative or other troubling responses you think might be issuing from your mental association of the patient with someone in your past or present relationships.

At the same time, total neutrality is not required. If you have served on a jury, you know that the lawyers try to select jurors whose past experiences and associations do not in any discernible way come into play when the facts of the case and the identification of the defendant and plaintiff are made known. A less rigorous standard is acceptable in the health professional and patient relationship. What is necessary for maintaining a respectful relationship with a patient is to be aware that transference and countertransference take place and try to be aware of how they might affect the interaction. It may not be possible always to identify the person whom the patient is "seeing" in you or you are "seeing" in the patient.[9]

Distinguish Courtesy from Casualness

You might think that showing common courtesy to patients is such an obvious component of respectful interaction that it need not be discussed. However, nothing is too basic or obvious to consider if it provides a support beam for you and the patient as you bridge the gap between you and define what your relationship will look like. You can begin to see its importance in the simple dictionary definition of *courtesy* as "courtly elegance and politeness of manners; graceful politeness or considerateness."[10]

It goes beyond "minding your manners" in a superficial sense because it requires doing so with dignity in the way you go about being polite. Patients take their initial cues about whether they matter as people from the courtesy they receive when they first come through the door (or, in the case of home health care, you go through theirs). Although we strive to go beyond courtesy to deeper understandings of care in the health professional and patient relationship, the patient's first, and often lasting, impression is connected to common courtesies they receive (or do not receive) from you. In this regard the work environment works best when it is a "consumer-friendly" environment.

As with many aspects of respect, you cannot generate a welcoming, courteous environment on your own. In almost every instance you will be a member of teams that schedule patient appointments, keep patients informed, collect fees, work toward making a diagnosis or carrying out a treatment plan, and conduct discharge or follow-up activities. But you can do your part, both personally and as a model for others. For example, common courtesies in an ambulatory care clinic include:

▶ greeting a person warmly and by name, introducing yourself and your role;
▶ providing a safe place for them to hang a coat or umbrella;
▶ offering assistance with mobility challenges and completing forms;
▶ keeping the patient (and family member) informed about delays or necessary changes;
▶ being sure privacy is honored; and
▶ providing reading material and other calming distractions.

The common denominator is that you pay attention to peculiarities and structure your approach so that the patient perceives you as one who cares about his or her well-being from the get-go.

⊚ REFLECTIONS

Take a minute to reflect on the last time you visited a physician, dentist, or other health professional. Picture the environment as you first entered.
• What did you find there that led you to believe that you were welcome and that the staff had given some thought to what would make you as comfortable as possible?
• How could the environment and conduct of the staff be improved to make it a more commodious place?
• Now try to picture yourself being visited in your home by a home health care provider during your recovery from a serious accident. List some courtesies you expect.

One can fall into some mistakes, even with good intentions. For instance, a too casual informality, if misinterpreted, may cause a patient to push back, become wary, be hostile, or show other signs that he or she is feeling disrespected. A common dynamic is that the health professional encourages the patient to establish a first-name relationship, suggesting they can be informal with each other but at the same time conveying consciously or subconsciously that the health professional should be treated with formality (Figure 10-3).

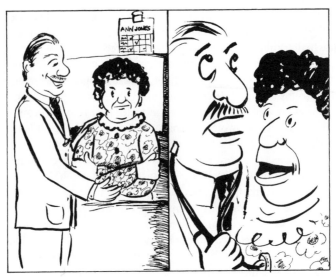

FIGURE 10-3: "Hello, Nancy. I'm Dr. Simon McGinnis." "Hi, Simon! I'm Mrs. Kittery."

⊚ REFLECTIONS

Take time, again, to reflect on your own experience.
- Have you encountered a situation in the setting you focused on a few minutes ago—or some other situations as a patient—when you found the environment and behavior of the staff too casual and therefore a "turn off?"
- List some ways that their attempts to establish a connection with you seemed superficial or in other ways were not working even though you knew the person had good intentions?
- What might you do to turn that behavior into more courteous conduct?

Your own experience can be a window into seeing more clearly why courtesy must be distinguished from an environment and conduct that substitute casualness for courtesy. In short, a caring professional person continually works at striking a balance between stiff reliance on correct manners and the imposition of a loose, casual physical and psychological environment that detracts from the seriousness of the situation for the patient. In other words, courtesy is one visible sign that the health professional "really cares" about the patient as a person.

Concentrate on Caring Behaviors

As we introduced in previous chapters, care is a concept so central to the identity of your role in the health professions context that your position is meaningless to others if you do not both profess and express it. Patient care sometimes is best achieved by sophisticated technology found in the intensive care unit (ICU), the surgical suite, or the diagnostic or treatment area of your workplace. *Technology* is the application of scientific findings and allows you to show care for the person's predicament by offering highly effective interventions from which everyone reading this book has benefited at some time. Only when any technology is substituted for a respectful demeanor or actions designed to show deep respect for the patient and his or her family has a weak bridge-beam been substituted for the extremely secure one crafted with other caring behaviors.

Understandably, behaviors that can be identified as caring behaviors are the subject of considerable attention in the health professions. As the authors have written elsewhere, the ultimate goal of your daily work is to find the caring response to each patient situation. A *response* is behavior based on experience, reflection, and knowledge. A response is different than a reaction, the latter being an immediate reflex when something catches one off guard. To what should you respond? To the two elements that comprise all caring relationships: an understanding of the situation of the other and a commitment to the good of the other.[11] Part of the recent impetus for identifying caring behaviors is the emphasis on measurable outcomes in health care interventions. Patient satisfaction scales, being used by institutions as one measure of a successful result, or outcome, are designed to capture the patient's interpretation of what is perceived as caring conduct.

Individualize Your Approach

Professional relatedness is dependent on individualized caring behaviors. Often this comes naturally when you are interested in the patient's well-being. Other times, such as in the following quote, the caregiver may show extraordinary attention to the patient and the effect it has on the loved ones can be immense. In this excerpt Caroline's best friend has been keeping vigil as Caroline dies of cancer, and when Caroline loses consciousness her friend Gail panics and calls the surgeon.

> I had found [Dr.] Herzog's home phone number and called him that evening from the hospital. He came into the room carrying a handful of lilies of the valley—he knew that whatever else had happened, Caroline would be able to smell and walked over to her and held them under her nose. It was a gesture that took my breath away with its exacting kindness. . . .[12]

Many previous discussions in this book have provided information, insights, and examples of how you and the patient, each of you individuals bringing your hopes, expectations, and goals to the encounter, can negotiate the appropriate terms of the relationship. You have learned that any attitude, action, practice, or policy that allows the patient's well-being to take second place to some other end is a threat to the respect the patient deserves in this relationship and that your role is to protect that respect with all your might. Dr. Herzog, a world-class surgeon, used his imagination to go beyond these essentials, paying close attention to a small detail that changed everything in terms of this loved one's ability to cope, and his awareness of the senses still available to Caroline in her condition allowed him to "touch" her as a human when so many of their usual ways to relate were challenged.

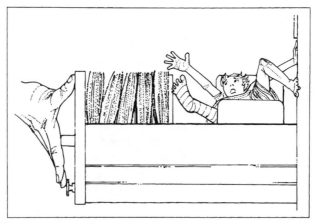

FIGURE 10-4: Nothing is more upsetting to a patient than to feel you are treating her as a "case" to be filed before you go on to the next "case" on your schedule.

Stay Focused—Completely

Almost everyone struggles with effective time management, and the environment of the health professions today provides every reason to become fragmented with competing demands on your time and attention. Your commitment never to cut corners in patient care unless it is absolutely necessary helps to keep you focused on fostering a relationship that goes beyond the mere minimum of caring behaviors. There is nothing more upsetting to a patient than feeling like you are seeing him or her simply as another case on the long list of cases, to be filed as "completed" at the end of the day (Figure 10-4). In contrast, consider the following quote. We do not know all the aspects of the exchange between Dr. Kris and the patient, but we do know she quickly became confident he was fully focused on her and not the last (or next) patient in his office waiting room.

> It would be difficult for me to come up with a list of competencies I look for in a doctor, but I know when I have met one I will trust. Mark Kris, who heads the thoracic-oncology service at Memorial, was this kind of doctor. The first thing Mark did, after looking at my medical records and having me carefully retell the story of what had happened to me over the past few months, was to give me a thorough examination. This was the first physical I'd had since this drama began; everyone else had just looked at the x-rays and scans. After he finished, he asked me how I felt. It was the only time in these months that anyone had asked me that question.[13]

When you must take shortcuts, a patient is likely to maintain his or her confidence in you if you explain why you must give that person short shrift in this unfortunate exceptional circumstance—and then make it an unfortunate, exceptional circumstance.

It sometimes helps at the outset to remind the patient of the amount of time you have to be with him or her, and work together regarding what you hope the two of you will accomplish in that time. Every health professional knows that on some days a particular patient needs some extra time to work through a problem, which can wreak havoc on a schedule. Then there are patients who for good (or poor) reasons are late or need to linger and make small talk, diverting your time and energy from other patients. Setting your compass of time management against a backdrop of patient needs will help to keep you on as clear a path through the day as possible. Although some patients you have kept waiting will become impatient, your focused attention on doing all that you are able to do for them when their turn comes will support their feeling that your behavior remains consistent with your caring for them.

Managing time with the goal of giving full attention to the patient can be aided by additional clues about how to act with the patient during the time you actually are together. Here are some hints:

1. Remove the person from areas where distractions are likely to impinge on your time together.
2. Sit down or in other ways convey your intent to give full attention to the person.
3. Approach the person slowly and graciously, even though you may have had to run to be on time for your appointment.
4. Look the person in the eye while conversing. A lack of direct eye contact communicates lack of interest.
5. Avoid looking at your watch. Place a clock at a place where you can be aware of the time without being obvious about it.
6. Let others know you are engaged and should not be disturbed. Turn off your cell phone or put it on vibration mode.

Little Things Mean a Lot

An important way to enhance a patient's feeling of self-worth and confidence in the relationship, thereby enhancing the conditions conducive to professional closeness, is to acknowledge little personal details that too often go unnoticed. The poet William Blake noted, "He who would do good to others must do it in minute particulars." One of the authors recalls a student's journal entry just before graduation when he was reflecting on his own developing professionalism:

> I'd say one of the most surprising things I've learned about being with patients is that little things mean a lot! For instance, I have learned the importance of pouring a glass of water for a thirsty patient, listening to a key play during the 9th inning of a baseball game between parts of a treatment, laughing at something the patient says, wiping a nose. Perhaps these things sound silly to you.

On the contrary, this observant student was learning early in his now successful career as a leader in his chosen field that "little things" count as expressions of deep respect for the patient. These little details take many shapes, but we remind you of a few common ones here:

Personal Hygiene

When a patient has a hygienic need, attention to it before any other activity or exchange will make him or her grateful. This is not to suggest that you need to wait on the patient with toothbrush, deodorant, and nail clippers in hand or that hygienic activity should in any way compromise time that should be spent using your workplace skills. However, sometimes a simple act, such as providing a tissue when the patient needs one, makes the difference between an embarrassed and an attentive person.

Personal Comfort

A person sometimes experiences a certain amount of physical discomfort in a treatment, diagnostic, or testing situation. It is easy to forget how often we shift posture, scratch, blink, swipe, or shrug just to get comfortable, yet there are conditions or techniques that prevent persons from performing these basic comfort functions. An extreme but instructive example is offered by Jean Dominique Bauby, the former editor of the magazine *Elle,* who suffered a brainstem injury that prevented him from any bodily movement whatsoever except to blink but left intact all of his sensations. This severe condition is called *locked-in syndrome.* Mr. Bauby leaves an incredible memoir of his experience, achieved by blinking words with his left eye while a speech therapist wrote down each word. Imagine his situation:

> This morning, with first light barely bathing Room 119, evil spirits descended on my world. For half an hour, the alarm on the machine that regulates my feeding tube has been beeping out into the void. I cannot imagine anything so inane or nerve-racking as this piercing beep beep beep pecking away at my brain. As a bonus, my sweat has unglued the tape that keeps my right eyelid closed and the stuck-together lashes are tickling my pupil unbearably. And to crown it all, the end of my urinary catheter has become detached and I am drenched. Awaiting rescue, I hum an old song by Henri Salvador: "Don't you fret, baby, it'll be all right."[14]

There are many ways a patient, even one with severe physical limitations such as Mr. Bauby, can be made more comfortable; they may involve straightening or cleaning the patient's glasses, wiping away sweat, supporting the person's arm while drawing blood, or running for an extra towel.

Many times patients are not asked simple questions such as whether the room temperature is OK, and if not, what can be done to make the person warmer (or cooler). Cold, clammy hands unexpectedly placed on a patient can be extremely unnerving.

◎ REFLECTIONS

- Have you been stuck in a situation where you could not get comfortable?
- What did you have to do to get assistance in remedying the situation?

You can remember that situation as a starting point of your own imagination when you are with patients. Asking, "Are you comfortable?" or "Is there anything else I can do for you while I am with you to make you more comfortable?" will always be appreciated.

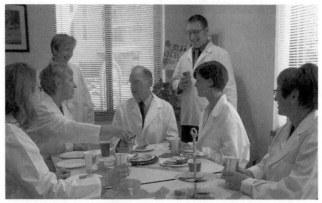

FIGURE 10-5: A birthday is often an important opportunity to recognize a person, whether a colleague or patient.

Personal Interests

Almost everyone has some area of interest, whether it be a hobby, job, family, or other focus. Showing interest in the person does not require probing unduly into his or her personal life, something we warned against in Chapters 6 and 7. Some patients will want to chat about life outside of the moment, and others will not. At the same time, asking an inpatient about the noon menu, complementing an ambulatory care patient on something he or she is wearing, reminding a teenager that her favorite rap artist has a special show on TV that night, and spelling Mr. Schydlowski's name correctly on his appointment slip count as appreciated attempts to personalize care. Birthdays and holidays are important occasions to recognize a person (Figure 10-5). If you think that he would enjoy the attention, on Mr. Arnold's birthday, write "HAPPY BIRTHDAY, DICK ARNOLD" in bold letters in the treatment booth or let other staff know so that they can acknowledge it, too. You will think of other expressions of this type of respect to put into everyday action.

Expanding Patients' Awareness

If you have been confined to a home, hospital, or other institution, you know how quickly one loses track of time and becomes out of touch with the rest of the world. By sharing an incident observed on the way to work, reviewing a play seen the evening before, or taking the patient to a window to see a child and dog playing together, you can extend the patient's environment beyond the immediate area, bringing him or her into contact with the outside world. One of the authors once brought apple blossoms into a four-bed room in an extended care facility only to have two of the residents burst into tears, saying they missed the smells of spring more than anything since being forced to make this their permanent home. This simple act opened the door to a discussion about springtime memories and moved the health professional into more of a position conducive to developing professional closeness.

None of the types of detail discussed earlier legitimately can be substituted for your provision of the technical professional services you are uniquely qualified to offer the patient.

Caring Behaviors: Taking the Patient's Perspective

A patient's perception of the difficulty he or she is experiencing is often quite different from that of the health professional. Earlier in this chapter we introduced the problem of "thinging" and how it undermines patients' trust. Patients are concerned primarily with what the problem signifies in terms of their daily lives, loves, and activities. Hardly ever is the technical aspect of what is wrong the governing factor. Health professionals are taught to look for the abstractive meaning of a condition: the chest sound, laboratory findings, x-ray films, the sight of the skin or tone of the muscle, and so forth. Contrary to this, the patient assigns a deeper *personal* meaning to the condition on the basis of his or her understanding of the broader experience and effects of the condition. This is a good time to remind you that Chapter 8 describes how the patient's story (or stories) is the narrative he or she brings to the relationship and provides the clues to what this deeper personal meaning might be.

In John Updike's short story "From the Journal of a Leper," a young man begins his journal as follows:

> Oct. 31. I have long been a potter, a bachelor, and a leper. Leprosy is not exactly what I have, but what in the Bible is called leprosy (see Leviticus 13, Exodus 4:6, Luke 5:12-13) was probably this thing, which has a twisty Greek name it pains me to write. The form of the disease is as follows: spots, plaques, and avalanches of excess skin, manufactured by the dermis through some trifling but persistent error in its metabolic instructions, expand and slowly migrate across the body like lichen on a tombstone. I am silvery, scaly. Puddles of flakes form wherever I rest my flesh. Each morning, I vacuum my bed. My torture is skin deep: there is no pain, not even itching; we lepers live a long time, and are ironically healthy in other respects. Lusty, though we are loathsome to love. Keen-sighted, though we hate to look upon ourselves. The name of the disease, spiritually speaking, is Humiliation.[15]

◎ REFLECTIONS

- What physical and psychological experiences of the patient lead him to conclude that "the name of the disease is Humiliation"?
- What might you, in the name of care, do to begin to address his humiliation within the context of your professional relationship with him?
- What parts of his suffering seem beyond your reach?

His example is just one powerful reminder that in lived experience, a patient takes the clinical condition and places it into the larger context of meaning for his or her life. Your job is to address the condition, but always with the goal of building or maintaining the bridge beam that brings the patient to the place of hoping for and needing your care.

Respect, Contract, and Covenant

Although a patient must successfully carry his or her share of responsibility for developing a flourishing relationship with you, the health professional must take leadership in the process of building support beams that encourage the patient to exercise authority and autonomy in your relationship. Respect for the patient is partially realized through your acknowledgment of the patient's authority as the key decision-maker. Decision-making must be a shared decision-making. In the United This States and increasingly in other countries, the mechanism of informed consent is a useful legal and ethical tool. *Informed consent* formally acknowledges a difference in power between you and the patient and places the onus of responsibility on you to level the playing field between you through a process of "informing" and being sure the patient understands and consents to a proposed course of action. A starting point is the guidelines of respectful communication addressed in Chapter 9. This contract between you and the patient is just the beginning.

Everything you do either reinforces or sets up barriers to the person's ability to participate in this part of life. An ethicist, Bill May, suggests that thinking of ourselves as health professionals as being bound by a covenant includes the contract elements of a mechanism such as informed consent with its mutual expectations and agreement, but goes further. *Covenants* place the parties in a situation of mutual benefit. This requires the professional to acknowledge all the benefits derived from health care practice and from the opportunity to be with a particular patient who arrives not only with signs or symptoms but also with talents, gifts, and histories. Therefore, an element of professional gratitude enters the relationship, empowering patients to do their best and encouraging professionals to go beyond the bare minimum of expectations that are agreed upon in a strict contract approach.[16]

A patient who is institutionalized and has lost control over many decisions in his or her life may still be able to command small details such as what to wear that day or when to eat, therefore expressing his or her individuality. Sometimes the loss of so many areas of decision-making is taken as a signal to both parties that the patient really should be treated like a baby, having everything done for him or her. This is just plain nonsense, but it is easy for everyone, including the family caregivers, to fall into that mode, and to do so out of a good faith attempt to help the patient. Family and friends also can be agents encouraging the patient and augmenting the health professional's efforts to counter unnecessary pampering. After a severe back injury, one of the authors suddenly realized how passive and discouraged she had become about the need to remain bedridden. This attitude was turned around by a close friend who sent a card with the following note:

NOBODY HAS EVER SAID THE
UNIVERSE CANNOT BE EXPLORED
FROM A RECUMBENT POSITION.

Obviously this friend was tuned into the patient's growing sense of despair and feeling of powerlessness due to the persistent back pain and fear of reinjury. A simple gesture was enough to give her a new perspective on her period of being in a recumbent position! A patient who loses confidence in what he or she can still do is at risk of becoming immobilized more by discouragement than by the condition itself. The good news is that in your role you can serve as a bridge builder so that the patient can meet you halfway or more in meeting realistic goals as a result of the relationship.

SUMMARY

This chapter highlights conditions under which the patient's confidence can remain high in partnering with you to help achieve his or her health-related goals. Your integrity is one essential component. The test of all of the ideas presented in this chapter is the extent to which any of them support genuine respect toward patients, their families, and the ideals of the health professions. Professional relatedness builds on basic human relational characteristics such as trust (and how reassurance fosters it), sensitivity to the effects of transference and countertransference, and your behaviors that engender the patient's feeling that he or she is seen as a person, cared for and deserving of attention even down to fine details that may seem mundane to others. Each is a necessary respect-beam that helps construct a bridge that can confidently stand up under the weighty decisions and situations that patients, their families, and you must traverse in your relationship.

REFERENCES

1. Sarton M: *A reckoning*, New York, 1978, Norton.
2. Secundy MG, Jackson RL: Engendering trust in a pluralistic society. In Thomasma DC, Kissell JL, editors: *The health care professional as friend and healer*, Washington, DC, 2000, Georgetown University Press.
3. Schwartz MC: Trust and responsibility in health policy, *Int J Feminist Approaches Bioethics* 2(1):28–40, 2009.
4. Rogers W, Ballantyne A: Gender and trust in medicine. Vulnerabilities, abuses and remedies, *Int J Feminist Approaches Bioethics* 1(1):48–56, 2008.
5. Beauchamp H, Childress J: *Principles of biomedical ethics*, ed 6, New York, 2009, Oxford University Press.
6. Greene H: *I never promised you a rose garden*, New York, 1964, Holt, Rinehart & Winston.
7. Burck R, Lapidos S: Ethics and cultures of care. In Mezey M, Cassel CK, Botrell M, Hyer K, editors: *Ethical patient care: a casebook for geriatric health care teams*, Baltimore, 2002, Johns Hopkins University Press.
8. Freud S: *The ego and the mechanisms of defense*, New York, 1966, International Universities Press.
9. Northouse PG, Northouse LL: *Health communication: strategies for health professionals*, ed 3, Norwalk, CT, 1998, Appleton & Lange.
10. *The compact edition of the Oxford English dictionary*, vol. 1, Oxford, England, 1971, Oxford University Press. (A–O).
11. Purtilo R, Doherty R: *Ethical dimensions in the health professions*, St Louis, Missouri, 2011, Elsevier.
12. Caldwell G: *Let's take the long way home: A memoir of friendship*, New York, 2010, Random House.
13. Trillin A: Personal history: betting your life, *New Yorker*, January 29, 2001.
14. Bauby JD: *The diving bell and the butterfly*, New York, 1997, Alfred A. Knopf (Translated by J. Lagatt).
15. Updike J: From the journal of a leper, *New Yorker*, July 19, 1976.
16. May WF: Code and covenant or philanthropy and contract? *Hastings Cent Rep* 5:29–35, 1975.

CHAPTER 11

Professional Boundaries Guided by Respect

CHAPTER OBJECTIVES

The reader will be able to:

- Describe why the idea of professional boundaries is relevant to respect
- Distinguish a respectful, professional approach from one based on objectivity and efficiency alone
- Identify and discuss appropriate physical boundaries in relation to unconsented touching, sexual touching, and sexual contact
- Describe three types of situations in which maintaining emotional boundaries are crucial to avoiding enmeshment
- Identify clues that may alert you that your sympathy is becoming pity
- Define overidentification and its negative effects
- Describe what it means to care too much
- List some ways that honoring professional boundaries serves the positive goals of the health professional and patient relationship

I remember the wintry day she called from a phone booth not too far from the office, barely hanging on. I got somebody to take me out to find her and bring her back to the office. I remember the moment when I realized that the absurd choice before me was to do grief work or find insulin. After a frustrating morning on the phone trying to find some public or private source of help—a struggle she was in no shape at the moment to handle—I took her to a drug store and bought the insulin myself.

I was feeling a bit of shame. There's an emphasis in our field now on maintaining proper boundaries, with the implication that those who do not are overfunctioning, codependent, and other compound words even more dreadful. Emotional disengagement was expected. Technically—though no one forbade it—it was not part of my job to go find people in phone booths or pay for their medicine. I was aware of stretching the limits of what I usually do.

—B. Jessing[1]

The health care provider in the quote is struggling with the appropriate limits of her involvement with her homeless patient. She is experienced and knows she could overstep an appropriate boundary in their relationship and in so doing may cause more harm than good in the long run. Still, almost everyone can sympathize with her attempt to be respectful of her patient's desperate situation. As she suggests,

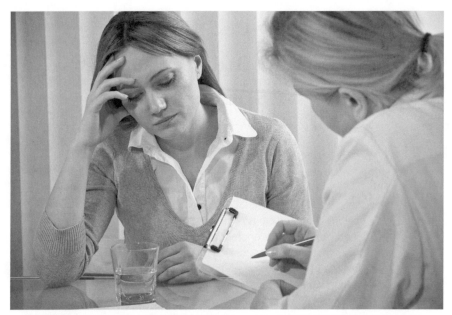

FIGURE 11-1: Maintaining professional boundaries helps put the goal of facilitating a patient's well-being at the forefront of the professional and patient relationship. *(©iStockphoto.com.)*

her challenge is not only to show respect by honoring the bonds of the relationship but also its boundaries.

A good general rule is that the physical and emotional boundaries between you and patients must always be guided by the goal of facilitating a patient's well-being and maintaining profound and caring respect in the interaction (Figure 11-1). But knowing the general rule does not necessarily help one with the complex human stories that face you in the line of work you have chosen. For one thing, relationships are dynamic, and there are changes in them with every encounter. As the authors of one article critical of boundary language correctly noted, " 'Boundaries,' for us, is a metaphor that, like 'resources,' leads to images of people as skin-bound containers with fixed contents or identities. This metaphor has implications for how subscribers to it view people and change."[2] Still, one has to appreciate the large body of literature that exists and the long tradition of behaviors that are considered appropriate for the type of relationship we are exploring here. As you read on you will see our attempt to provide some more details and examples of what it means to maintain professional boundaries and why.

What Is a Professional Boundary?

A *professional boundary* is the usual way of talking about physical and emotional limits to intimacy, the general contours of which were introduced in Chapter 5 when you were considering the differences between personal and therapeutic relationships. An extreme example sometimes is reported of health professionals losing their licenses or in other ways being sanctioned for engaging in sexual intercourse with patients or clients. We will briefly discuss this type of concern in a section that more broadly describes physical boundaries. Guidelines regarding emotional boundaries are designed to prevent psychological dynamics that are harmful to the patient or to you during the relationship. We will discuss these, too. While studying this chapter bear in mind that some boundaries come from external sources (e.g., the time you spend in the encounter), whereas others are internal (i.e., characteristics you and the patient bring to it).

The guidelines for physical and emotional boundaries are derived from several sources. Some are from professional ethics codes; others are from laws. These in turn have grown out of the experience of health professionals and patients in the past. Sometimes the guidelines change on the basis of insights from psychology regarding tensions that may arise from human needs for privacy, intimacy, and acceptance. Today studies of power differentials among persons within institutions and relationships add another component of understanding.

One way the wisdom of maintaining boundaries has been dramatized in the past is through the erroneous idea that being professional requires one to be aloof, objective, and efficient *at the price of personal warmth and affectionate conduct*. But to suggest that respect entails aloofness is a distortion of the highest goals to which we aspire and is often substituted for, rather than a sign of, competence.[3]

Recognizing a Meaningful Distance

In human interaction, psychological and physical distances take on deep meaning, determined by the degree of intimacy it represents for both parties. At one pole, there may be a complete sense of separateness, and at the other there is the realm of togetherness that is highly personal, informal, and familiar (i.e., intimate). At any point along this continuum, certain behaviors are put into play, whereas others remain in the background. In Chapter 8 you learned that a patient's narrative unlocks doors to what the patient thinks and feels. Listening with care to this information will help you to be sensitive to the patient's needs, including those that may go beyond what you can respond to in your role. A health professional dare not place too great an expectation on the patient or his or her family for emotional support in times of the professional's own crisis. The delicacies with which the boundaries of respect must be maintained are the impetus for many of the reflections on this topic, some of which we share here.

Physical Boundaries

As a general rule Western societies do not condone much touching, especially among strangers. You may find a clerk in a store who physically touches the palm of your hand in returning change. You may be jostled in a crowd. You may shake a stranger's hand in meeting. Among some a formalized form of kiss or buzz on the cheek is expected. Strangers may impulsively hug the man or woman next to them in the midst of an important sports event. However, the occasions when touching among strangers is socially sanctioned can probably be counted on the fingers of one hand. At the same time, many tasks in the health professions environment require caregivers to be in close physical contact with strangers who are their patients, and to do so respectfully. In addition, displays of affection expressed by a pat on the shoulder, a gentle hug, or other signs of support are behaviors you may be comfortable engaging in as a part of your interaction.

⊚ REFLECTIONS

We all experience a stranger's touch on a regular basis.
Think of a time in the past couple days that you and a stranger came into physical contact.
Was it comfortable? If so, what made it so? If not, what happened that you had a flash of discomfort?

All cultures and their subcultures have socially constructed rules about when and between whom touching is condoned. Such rules and mores often extend to the acceptable conduct between health professionals and patients. For example, in some a male caregiver may not touch or even look at a woman's body. At the same time, when taken seriously appropriate touch can be an effective means of establishing rapport or showing reassurance—and may be required for diagnostic or treatment regimens. In short, acceptable contours of physical contact between health professional and patient deserve your attention.

Unconsented Touching

Informed consent mentioned at the end of Chapter 10 is one of the most basic societal acknowledgments that professional contact may permissibly depart dramatically from general accepted social norms of physical contact. Informed consent arose in part from the legal concept of battery. *Battery* is a legal term acknowledging society's deep prohibition against unconsented touching. By giving informed consent the patient is saying, in effect, I give you—and others involved in my care—consent to hold, stroke, rub, poke, or even puncture or cut me, depending on the scope of practice in your professional role. Obviously the permission to make physical contact already puts the health professional and patient relationship into a special category where usual, socially acceptable distances are breached on a regular basis.

Your right to make physical contact does not give you permission to impose on a patient's sensitivities or dislikes regarding physical contact. Many cultural, social, and personal factors will come together to create a patient's comfort zone regarding physical contact, and you should be guided by a sensitivity to individual differences.

Sexual Touching

Some types of physical contact are deemed unacceptable in the health professional and patient relationship under any conditions, even with the consent of the patient or client. Under law you cannot make contact with a patient with an intent to harm him or her physically or psychologically. If you do, you will be charged with abuse.

The type of touching that has received the most attention is physical contact delivered with an intent to excite or arouse the patient sexually. Although sexual intercourse is the most verboten, the prohibitions are not limited to it. For example, the American Medical Association's 2010–2011 *Code of Medical Ethics: Current Opinions with Annotations* addresses the broader notion of sexual misconduct.[4] Why should it be forbidden if a competent, adult patient consents to or even seems to invite sexual contact? The strongest argument against this type of contact is that it betrays the reasonable expectations built into the essence of the health professional and patient relationship. Patients have a right to receive the best care possible without having to satisfy the professional's needs.

However, what about the idea that sexual activity between professional and patient may be taking place between two consenting adults? An objection to this argument is that sexual activity is never free from other types of claims on the other person, so both patient and health professional may begin to alter the conditions of the relationship in light of the power of its sexual dimensions rather than the conditions under which a patient sought professional care in the first place. In short, it is never considered fair that the patient would have to meet your need for sexual pleasure, sexual intimacy, sexual fulfillment, dominance in a relationship, or any other gain, no matter what the patient might believe will be gained.

Sexual Harassment

The importance of the idea that sexual distance must be maintained in public settings is being aired today in the notion of *sexual harassment.* The U.S. Equal Employment Opportunity Commission (EEOC) defines harassment as unwelcome sexual advances, requests for sexual favors, and other verbal or physical conduct and includes activity that creates a hostile or unwelcome work environment for the person who feels "harassed." A more specific description follows:

> Sexual harassment is a form of sex discrimination that violates Title VII of the Civil Rights Act of 1964. Unwelcome sexual advances, requests for sexual favors, and other verbal or physical conduct of a sexual nature constitute sexual harassment when this conduct explicitly or implicitly affects an individual's employment; unreasonably interferes with an individual's work performance; or creates an intimidating, hostile, or offensive work environment. Sexual harassment can occur in a variety of circumstances, including but not limited to the following: The victim and harasser may be a woman or a man. The victim does not have to be of the opposite sex. The victim does not have to be the person harassed but could be anyone affected by the offensive conduct. The harasser's conduct must be unwelcome. It is helpful for the victim to inform the harasser directly that the conduct is unwelcome and must stop.[5]

Most state licensing acts have provisions prohibiting such behavior by professionals, and many institutions include prohibitions in their policies. You will have ample opportunity to learn more about the particulars of the legal issues involved in this evolving area of the law. An important aspect of sexual harassment that has not been explored deeply enough involves sexual behaviors that issue from patients or their family members toward professionals. One of the only studies we found was of physical therapists: 63% of respondents reported having experienced some form of sexual harassment perpetrated by patients.[6] At the heart of the discussion is the degree of distance and quality of exchanges that must be maintained for respect to be expressed and for human dignity to flourish for everyone involved.

What about Dual Relationships?

Dual relationships are defined as those in which "[a] professional . . . assumes a second role with a client, becoming . . . friend, employer, teacher, business associate, family member, or sex partner." In the past the typical belief has been that once a health professional and patient relationship formally has ended, two consenting, competent adults ought to be free to do whatever they please. This makes good intuitive sense on the face of it. We call your attention, however, to insights from literature on the dynamics of dual relationships. It may begin before, during, or after the [professional] relationship. Dual relationships in the professions for the most part involve professionals who often rationalize their behavior, arguing that the situation is unique. "However, dual relationships are potentially exploitative, crossing the boundaries of ethical practice, satisfying the practitioner's needs and impairing his or her judgment."[7]

Friendships initiated after the termination of a professional relationship can be injurious to a former patient. Others warn that other relationships, such as business partnerships, can interfere dramatically with the professional's ability to be sensitive and appropriately objective in the professional and patient relationship.[8]

More research in this general area is necessary. Current thinking about dual relationships is not conclusive. Not even all major health professions caution against it, especially once the formal therapeutic relationship has ended. To take seriously the potential for harm to a patient or former patient is to err on the side of better judgment. Although an exception may present itself, a good rule is to honor physical and emotional boundaries with great thoughtfulness and care.

We turn, then, to three types of experiences in which maintaining emotional boundaries become a tool of respect in the health professional and patient relationship.

Psychological and Emotional Boundaries

Some specific ways the emotional responses and psychological attachments of the health professional or patient can interfere with respect for the patient can be summarized in the term *enmeshment:*

> . . . the nurse who has become enmeshed often develops an emotional connection with or an emotional availability to the client that may be impossible to maintain over the life span of the client. This can ultimately lead to client feelings of anger or emotional pain and to a sense of abandonment. The process of enmeshment may also complicate provision of adequate care at a later time. This can occur if the patient sees the other care team members as not caring sufficiently or as providing inadequate care, in comparison with the nurse who is enmeshed.[9]

In these situations a self-conscious distance zone should be created to enable each person to gain or regain perspective on the appropriate nature of this public-sector relationship and the expectations each can reasonably have of it. Challenges include tendencies for sympathy to slip into pity, to overidentify with the patient's plight, and to misjudge the scope and type of caring behaviors you should exhibit toward the patient.

Slip from Sympathy to Pity

Emotional boundaries may have to be clearly set to maintain full respect for the patient if, in your attempt to respond well to her or him, you become so entangled in the apparent tragedy of the patient's plight that you begin to pity him or her. In pity one looks down on the other person. Once that happens it is impossible to think about the patient or act in a way that really serves the patient's best interests.

Most health professionals can name at least one type of illness or injury that profoundly affects them emotionally.

◎ REFLECTIONS

Can you name one thing that would be horrendous if it were to befall you?
What symptoms or other aspects of that condition would be the most difficult
   to accept?
Would you want people to have pity for your plight? Why or why not?

Looking inward at your own strong reactions can provide insight into a block you may feel when faced with treating such a person. Recognizing that such a block exists does not mean you are unfit to be in your field, but it may guide you into some arenas of service rather than others.

Sometimes feelings are so strong that the health professional cannot bear to treat patients with that particular condition without feeling sorry to the point of pity for a person who has that condition. In chapter 5 you learned about referral and it is appropriate in this case.

It is not at all unnatural for you to become periodically so involved in patients' situations that you take these problems home with you. Almost any health professional can recall the time he or she had trouble falling asleep or was moved to tears or laughter by a sudden tragic or joyful announcement touching a patient's life. There is, however, a significant difference between this depth of professional caring, which stimulates a purely human response, and fruitless or destructive enmeshment. The difference can be illustrated with the following case.

Michael Anderson was admitted to the psychiatric ward of City Hospital after the police brought him there from the streets. The police found him unconscious in a doorway of a downtown office building. Michael is a 64-year-old alcoholic who periodically holds down part-time jobs and has lived in various boarding houses until evicted for his drunken behavior or failure to pay his bill. His mother died when he was 15 years old, and he left home shortly after that. He recently learned that his father died of a heart attack while Michael was serving a stint in the military as an enlisted man in his early 20s.

Craig Hopkins is a little younger than Michael but only by 4 years. His similarity to Michael Anderson, however, ends there. Craig Hopkins grew up in an upper-middle-class home and served as an officer in the Marines before entering professional school when he retired from the military at age 57. Some of the officers in the military certainly had alcohol dependencies, but being a teetotaler

Continued

himself he tended not to hang out with them much. He tells his wife that he is fascinated with Michael. He finds Michael very warm and human, and they enjoy sharing what they call "war stories." Michael is admitted to the detoxification unit on the ward, where he will spend some weeks drying out. Craig asks to remain one of his caregivers, and the supervisor initially is happy to comply. The two men chat when Craig has a few minutes, and, over the next few days, Craig arrives at the conclusion that Michael has had more than his share of misfortune.

One day when Craig goes into Michael's room, he finds Michael doubled up, writhing in agony. With a trembling voice, Michael tells him that the doctor has not given him anything to take the edge off his withdrawal from alcohol. To Craig's surprise, Michael grabs him by the wrist and pleads, "Please, please, I can't stand this agony. If you will just get me something to drink, just enough to make it over the hump, I swear I'll never touch another drop. If I can't get a little relief, I will kill myself. The doctor is a sadist."

Craig Hopkins tears himself away and leaves the room. That night, however, he cannot sleep. He is haunted by the picture of this man who has survived the death of his parents, claims to have been divorced three times, and has "some kids somewhere who don't want anything to do with their old dad," been on the front lines as an enlisted man "with a few notches" in his belt, but has succumbed to the bottle. Craig sees clearly the beads of sweat that clung to Michael's face as he spoke, thinks that Michael is clearly all alone in the world, and realizes he is irrationally angry at Michael's physician for not making detox a little easier for Michael.

The next morning the unit supervisor motions to Craig to step into a quiet area of the unit. She says that Michael is in a restless sleep and experiencing some visual hallucinations. She adds, "I see you are spending quite a bit of time with him. I don't know how much experience you have in this area but you've got to watch these alcoholics. They're all liars. They'll do anything to manipulate the staff to give them more of the stuff, so be on your guard."

Craig remembers Michael's pleading eyes the day before and is overcome with a desire to make a sharp retort to the supervisor's statements. He goes instead to Michael's room and deftly slips a half pint of whiskey he bought the night before into the drawer of the bedside stand and makes enough noise so that Michael stirs from his tortured sleep and sees what he is doing. As he leaves he suddenly thinks, *"What* am *I thinking*?!" But he continues hurriedly out of the room.

We can see that Craig has reached the point where he is responding impulsively out of pity, rather than with genuine caring because the situation has become so painful to him. Because pity distorts what he can do that is consistent with the appropriate boundaries of this relationship, he errs. In fact, he may include himself among the patient's many problems, as well as jeopardizing his own position.

⑨ REFLECTIONS

What details of this story do you think contributed to Craig's sympathy turning to pity? What else could Craig have done to help alleviate the patient's suffering? Was it his professional duty to do anything? Why or why not?

You cannot solve the type of problem arising from pity simply by enmeshing yourself more deeply into the patient's personal life, as Craig did. Of course, your pity is in response to a genuinely felt need of a patient. Michael may be manipulative, but Craig saw the depth of his suffering. What was called for was sympathetic acknowledgment of the person's problem but also clarity that his professional role required him to put boundaries on what he could do professionally to intervene constructively in Michael's plight.

Many patients who become objects of pity are suffering and do not know how or when to limit personal revelations when they find a professional person with a sympathetic ear. Health professionals in general are in no position to solve most of the patient's personal problems. As one colleague commented, "Overall we are really just a flash in the pan of a patient's life!" He is right. Craig went beyond even his best considered judgment to try to become more.

Pity is a powerful emotion. It can be communicated to the patient in one meeting and over a period of time. Facial expression can instantly convey one's feelings. Quick nervous movements, coupled with a sudden departure, are sometimes correctly interpreted as expressions of pity. The desire not to talk about the patient's problem and trite comments such as, "It'll be *fine*, I'm sure," can also be interpreted to mean, "Poor, poor you." More often than not, patients abhor pity, even if it serves some small immediate purpose. Pity is destructive and belittling to the patient, who will eventually recoil from it.

We can assume that Craig, with a life as an officer in the military, had encountered other difficult situations, but something about Michael hit him deeply. We do not know for sure what it was.

Checking one's feelings with trusted other professionals in such situations can be helpful. Craig bristled when the supervisor confronted him and responded antagonistically. However, if he had listened to what she said, he might at least have taken it as a signal to back off a little and discuss his feelings with someone else on the ward. This might have given him a clearer insight into this patient, into others like him, or into himself, providing a chance to reset his own professional compass.

Overidentification with the Patient's Predicament

Emotional boundaries and psychological distance can become a challenge when you have had an experience so similar to the patient's that you believe your experiences to be identical. Such a reaction of *overidentification* is another variety of enmeshment.

At first it seems a mistaken idea that having had similar experiences may actually hinder the effectiveness of a respect-based health professional and patient relationship. But everyone has had the experience of beginning to relate a traumatic (or exciting) event only to have the other person interrupt with, "Oh! I know *exactly* what you mean!" and then go on to describe his or her own story. One feels cheated at such times, thinking, "No, that's not what I meant, but you are more interested in telling me about yourself than in listening to me!" The way such overidentification works within the health professions can be illustrated in another case:

Mrs. Garcia, an elementary school teacher, became interested in teaching language skills to hearing-impaired children after her third child, Lucia, who was born deaf, successfully learned to communicate by attending special classes for those with hearing impairment. Mrs. Garcia enrolled in a health professions course directed toward training teachers of hearing-impaired persons.

In her first position she was surprised and alarmed that some of the mothers requested that she not be assigned to their children. Finally, she approached one of the mothers whose child she had been working with and with whom she felt comfortable. "What's wrong?" she asked. "Do they think I'm incompetent because I was older when I went back to school or am new in my field? Is it my personality? I want so much to help these children, and I can't understand what I'm doing wrong." The embarrassed mother replied, "Well, since you asked, I'll give you a direct answer. I don't feel this way, but some of the mothers think that you don't understand their children's difficulties because every time they start to tell you something about their children, you immediately interrupt with an experience you have had with your own child."

Unfortunately, Mrs. Garcia's effectiveness as a teacher was hindered by her own intense experiences and, likely, her need to share what she had been through. She would benefit from recognizing that the tendency to overidentify is bound to be present because of her own situation. It will also be helpful to remind herself periodically that attempts to relate to the patient (or in this case the parent of the patient) by pointing out superficial similarities between her own experience and theirs may be interpreted as her desire to talk about her own problem, even though that is not her intent. Overidentification, once it becomes a part of the caregiver's thinking, cannot be easily erased. But giving the other an opportunity to fully describe his or her unique experience and express the feelings attached to it before superimposing any similarities can help to decrease the deleterious effect on the relationship. Co-workers can also be valuable when a health professional's close relationship with the patient prevents him or her from seeing the patient's situation clearly. They may see what is happening and thus provide insight into the trouble. When you refer a patient to someone else or share disturbing feelings with co-workers about your assessment that your therapeutic relationship is being compromised by something, you are maintaining a healthy, respectful boundary between you and the patient by bringing other colleagues' reflections into what seems to be going awry.

REFLECTIONS

How might Mrs. Garcia have become better prepared to overcome the natural tendency for her to use her own child as a reference point to bond between her and the parents of her clients?

As you think about your own situation, what types of clients or families might be in your care that would pose a challenge to you not to overidentify with them?

The task for all who encounter patients' situations that lend themselves to overidentification is to be on the lookout for and honor the unique details and differences as well.

Caring Too Much

A third situation addresses the awkwardness that ensues when a relationship that began with appropriate boundaries has still led to circumstances signaling to you that a new set of boundaries must be established. This type of situation is often precipitated by genuine affection many people in health professional and patient relationships learn to feel for each other. The affection may spill over to, or be primarily directed toward, the patient's family or other loved ones, too. One study suggested that professionals who have been brought up to view themselves as "caregivers" in the family may be more susceptible to overstepping this boundary than others because they become sensitively drawn into the other's life situation.[10] We identify some signs that affection, a positive component of the relationship, has spilled over into enmeshment and make some general suggestions about what can be done to rectify the situation.

Obviously, affection is more likely to develop in health care settings where longer-term professional relationships exist. One example of how a problematic dynamic can arise is illustrated in the following story

Jack Simms has been an ambulatory patient at University Rehabilitation for 6 months. His affable, optimistic spirit has made him popular with the staff. At 23 years of age, he was involved in a car accident in which his fiancée was killed, and he suffered a traumatic brain injury. Some health professionals have long suspected that Jack's optimism is a veneer for the deep grief and frustration resulting from this sudden, dramatic change in his life. However, attempts to encourage him to visit with the staff psychiatrist have been largely unsuccessful, a problem exacerbated by the fact that his insurance plan covers only 6 hours of psychiatric evaluation and treatment anyway. One day he tearfully tells Karen Morgan, a health professions student who has been treating him, that he is depressed and desperately lonely. Up to this point, their interaction has been full of banter and they have felt quite comfortable with each other. Karen does not divulge to the rest of the staff Jack's expression of depression and loneliness, but that night on the way home, she stops by a local pub where he has invited her to "come and have a drink" following work.

In the following weeks, she begins to visit him more often. She finds him attractive, they share common interests, and he is obviously happy in her company. During this time, however, Karen also leads her own private life, going on dates and interacting with a world of other people. However, Jack hangs around the clinic before and after treatments, and he counts the minutes until she arrives at the pub.

During her Christmas vacation Karen visits friends in a distant city and has a marvelous time. When she returns, bursting with enthusiasm and eager to share her stories, she finds Jack sullen and angry at her for staying away from him for so long. He has arranged for her to receive a present from him, which he plops angrily on the clinic desk. He says, "That's for you. Take it if you want." Then he leaves the clinic angrily.

Jack's reaction indicates that he feels Karen has betrayed their growing personal relationship and abandoned him. He has now reached the point where someone he thought was a friend has rejected him. Karen, who acted in good faith on her feelings of warmth and affection for Jack, has thus unwittingly fostered a dependence on her that is detrimental to his well-being. Her subsequent attempts to explain her sudden withdrawal may have profound, lasting negative effects on Jack. Instead of being a friend and confidante—maybe eventually a lover—as he had hoped, she will become just another of a long line of rejections he has experienced. He has relied on her more than she had intended or was able to manage.

⊙ REFLECTIONS

As you may know from your own professional or personal experience, it is easy to get more involved with a person than you intended at the outset or not take the clues that the other is becoming more attached than you.

In Karen's situation, in retrospect were there any junctures that would have served as a warning to her that Jack's expectations were growing more intense than hers?

What might she have done then?

What can she do now to help ensure that the professional goals appropriate for him are met optimally?

In retrospect, Karen paid too much personal attention to this patient, meeting with Jack in an environment that invited more involvement than she apparently wanted. With rare exceptions it is always wise for the health professional to refrain from visiting the patient in a social setting until absolutely certain that the patient's feelings and life situation are such that an injury to the patient's feelings and dignity will not result.

Another way to maintain constructive physical and emotional boundaries is to remind the patient of the real situation between them. A young man, for instance, should know that the health professional he adores is engaged to someone else. By discreetly sharing with the patient personal incidents from everyday life, you will be better able to maintain the "reality testing" addressed in Chapter 10. It is the health professional's responsibility to give and receive pertinent personal information in such a way that workable limits are maintained in the relationship.

There are no hard and fast rules about how to proceed when genuine affection and enjoyment of the other is present in the therapeutic relationship. Many of the caveats regarding dual relationships discussed earlier in this chapter can be useful if a relationship seems to be becoming sufficiently intense to cause you to question. Periodic reexamination of your own motives and conduct or others' assessment of your relationship is essential. Although it is important to maintain a professional demeanor, you will best be served by showing genuine warmth and affection but always tempering that with awareness that the other person's needs and wishes may exceed or differ from your own. In fact, a powerful antidote to enmeshment of this type is the health professional's strong personal identity and the presence of a satisfying personal life.[11]

Maintaining Boundaries for Goodness' Sake

The three cases described earlier illustrate that trying to maintain respectful boundaries will serve everyone's interests well. The good news is that although an emphasis on boundaries taken alone leaves everyone feeling hemmed in, the reverse is true when it is understood that respect for boundaries simply are instruments for everyone being able to fully flourish within the unique goals of a therapeutic relationship.

People who seek your services to remain well or who become ill or injured are thrust into a new, unique relationship when they begin their encounter with you. The starting point for a flourishing relationship is to once again reflect on how different your two roles are. Most patients probably do not fully understand their feelings toward you; they may be expressed as awe or deference, as vague admiration, as infatuation, or as resistance and hostility. Some patients may not have a good idea of how to be in their role as a patient or client or honor yours. The whole environment is strange. To a large extent you can alter the patient's attitude and expectations by learning about the basis of their feelings and by consciously keeping your own focus on your role as a health professional.

Anything beyond that ceases to be mutually beneficial. This understanding about the terms of involvement is usually easily established at the first meeting with refinements along the course of the interaction. If the relationship is more sustained, rough spots must be navigated, aware that adherence to the goals must continue to inform attitudes and conduct toward each other. Because limits of the relationship are also understood by both, there is no fear of rejection. At the core of the relationship lies a paradox: The people who respect each other find that in their closeness they are able to provide each other freedom and mutual benefit as it applies to the health professional and patient relationship. What often occurs is an acknowledgment (though seldom spoken) that the health professional has found satisfaction in applying professional skills optimally for this person, and the patient has benefited from the services of a skilled professional.

Their involvement is personal to a degree and not merely a business transaction; they express to each other those feelings and opinions that can be shared within the limited professional setting.

When the patient no longer requires the services of the health professional, there will be no regret about ending their relationship because each one has benefited from it, whether it lasted for 10 minutes or 10 months. This is how goodness itself is served in the work we are privileged to do.

SUMMARY

This chapter promotes respectful interaction through your being aware of, reflecting on, and willingly and intentionally acting within the constraints of the therapeutic relationship. We have shown that maintaining professional boundaries is not achieved by employing a cold or impersonal approach. Indeed, such an approach may only increase a patient's conviction that he or she is not respected or understood by you. At the same time, the line between behaviors and expectations in your personal and professional relationships can be stretched thin in some situations. Moreover, your physical attractions (and those of patients towards you), your emotional responses, and your personal experiences sometimes present themselves as challenges. You are faced with the opportunity to respectfully structure the individual situation to uphold the dignity of both you and the patient.

REFERENCES

1. Jessing B: Back to square one. In Haddad A, Brown K, editors: *The arduous touch: women's voices in health care*, West Lafayette, IN, 1999, Purdue University Press.
2. Combs G, Freedman J: Relationships, not boundaries, *Theor Med Bioeth* 23:203–217, 2002.
3. Swisher LL, Page CG: *Professionalism in physical therapy practice*, Philadelphia, 2005, Saunders.
4. American Medical Association: Section 8:14, sexual misconduct in the practice of medicine. *AMA code of medical ethics with current opinions and annotations*, Chicago, 2011, American Medical Association.
5. Equal Employment Opportunity Commission: *EEOC-FS/E4: Facts about sexual harassment: EEOC guidelines on sexual harassment 29 CFR 1604 11a*. 93, January 1992 (website) http://eeoc.gov/types/sexual_harassment.html. Accessed January 12, 2012.
6. deMayo RA: Patient sexual behaviors and sexual harassment: a national survey of physical therapists, *Phys Ther* 77:739–744, 1997.
7. Kagle JD, Giebelhausen KB: Dual relationships and professional boundaries, *Soc Work* 39(2):213–220, 1994.
8. Nadelson C, Notman M: Boundaries in the doctor-patient relationship, *Theor Med Bioeth* 23:191–201, 2002.
9. Rich RA, Hecht MK: Staffing considerations. In Haddad A, editor: *High tech home care: a practical guide*, Rockville, 1987, Aspen.
10. Farber NJ, Novack DH, O'Brien MK: Love, boundaries and the patient-physician relationship, *Arch Intern Med* 157:2291–2294, 1997.
11. Davis C: *Patient-practitioner interaction: an experiential manual for developing the art of health care*, ed 3, Thorofare, NJ, 1998, Slack.

PART FIVE

Questions for Thought and Discussion

1. Everyone who treats patients sometimes gets into a time bind for one reason or another. Cecilia has been caught short today because so many of her patients needed a little extra time with her in order for her to feel she has done what they needed done. At the same time, she is getting more and more behind and is aware that three patients are waiting in the outer area. She must find a solution to fit three into a time frame usually reserved for two before the unit closes. None of them knows the time when the others were scheduled to be seen.

   What are her best choices for how to handle this situation, showing respect for the patients?

   a. Tell all of them what the situation is and let them decide among themselves what order they will be seen.

   b. Make an independent "triage" decision about who is the neediest of care and take them in that order, telling all three of them what you are doing and apologizing for what has happened.

   c. Make an independent "triage" decision but do not announce it, letting the chips fall where they may by the time the unit closes.

   d. Continue to go on treating them in their scheduled order, but giving each less time than usual, explaining what happened.

   e. Continue to treat them in their scheduled order, cutting the pie thinner for each one, so to speak, and say nothing.

2. You have become friends with another person who works closely with you. Your friend tells you that he is thinking of going on a date with a male patient who was discharged from your institution a week ago. Everyone thought the patient was progressing sufficiently not to have to continue, but it is now apparent he will be coming in as a rehabilitation patient in the ambulatory care clinic. Your friend wants your advice. Both of you were part of his treatment team, so he is aware you have been treating this man and know what a fine person he seems to be. Also, you know your colleague will be rotating into the ambulatory rehabilitation unit in about 3 months. He asks you, "Do you think there is any reason I shouldn't go out with him? I suppose he could become my patient again. But I really like him. Actually, he asked me out before he was even discharged. I told him we should wait. And now this . . ."

   As a friend and as a co-worker how would you respond to your colleague's question? Why?

PART SIX

Some Special Challenges: Creating a Context of Respect

In this section of the book we explore two types of special challenges we believe warrant your attention. Chapter 12 addresses relevant considerations you will want to bear in mind while working with patients who are dying and with their loved ones. Patients and their families almost always show evidence of the disruption of their present lives and future dreams. The news may also bring challenges, unleash new hopes, and expose as yet unexercised strengths during this time. You have an opportunity to examine these issues and how they affect patients and their families. You will learn about priorities that you as a health professional can set for such patients and their families to show them respect.

In Chapter 13, we examine some situations that health professionals sometimes identify as difficult. Now that you have read and thought about different types of patients and situations, you have a good basis for thinking about disparities of power or status in the health professional and patient relationship and how role expectations may affect your interactions. In each of the examples our goal is for you to think expansively about your potential for respectful interaction when you encounter such situations.

Respectful Interaction when the Patient Is Dying

CHAPTER OBJECTIVES

The reader will be able to:

- Discuss the dying-death relationship and some sources of understanding about dying and death
- Discuss denial in regard to its effects on respectful interaction
- List several factors that have a bearing on a patient's response upon learning that he or she has a life threatening illness
- Explain several areas of consideration in setting treatment priorities when a patient is dying
- Discuss ways to help maintain hope when a patient's condition is irreversible and will result in death
- Identify some important changes in focus that health professionals should seek when a patient is near death

The newspaper near his chair has a photo of a Boston baseball player who is smiling after pitching a shutout. Of all the diseases, I think to myself, Morrie gets one named after an athlete.

You remember Lou Gehrig, I ask?

"I remember him in the stadium, saying good-bye."

So you remember the famous line.

"Which one?"

Come on. Lou Gehrig. "Pride of the Yankees?" The speech that echoes over the loud-speakers?

"Remind me," Morrie says. "Do the speech."

Through the open window I hear the sound of a garbage truck. Although it is hot, Morrie is wearing long sleeves, with a blanket over his legs, his skin pale. The disease owns him. I raise my voice and do the Gehrig imitation, where the words bounce off the stadium walls: "Too-dayyy . . . I feeel like . . . the luckiest maaaan . . . on the face of the earth. . . ."

Morrie closes his eyes and nods slowly.

"Yeah. Well. I didn't say that."

—*M. Albom*[1]

This excerpt, from a book titled *Tuesdays with Morrie*, chronicles the last months of a man's dying as it is recorded through the pen of his friend and former student. Here you catch them in one of their many exchanges, the young man trying to make conversation and the dying one bringing the narrative back to the heart of the matter—his own unique experience of dying. Of all the challenges you will face, your work with people who are dying will provide some of the greatest opportunities to use your skills in the health care environment.

Terminally ill is a term that is commonly seen in the literature to describe people who are dying. Like all labels, it allows people in this group to be identified easily according to their special needs. At the same time, we refrain from using it in this chapter. One difficulty with the term is its generality. Persons such as Morrie, who suffered from amyotrophic lateral sclerosis (commonly known as *Lou Gehrig's disease*), may live for many months or years. Another person with a different condition may die within days or weeks. Still, both are labeled terminally ill.

Many health professionals, as well as others, tend to place people on the "critical list." One of the authors remembers a friend who had lived for more than 10 years with a diagnosis of malignant lymphoma. He went into the hospital for his periodic blood test. A health professional who had come back to work after a 5-year hiatus greeted him cheerfully, "Are *you* still around?"

She was apparently astonished that this "terminally ill" patient had not died long ago! The patient recalled that although he knew her intentions were good, her greeting led to the most severe depression of his entire illness. As with all types of patients, the key is to look for the distinguishing factors that make this person's situation unique and respond respectfully to the needs that arise out of that individual person's experience. Toward achieving that goal, a first step toward any health professional's understanding of a patient's situation is to gain some general idea of how the dying process and death are viewed within the larger society.

Dying and Death in Contemporary Society

Dying is first and foremost a personal experience. All persons share some awareness that the end of the dying process is the death event. What does this mean to a person? In the minds of some patients or their families, a known diagnosis and somewhat predictable range of symptoms make them feel robbed of the "natural" flow of life. The dying process feels unnatural, an imposition.

A life-threatening condition generates new fears and concerns. Fortunately, for others it is also an opportunity to conduct long-neglected business, put one's affairs in order, or pursue a postponed adventure. Anticipation of the death event, too, creates its own concerns, fears, and hopes. For most people death remains perhaps the ultimate mystery.

Dying as a Process

How do we gain an understanding of the relationship of the process of dying to the end point of death?

In almost all cultures, stories passed down from childhood onward in fairy tales or, in some cultures, the mythic stories deeply inform our understanding from childhood—or lack of it. Note how in the following popular Western fairy tales death is something that happens to the bad guys, and a notable goal is to help bring it about:

Down climbed Jack as fast as he could, and down climbed the giant after him, but he couldn't catch him. Jack reached the bottom first and shouted out to his mother, who was at the cottage door. "Mother! Mother! Bring me an axe! Make haste, Mother!" For he knew there was not a moment to spare. However, he was just in time. Jack seized the hatchet and chopped through the beanstalk close to the root; the giant fell headlong into the garden and was killed on the spot.

So all ended well. . . .[2]

Then Grethel gave her a push, so that she fell right in, and then shutting the iron door she bolted it. Oh how horribly she howled! But Grethel ran away, and left the ungodly witch to burn to ashes.

Now she ran to Hansel, and opening his door, called out, "Hansel, we are saved; the old witch is dead!"[3]

Many Western childhood portrayals show no connection between the process of dying and the final death event. Both the health professional and patient may share beliefs about the "unnaturalness" of death rooted in many Western childhood stories. Of course, not all cultures have the same understanding of life and death. How might your relationship with a patient be different if, say, he or she grew up with the deep memory of this childhood story recounted by Mitch Albom, the author of *Tuesdays with Morrie* (whose conversations with his dying friend led him to read about how different cultures view death)?

There is a tribe in the North American Arctic, for example, who believe that all things on earth have a soul that exists in a miniature form of the body that holds it—so that a deer has a tiny deer inside it, and a man has a tiny man inside him. When the large being dies, that tiny form lives on. It can slide into something being born nearby, or it can go to a temporary resting place in the sky, in the belly of a great feminine spirit, where it waits until the moon can send it back to earth.

Sometimes, they say, the moon is so busy with the new soul of the world that it disappears from the sky. That is why we have moonless nights. But in the end, the moon always returns. As do we all. . . .[1]

In today's rich diversity of patients an essential step in creating a therapeutic relationship based on care is to try to gain some understanding of dying as a process to be viewed apart from death itself. This provides a starting place for further deliberation about how to respect what a patient or family says, how they behave, and what their attitudes are toward various aspects of their interaction with you and others during the dying process.

Denial

It is often said that Western societies are death denying. What can that possibly mean when all around us people are dying every day from illness, accidents, violence, old age, war, and other causes? Probably the best explanation is that although there is evidence everywhere of our mortality, we do our best to hold the inevitable at arm's length.

In many parts of Western culture, treatment of the dead body is one expression of a need to deny death its power. The dead body is painted and dressed to make it appear alive, although a sign of life, such as a sigh or fluttering eyelash, would cause most people to rush screaming from the room. For the most part, however, denial has simply become more subtle. For example, a subtle denial that death is the end point of the dying process is manifested in the incredible scenes of violence and killing viewed in films and on television, as Figure 12-1 illustrates. People of all ages see the culprit killed, but the same actor appears on next week's show, having adventures in dangerous places. Another response is a distancing that keeps death at arm's length for as long as possible even during one's dying process. This attempt to stave off the inevitable is also experienced by loved ones and poignantly is conveyed in the following quote of a 51-year-old woman who learned that her best friend was dying of cancer:

> Before one enters this spectrum of sorrow, which changes even the color of trees, there is a blind and daringly wrong assumption that probably allows us to blunder through the days. There is a way one thinks that the show will never end—or the loss, when it comes, will be toward the end of the road, not in its middle . . . I meant that I might somehow sidestep the cruelty of an intolerable loss, one rendered without the willful or natural exit signs of drug overdose, suicide, or old age.[4]

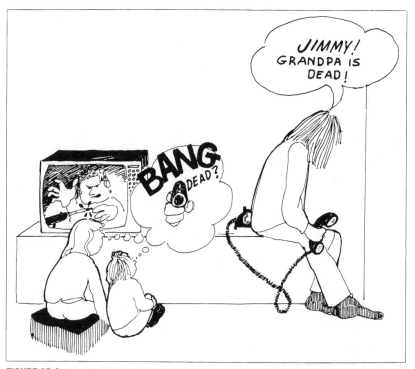

FIGURE 12-1: TV's influence on the viewers' perception of the reality of death. *(From the Swedish translation of Health Professional and Patient Interaction: Vård, Vårdare, Vårdad, p. 242.)*

At the same time, the health care team can be helpful in assisting both patients and loved ones not to become stuck in prolonged denial such as happened in the following:

> My husband, John, age 55, was handed his diagnosis of liver cancer by a newly graduated doctor—John's own had just retired. "As I'm sure you know," the young man had blushingly begun, and John said simply, "Yes." We walked out of the office holding hands and cold to the marrow.
>
> Near the end, I started looking for signs that the inevitable would not be inevitable. I watched a few leaves that refused to give up their green to the season. I took comfort in the way the sun shone brightly on a day they predicted rain—not a cloud in the sky! I even tried to formulate messages of hope in arrangements of coins on the dresser top—look how they had landed all heads up . . . what were the odds? I prayed, too, in a way that agnostics do at such times. Sorry I doubted you "dear God, help us now." I stood shivering on our back patio in the early morning with my mug of coffee and told whatever might help us that now would be the time . . . but my dreams betrayed me: John, shrunk to the size of a thumb, fell from my purse where I'd been carrying him and was stepped on. In another dream, I took a walk around the block and when I came back, my house was gone.[5]

⊚ REFLECTIONS

What, if anything, do you think the doctor could have done at the outset to help set this bereaving wife on a different course?

Denial mechanisms are so widespread in almost all Western societies that we gave special attention to it, but obviously there are other considerations and responses that we turn your attention to now.

Responses to Dying and Death

Because nearly all of us dread the thought of gradual and certain loss, the news of a life-threatening diagnosis is almost always disquieting. In this section you have an opportunity to think about what this state of affairs gives rise to.

Common Stresses and Challenges Demanding Response

What would be your biggest challenges if you learned that you were dying? Most people can vaguely imagine and project what they would dread most; once the diagnosis is made, however, the reality of their specific situation intrudes. Then a patient's previous notions about a particular disease or injury and the known experiences of others who have had it combine to create a vivid picture of what the patient believes to be ahead. The following are some of the most commonly expressed concerns.

Anticipation of Future Isolation

As you learned in studying Chapter 6, separation from the routine and regularity of life has a profound disorienting effect on many people. Often a prolonged dying process involves gradual loss of habits, acceptance by others, and familial, social, and societal roles.

The fear of separation from the familiarity of home and routine as a way of ordering one's life becomes a reality for many. At the heart for most is a deeper fear of abandonment by loved ones and caregivers. Anxiety about this may be expressed in comments such as: "They are starting to ignore me"; "My family is busy with other things"; "The nurses skipped my medication this morning, so they are probably giving up on me"; and "They spend more time with the woman in the next bed, but of course they know I'm dying." Many persons are aware of the practice of being admitted to the hospital to die or of having to spend the final period of their lives in a care facility, and some contribute to their isolation by rejecting visitors or others who come to visit, fearing that visitors have come to "hang the crepe," an expression referring to an old custom of hanging a lightweight fabric above their doorway as a sign of mourning, or worse.

You can "treat" (allay) the patient's fears of isolation by your own presence. You cannot always ensure patients that their loved ones will not "jump ship" when the going gets rough, because sometimes families or friends do. Observing this tapering off of supportive relationships is often trying for you, let alone the patient. Relationships are bound to be altered during this time; some friends and relatives disappear because of indifference, despair, or exhaustion, and those who do not become more cherished. Health professionals are often eventually able to ascertain who, among the many at the onset, will endure. Often, it is wise to begin providing your own support to those whom you judge to be the most enduring so that the patient will continue to have a community of support as the condition progresses.

Prospect of Pain

Those who have known others who experienced a distressful end to life cannot be sure that their own dying will not be equally painful or worse. Fortunately, modern modes of health care intervention for pain today have the potential to nearly obliterate the physical pain of dying, though it is still a challenge in some settings to get positive pain relief.[6] Anxiety and depression can have a heightened effect on pain, whereas distraction and feelings of security tend to diminish the suffering associated with pain. These patterns of response, first characterized by Kubler-Ross several decades ago, have since been shown to better being understood as the range of responses that come and go from time to time.[7] Therefore the patient's suffering may be decreased by your reassurance, presence, compassion, and caring discussed in Chapter 10 and elsewhere.

Resistance to Becoming Dependent

Real or feared loss of independence during illness or injury is often a challenge, as also described in previous chapters. Continued independence within whatever sphere of decision-making a person can exercise when in the dying process usually remains a high priority. Proof that they have thought about this is shown in their expressions of astonishment at having reached a point in their symptoms they had previously believed would be totally unbearable. Indeed, everyone has ideas beforehand of what he or she believes to be the "outer limits" of what one could bear: loss of bowel and bladder control; sexual impotence; inability to feed oneself, to communicate verbally, or to think straight; unconsciousness; or other loss. Often (though not always) patients' acceptance changes after a period of fighting the specific loss.

Patients' experiences of real or imagined isolation, pain, and increasing dependence are basic, but there are other concerns as well, such as the dread of suffocation and the fear that one's loved ones will not be adequately provided for. A person who dies suddenly in a car accident or plane crash or from a myocardial infarction may have long harbored these fears but did not have a period of prolonged illness during which these concerns surfaced. For instance, a man who has had trouble openly expressing affection to his wife may be able to do so by sharing his sorrow that he fears she will not be adequately provided for. An indirect means of communication, such as writing a letter or telling a friend how wonderful she is, serves a similar purpose. You can be instrumental in making suggestions to help such a patient carry out his or her wishes if you get a hint that the patient desires to do so.

In summary, during their dying process, people must rely on their own best inner resources and the support of family, friends, and health professionals to sustain them as they face their challenges. Any hesitance, embarrassment, or disdain you show when a person expresses a concern, even one that seems unfounded to you, will exacerbate the suffering associated with it.

Reckoning with What Death Might Mean

Different cultures and individuals treat the moment of transition from alive to dead differently, but for many it is not something to relish. What is the range of expressions about what will happen when death comes?

Many people believe that after this life there is something else. The varieties of religious or philosophical beliefs are many, regarding the relationship of this life to the next.[8] Predominant beliefs in many religions, especially but by no means only those associated with Eastern religions such as Hinduism, propose that "death" is a process of birth and rebirth (e.g., reincarnation). The last step is not extinction but perfection, at which time one is absorbed into a "place" or into a "being" where complete unity of all beings is realized. Depending on the religion, the type of being one will become after physical death and the opportunity for the final step into ultimate unity may or may not depend on the type of life one lived on earth during an embodied human lifetime. In Islam one may be transported through several levels of paradise depending on the type of life one has lived.

Some people believe in the resurrection of souls only, whereas others believe that the actual human body will be restored, usually in an improved form. There is one version of a literal, sudden bodily resurrection (sometimes referred to as the "rapture") in which those—both dead and still living—who have lived holy lives will be immediately transported to heaven, whereas others will be left behind forever to suffer the consequences of their sins. Other Christians have different versions of what it means to be "resurrected," although all share this basic belief.

You will meet individuals who talk with anticipation about "going to meet the Lord," whereas others are sure their lives will not meet the standards of acceptability and they will be consigned to suffering of some kind. Knowing that any of these beliefs about immortality may influence the way an individual interprets the impact and meaning of his or her own impending death, you can be better prepared for comments from the patients or for rituals a patient and family engage in during the dying process.

⊚ REFLECTIONS

Before proceeding, think about conversations you may have had with patients or others who hold these positions. Which ones do you hold, if any?

A significant number of people in today's society do not view death as a precursor of immortality in any form. This view finds artistic expression in Tom Stoppard's play, *Rosencrantz and Guildenstern Are Dead*. The two attendants, who believe through most of the play that they are accompanying Prince Hamlet to his death in Denmark, find out that, instead, they are going to be put to death. Upon realizing their fate, one of them reflects: "Death isn't romantic, death is not anything. . . . Death is . . . not. It's the absence of presence, nothing more . . . the endless time of never coming back . . . a gap you can't see.[9]

⊚ REFLECTIONS

Try to construct a conversation you might have with a patient or family who does not believe in immortality.
• What kinds of comments might such a person make?
• How would you respond to the person in ways that would be affirming or comforting?

All of these concepts about death can help you understand patients and their families when they share their feelings and ideas about death and how to prepare for it. When you can enter into such conversations with equanimity and express genuine interest in what the person wants or needs to say about death, you will be showing respect for that person.

Coping Responses by Patients

Although denial is initially a common coping response, the aforementioned concerns associated with dying and the death event usually become more sharply focused over time and you can anticipate other emotional-psychological responses as well. For many, the first response is acute shock or disbelief. Effective coping also may take many other forms, such as periods of depression, anger, and hostility, bargaining behavior, or acceptance.[10] Patients who undergo a long process of dying are likely to feel all of them from time to time, and many times over. On one day, a woman denies her impending death; on another, she makes secret bargains with God about how long she will live; on the following days she feels the relief of acceptance followed by a deep depression; and so on. Although the danger with any such framework is that you or your colleagues may tend to pigeonhole a patient according to the categories provided, we have found them to be a useful general set of benchmarks for thinking about what a patient is experiencing.

The patient's basic personality structure is an important factor in determining which kind of responses will predominate, too. How did the person deal with stress before learning that he or she had a life-threatening condition? Similar coping responses will probably surface in his or her present situation.

To further prepare yourself for working with such patients, we suggest you pause here to engage in a reflection on your own life.

⊙ REFLECTIONS

Try to think about how you respond to stressful situations in your life.
- Can you imagine what you might be like as a patient or family member faced with the challenge of a dying loved one?
- If you have, in fact, had to face it, try to recall your major types of responses.

Another resource you can use was mentioned in Chapter 8, in which we highlighted how useful the writings of novelists, poets, essayists, and others can be. Many have recorded their experiences in this powerful period of life, and it is to your advantage to avail yourself of these narrative accounts in preparation for your professional encounters with people who are dying.

Coping Responses by the Patient's Family

The best and worst aspects of family relationships are exposed when a family member is gravely ill or dying. You will witness lifelong destructive patterns and the most intimate, loving characteristics of family relationships. The great majority of families are brought closer together by the experience, and their mutual support during this time is touching to observe. Despite this, for some health professionals, the members of the patient's family are viewed as intruders to be tolerated rather than as important people to be included. The experienced health professional knows that the family's presence may complicate the situation. At all hours of the day and night, they may ask questions, peek in on the patient, disrupt schedules, and aggressively offer suggestions. If the patient has not been told of the life-threatening nature of the condition, family members may whisper to you in doorways, trying to involve you in elaborate schemes to ensure continued deception. At the busiest time of day, they may stop you to tell you something, only to burst into tears. Why is it important for them to be there?

▶ It allows them to cope more effectively with their own stresses.

▶ *Anticipatory grief* that parallels the symptoms usually seen in the acute grief that follows a death can be dealt with at closer range. Symptoms of acute grief may take the forms of a tendency to sigh, complaints of chronic weakness or exhaustion, and loss of appetite or nausea. In addition, a family member may be preoccupied with what a person looks like, express guilt or hostility, and change his or her usual patterns of conduct.[11]

▶ Except in extreme situations, family members are so integral to the ongoing life and preferences of the patient that the patient feels lost without this support.

▶ They can be an essential element of communication for and about the loved one.

In many instances institutional resource personnel such as social workers, counselors, and chaplains can make themselves available to the whole team of decision-makers in this unique moment of their lives. Your willingness to access these personnel can extend your own effectiveness considerably.

Setting Priorities in Respectful Interaction

In addition to your role as one who respects the patient and family through listening and responding caringly to them, two additional priorities are appropriate when a patient is dying. They include information sharing and helping patients maintain hope.

Information Sharing: What, When, and How?

What types of information do patients and families need to know? Start with the patient's diagnosis. The key is for the entire team to try to be attentive and ready to communicate those things they each have a right to, and are ready to, know. For the most part today in the United States, Canada, and many European countries, medical policies and practices support the position that a patient has a right to information about his or her health status. There is also a conviction that the duty not to harm is best realized by disclosure—the truth "sets free." In support of this, some states in the United States have passed laws that allow a patient to read the notations on his or her own medical record in the presence of the physician, whereas other states permit the patient's lawyer to do so.

This trend toward openness is by no means shared universally or even by many of the cultures within the changing U.S., Canadian, and Western European populations. At the very least, you can be attentive to clues you are receiving from the patient and family as to whether directly sharing this information with the patient is a culturally competent way for members of the health care team to proceed. Do patients figure it out? Probably some do, and some do not.

Whatever combination of considerations make up the physician's decision, many are now telling patients with life-threatening conditions their diagnoses, usually in direct terms with emphasis on keeping communication channels open after the initial discussion.[12] In the end, there is no substitute for personalized, sensitive communication by all members of the health care team, initially and throughout the patient's course of interaction with them. Key to such communication is determining what information is shared, along with how and when it is shared.

ⓢ REFLECTIONS

- Do you think you would want to be told the news that you have a life-threatening condition that the physicians have just discovered? If yes, try to imagine the physical setting, people you would hope were (or were not) present, and key points you would want to know in this initial exchange.
- What would you like to have happen over the course of your dying that would most help you feel that you were being treated with respect from the start of your ordeal?
- What (if any) role would health professionals play in this process?

Seldom will it be within the boundaries of your role personally to directly communicate a diagnosis or prognosis, but you can always encourage this course of action with the physician or others whose legal/ethical responsibility it is. And you can always listen to the patient's story with focused attentiveness. Your attention to their questions will provide some relief to their anxieties because it will show that you care and respect even their most unusual concerns. It also conveys your willingness to keep communication channels open.

Using words the patient really understands is imperative. Without this translation from medical/clinical terminology to everyday language, nothing will make sense in the conversation.

For example, in *Endings and Beginnings,* a young woman's account of her husband's terminal diagnosis and eventual death, the author recalls that after exploratory surgery the doctor tried to be reassuring by saying they had found a "lymphatic tumor" but did not go on to tell them that it was an aggressive, life-threatening malignancy. In fact, that evening her husband reassured her that, because it was "lymphatic," at least it was not cancer. Their reassurance was short lived:

> That evening, as I left the hospital elevator I was startled to have the head resident under Dr. C. (the surgeon) turn to me and say, "Try not to worry; we'll do everything we can." It was clear there was much more going on than any of us was admitting.[13]

Following her encounter the young couple spent many days trying to verify the simple truth that the husband had something serious. In reflecting on the whole course of his dying, the author remembers that period of unclarity as one of the most painful for both of them.

Talking with a patient and family about the patient's prognosis has its own challenges because almost always the prognosis is not known with absolute certainty. Today physicians often talk about probability: "You have a 50% chance of a 5-year survival." This approach allows certain information to be transmitted to the patient and may permit the patient to learn what usually happens to people in similar situations. At the same time, probabilistic information does not answer the key question of "what, exactly, does this mean for me?"

Attending to the Patient's Strengths and Needs

In the first part of the chapter we emphasized the importance of recognizing and understanding the patients' challenges during this unique period of their life. Those experienced by people with life-threatening conditions can span the whole range discussed in Chapter 6.

Many life-threatening conditions are accompanied by a gradual or quick diminution of strength, endurance, control of movement, or sensory acuity. Helping the person and family adjust to each of the "little deaths" as they are experienced is a continuing challenge. Your respectful caring requires being attuned to the losses while affirming the patient's remaining strengths.

Helping Patients Maintain Hope

When a patient is dying, the focus of hope will change over time, from a hope for cure to a hope for meaningful activities in the remaining life left to this person. His or her hope may be directed toward events such as seeing a loved one or pet another time, visiting a favorite place, or hearing a familiar piece of music played.

Some hopes are less tangible: that one will be able to keep a positive spirit or sense of irony to the end, that one will be remembered and missed, or that a particular tradition will be carried on in one's absence. Previously sought long-term goals are put into perspective, and the patient focuses his or her hopes on the most important ones, knowing that some will no longer be attainable.[14]

Families also adjust their hopes for what is possible given the new circumstances. As one husband wrote when he learned that his wife was not going to recover from her early bouts of ovarian cancer:

> There is a transition between the certainty of living and the acceptance of dying. When there is such acceptance, there is a kind of emotional purgatory. The cartoon character stands still in space beyond the edge of a cliff and awaits the fatal fall. That is where things were for us in early October. There were choices, however, even in this purgatory. They remained a moment to live in . . . if only a moment. After that we will go on with our lives. Before it was over and before I began my desperate search for a new life, there would be a time for us as a family that was like none other. Most important was that we manage the pain. The first priority was comfort. The second priority was to get Lezlie back home not so much so that she could die there as that she could live there before she left.[15]

How can you show respect in terms of supporting hope? Hope itself depends significantly on the attitudes of health professionals, as well as on those of family and friends when the patient dares to disclose a hope. We have witnessed tender scenes between family or friends and the patient when one dares to say "I was hoping . . . ." Your listening for clues can help to maintain the person's feeling of worth and provide a human context into which hopes may be more freely expressed. Health professionals can also often play a significant role in actually helping the patient realize some specific hopes by making a few important telephone calls to the right people, by mentioning the patient's wishes to the family and others, or by other similar means.

People faced with dying all hope that they will be treated kindly, that everything clinically reasonable will be done for them, and that meaningful human exchange will not disappear. You can do your best in your role to support those general hopes.

Care in the Right Place at the Right Time

The site, timing, and focus of caring interventions have been the source of discussion and policy. An important factor is considerations arising from an improved understanding of physiological and other responses to pain or other disturbing symptoms associated with many life-threatening conditions, and where the interventions can best be delivered.

Hospital, Hospice, or Home Care?

Hospital

Many patients who are dying still do so in the hospital, though the actual figures will vary according to the number of hospital beds and general demographics of the area's population. This is usually the appropriate site for interventions that require complex technologies and specialties available in the hospital setting. However, today the hospice and home care settings have become viable alternatives for many patients during their dying. The most dramatic changes from the past century have taken place due to the rise of the *hospice* movement.

Hospice

The modern hospice, which began in England and has spread to Canada, the United States, and many other countries today, has been a commendable attempt in recent years to provide treatment and care expressly designed to meet the needs of patients with life-threatening conditions and their families. Initially, hospice care was geared to the treatment of patients with cancer, but it is available for many other types of patients with irreversible conditions such as Alzheimer's disease, progressively deteriorating neurological conditions, and AIDS.

Hospice focuses on comfort measures when cure or remission is no longer possible. The hospice setting is characterized by interdisciplinary health care approaches. When there is a family, it (and not the patient alone) is the unit of care. A large study of family perspectives on end-of-life care in different settings showed significantly more favorable experiences of their loved ones dying in hospice than those whose loved ones died in hospitals. The authors concluded that this setting is far better equipped to provide symptom relief, communication with health professionals, emotional support, and the perception of being treated with respect.[16]

Home Care

In some locations, home care is supported sufficiently by government and/or insurance plans to make this a viable alternative for families. Some hospices are actually "without walls"; that is, they are designed to provide services within the home with devices such as hotlines, care networks, and respite programs for caregivers. Churches and other organizations sometimes become involved in such home caregiving arrangements.

You and your patients will benefit if you take time to acquaint yourself further with the functions and structure of each of these settings in the communities where you work. This will prepare you to inform patients of their options when it becomes appropriate and to be active in their information-gathering process. You may even find yourself drawn to these aspects of health care and be one of the growing numbers of health care providers working in hospice or home health care.

Balancing Cure and Comfort Measures

From a clinical point of view, the treatment must always fit the situation. What constitutes "appropriate treatment" when a patient is dying?

Palliative care (or, as it is commonly called, *comfort care*) traditionally was thought of as what health professionals can do when cure no longer is possible. In other words, it becomes appropriate when all else has failed. From Hippocrates' time onward the suggestion was that if cure was no longer possible, the disease had gone beyond the "art of medicine" and should not be interfered with by the doctor. So all too often palliation meant that dying patients received little care. At the same time, you can understand that the idea of palliative care is important because, applied appropriately, it allows you to have better insight into how to respond well to patients' fears of abandonment, pain, and other distress associated with the dying process.

Today the growing focus on appropriate end-of-life care has shed new light on what palliative care entails. Comfort care goes well beyond the traditional "hand-holding at the bedside" so often portrayed in the pictures before modern medicine could offer so much. Comfort can be achieved for patients through many varieties of intervention, such as painkillers, ventilators, dramatic surgical procedures, and psychological counseling, to name some. Moreover, there has been a rethinking of traditional medical, nursing, rehabilitation, and other health care specialties to include palliative, as well as curative, aspects in their realm of expertise. Within medicine this may include anesthesiologists, physiatrists, internists, pediatricians, geriatric specialists, and surgeons, all of whom often address distressing symptoms associated with dying. Along with this heightened consciousness and technology focus, there has also been a rethinking about the traditional assumption of a progression from "treatment" to "palliation" as the patient's dying ensues. Using cancer as a model, the Institute of Medicine in the United States proposes that treatment geared to cure and treatment geared to palliation do not progress in a tidy, linear way (Figure 12-2). Different combinations of education about how to prevent deterioration or the appearance of new symptoms, responsiveness to rehabilitative needs, acute care interventions, and comfort measures all may remain appropriate from the beginning to the end of the patient's dying process.[17]

Other models that are fine-tuned to patients' and families' real needs are also being attempted. You are entering the health professions at a time when the attention devoted to these issues will assist you in doing a better job than your forbearers did in providing care for dying patients.

When Death Is Imminent

At some point in the course of an irreversible, life-threatening illness it becomes apparent that the person will die soon. Persons who do not suffer from a prolonged illness as such also face the moment of imminent death: the accident victim, the attempted suicide or murder victim, and the young person seriously injured in battle or other violence.

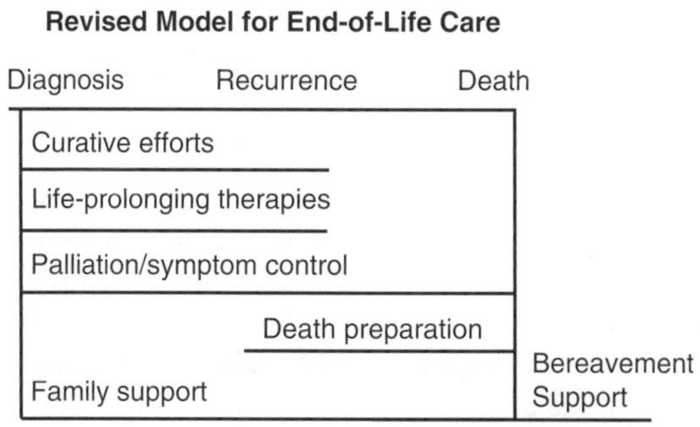

Revised Model for End-of-Life Care

FIGURE 12-2:   *(From M.J. Field, C.K. Cassel [Eds.]: Approaching death: improving care at the end of life, Committee on Care at the End of Life, Institute of Medicine. Washington, DC, 1997, National Academy Press.)*

Individualized Care

The patient whose death is imminent should not be barraged with routine requests and procedures that no longer matter. As one woman sitting by her dying father's bedside asked dismayingly, "Does it matter, really, if his bowels haven't moved on the last day he will probably be alive?"

Attempts to relieve pain by medication, massage, and other therapeutic means may have been started long before, and these should be continued unless the patient asks that they be withdrawn. Some people, knowing that they are experiencing the final days of their lives, find the torpor induced by heavy medication more troublesome than uncomfortable symptoms.

However, maximizing comfort goes beyond alleviating pain. It involves the relief of real or potential suffering. Suffering is a far more inclusive, personalized concept than pain, and your assistance in helping patients and their families have a final time together as free of pain and suffering as possible is a laudable goal. Families may do many things to try to provide a meaningful and peaceful transition. We have seen families who read to their loved one, bathe him or her, sing songs he or she loved, or fill the room with flowers. A friend of one of the authors sneaked her 2-month-old daughter up to the hospital room so that her husband could witness his wife nursing their child for one last time. A religious leader may be called in for instruction or rituals. The patient who has been nourished only intravenously for days or weeks may request that all medications and IVs be removed. Specific activities will vary from person to person influenced by personal preference and ethnic, religious, or other beliefs. When they exist, respect requires you to alter your treatment procedures to honor them.

Caregivers in the health care environment can be facilitators by allowing the family and friends their final day or days together, remaining "on standby" if needed. This might mean breaking hospital rules and readjusting one's schedule. It also means knowing whom should be called if the patient's condition worsens and death appears near.

Saying Good-Bye

Many people find it difficult to say good-bye to a friend or other loved one who is going away. It is often more difficult still when the person is dying—so much so that good-byes are seldom said, especially by the health professional to the patient and the patient's family. This is, however, something that you can do to show respect for the people and their situation when many other forms of interaction have been suspended. One psychiatrist offers this suggestion:

> What should be said is, I want you to know the relationship was meaningful, I'll miss this about you, or . . . it won't be the same, I'll miss the bluntness that you had in helping me sort out some things, or I'll just miss the old bull sessions, or something like that. Because those are things you value. Now what does that do for the other person? The other person learns that although it's painful to separate it's far more meaningful to have known the person and to have separated than never to have known him at all. He also learns what it is in himself that is valued and treasured by [you]. And some of those underlying, corrosive feelings of low self-esteem that plague people are shored up. . . .[18]

This encounter also allows the patient and his or her family to express similar feelings. There is often a real sense of closeness and gratitude felt toward the health professional, and to be able to show it is a great relief. In addition to what the exchange does for the patient and family, it is important to realize how much it can help in your own grieving. Giving patients and families an opportunity to express gratitude to you may sound odd, but it is one way in which some patients and families can be assisted in their own grieving. When they observe that the health professional receives his or her thanks humbly, they will appreciate this show of human caring.

However, you should also prepare for the patient and family to reject your attempts to show respectful caring during this intense period of their lives.

Sometimes when a person is close to dying, he or she shuts out many people. Such a patient may not want to have anything more to do with you. There are many possible reasons for this:

▶ Many have great difficulty saying good-bye under any circumstance.
▶ The person has accepted his or her death and no longer needs any people around, except the closest few of whom you are not one.
▶ The patient and his or her family may actually direct their anger about the death toward you and other members of the team.
▶ You are inextricably linked to the whole setting in which suffering and the dying process have taken place. So much anguish may be associated with you and your professional environment that it is painful for the patient to be in your presence.

In short, when your final efforts and good intentions are neither wanted nor welcomed, you may feel hurt by these sudden or unexpected rebuffs and can do little more than forgive the person responsible for them. At times when hurt is present, support from your professional colleagues may become vital. Sharing feelings of failure, rejection, or bewilderment with an understanding colleague can lend insights into the reasons listed earlier.

SUMMARY

This chapter takes into account some key considerations that can be helpful to you in your attempts to show respect in the extreme life situation in which death is approaching for a patient in your care. The patient needs your professional skills, compassion, and wisdom in this situation. At the same time you are confronted with your own uncertainties and fears about dying and death along with the irony that, no matter what you do, the end result for this patient will be death. Your part in making the remainder of life for a dying patient as rich and worthwhile as possible may be the motivation you will need to sustain that person and his or her loved ones.

REFERENCES

1. Albom M: *Tuesdays with Morrie*, New York, 1997, Doubleday.
2. Jack and the beanstalk (a traditional English fairy tale). In *The Arthur Rackham fairy book*, Philadelphia, 1950, Lippincott.
3. Hansel and Grethel (a Grimm's fairy tale). In *The Arthur Rackham fairy book*, Philadelphia, 1950, Lippincott.
4. Caldwell G: *Let's take the long way home*, New York, 2010, Random House.
5. Berg E: *The year of pleasures*, New York, 2005, Random House.

6. Brennan F: "Pain relief is a basic human right": the legal foundations of pain relief, *J Palliat Care* 20:236, 2004.
7. Kübler-Ross E: *On death and dying*, New York, 1969, Macmillan.
8. Burt RA: *Death is that man taking names: intersections of American medicine, law, and culture*, Berkeley, 2002, University of California Press.
9. Stoppard T: *Rosencrantz and Guildenstern are dead*, New York, 1967, Grove Press.
10. Balber PG: Stories of the living dying: the Hermes listener. In Corless I, Germino BB, Pittman MA, editors: *Dying death and bereavement: a challenge for living*, ed 2, New York, 2003, Springer Publishing.
11. Hodgson H, Krahn L: *Smiling through your tears: anticipatory grief*, North Charleston, South Carolina, 2005, Booksurge LLC, www.booksurge.com.
12. Veatch RM, Haddad A: *Veracity: dealing honestly with patients*, In *Case studies in pharmacy ethics* ed 2, New York, 2007, Oxford University Press.
13. Albertson SH: *Endings and beginnings*, New York, 1980, Random House.
14. Purtilo RB: Attention to caregivers and hope: overlooked aspects of ethics consultation, *J Clin Ethic* 17(4):358–363, 2006.
15. Surman O: *After Eden: a love story*, New York, 2005, iUniverse.
16. Teno JM, Clarridge BR, Casey V, et al: Family perspectives on end of life care at the last place of care, *JAMA* 291(1):88–92, 2004.
17. Field MJ, Cassel C, editors: *Approaching death: improving care at the end of life, National Academy of Medicine Report*, Washington, DC, 1997, National Academy Press.
18. Cassem NH: The caretakers. In Langone J, editor: *Vital signs: the way we die in America*, Boston, 1974, Little, Brown.

Respectful Interaction in Difficult Situations

CHAPTER OBJECTIVES

The reader will be able to:

- Identify three potential sources of difficulties that create barriers to respectful health professional and patient interaction
- Discuss how disparities in power within the relationship can lead to anger and frustration on the part of all involved
- Identify attributes and behaviors of patients, such as manipulative, sexually provocative, or aggressive behaviors, that may challenge the health professional's ideal of compassionate care
- Reflect on personal expectations of what it means to be a "good" health professional and how this affects interactions with patients
- Describe environmental factors that may contribute to difficulties in health professional and patient interaction
- List and evaluate guidelines for managing and, when possible, preventing difficult health professional and patient relationships

She asks for help and I have given it to her. She has been on various medications but nothing seems to work. She is a sad case really, and her anxiety seems to stem from a poor home environment. She gets anxious and then gets anxious about being anxious. I prescribe, but I know she will be back again in a short time. It would not be so bad if she tried to help herself.

I. Shaw[1]

Many health professionals view working with dying patients and their families as one of the greatest challenges they face in health care. However, as you read in Chapter 12, working with patients who are dying can sometimes be full of joy and sorrow. Even though you might experience loss and grief when a patient you have cared for dies, there is often also an accompanying sense of satisfaction that you were able to make his or her death a little easier, a little less painful, or less lonely. There are other patient care situations in which you will not come away with a sense of satisfaction, but one of profound frustration. This chapter focuses on difficulties inherent in the health professional and patient interaction that have not specifically been addressed elsewhere in this book or that bear reemphasizing. We suggest that you refer to Chapters 10 and 11 to review the content on establishing relatedness, recognizing boundaries, and creating professional closeness. You will need to use all of these insights and skills in your work with patients who challenge your conceptions of what it means to be a "good" health professional. Moreover, you will have an opportunity to think about other factors that can create great tension in the health professional and patient interaction, such as disparities in power and role expectations or an unsafe working environment that can cause harm to the health professional or patient. We devote this chapter to some summary statements about how to work more effectively with "difficult" patients and offer ways to effect change in "difficult" settings and situations.

Sources of Difficulties

Generally, when you enter a relationship with a patient, you have good reason to expect that things will go well, or if there are problems, you expect that they can be resolved. However, there are situations in which even your best efforts cannot make things right. When this happens, a common response is to look for a place to lay the blame. For example, you might wonder what else you could have done for the patient, or you might reason that the patient was not ready for treatment, or you may become defensive and decide that the patient was disruptive, noncompliant, maladjusted, or any number of other negative labels. Refer to the quote that opened the chapter regarding a patient who does not seem to be meeting the health professional's expectations for improvement. Especially note the last sentence indicating that the patient is at least partly to blame for the situation. Difficulty relating to a patient may originate in the health professional, in the interaction itself, or within the setting in which the interaction takes place.

Sources within the Health Professional

As emphasized throughout this book, you bring a wealth of experiences, education, prejudices, and values to your interaction with patients and their families. All of these factors can affect how you react to a particular patient. For example, recall the discussion on transference and countertransference in Chapter 10. A patient may remind you of your third-grade teacher whom you particularly feared and disliked. This past experience can arouse intense emotional reactions in the present relationship. In addition, your personality and how you deal with stress will play a large part in how you manage patient care situations that are interpersonally difficult.[2] In fact, your personality, more than your professional or demographic background, may explain why you react negatively to some patients and certain situations and have little difficulty with others.

For the health professional, the most reliable indicator of a negative emotional response is an unfavorable gut response or sense of discomfort in encounters with a particular patient.[3] If you are attuned to monitoring your feelings, then you can try to assess how much anger, fear, or guilt you bring to the interaction and try to manage those feelings before trying to manage the patient. After you identify the emotions you are experiencing, two questions often follow: "Why is this happening?" and "Where is this emotion coming from?"

Although it is a widely held belief, which has certainly been emphasized in this book, that health professionals should be nonjudgmental in their relationships with patients, it is a fact that we often find some patients more likable than others. More than 50 years ago, Highley and Norris[4] asked their nursing students to identify major "dislikes" related to working with patients. The types of patients the students said they disliked in 1957 can still be found in the clinical practice literature today. The students reported the following dislikes:

1. Patients who feel bad and complain after everything has been done for them
2. Patients who are not clean
3. Patients who will not do what the health professional asks them to do, will not cooperate, or will not obey the rules
4. Patients who are extremely demanding
5. Patients who can help themselves but insist on the health professional doing everything

The common denominator in these dislikes is that either the patients made the students feel guilty because of their dislike for the patients or, because they were never satisfied, the patients made the students feel inadequate as nurses. In general, patients who do not affirm the health professional's identity (i.e., accept and appreciate professional assistance) are considered bad patients. The patient's rejection of the health professional's help can easily be misread as rejection of the health professional. This rejection can take many forms, ranging from complaints to incessant demands, manipulative behavior, ingratitude, or basic noncompliance with advice or treatment.

Because this study was conducted in the 1950s, the students might not have mentioned some problems people are more self-consciously aware of today, such as patients who make sexually explicit remarks that cause embarrassment or aggressive patients who frighten or sometimes even threaten or physically harm health professionals.

These findings lead to another factor that is characteristic of health professionals and can cause difficulties in patient interactions: high expectations regarding the ability to help. As you progress through your program of study to become a health professional, the ideal is reinforced: You should be able to function effectively in all patient situations, and you are solely responsible for the success or failure of these interactions. This may not be what your teachers or we want to convey, but it is often what health professionals feel at the beginning of their careers. Thus, long before you have a full complement of skills with which to deal with difficult situations, you may blame yourself for failing to meet the needs of a challenging patient. Before jumping to self-blame for not meeting these unrealistic expectations, you need to recognize that many missteps occur before full competence is attained. Even then you should continue to work at establishing realistic expectations of yourself as a health professional.

Your perception of the patient's socioeconomic status can also influence your reactions to a patient. You are encouraged to review the content of Chapter 3 regarding appreciating differences and recognizing discrimination. A perceived difference in socioeconomic status can have a profound effect on the health professional and patient interaction. Papper noted:

> The very poor may be viewed as undesirable unrelated to their ability to pay. Even when the physician has genuine concern for the economically disadvantaged, he may because of his own background, unwittingly regard the extremely poor as different, with a flavor of inferiority included in the difference.[5]

Papper's personal observation of his medical colleagues was substantiated in a research study by Larson, who presented nurses with case studies in which the patient was identified as middle or lower class, with a more or less serious and more or less socially acceptable illness. The specific findings of Larson's study indicate that persons ranked as "lower class" regardless of other social variables were perceived as relatively passive, dependent, unintelligent, unmotivated, lazy, forgetful, noncomprehending, uninformed, inaccurate, unreliable, careless, and unsuccessful.[6] We return to the findings related to socially unacceptable illness later in this chapter because this also leads to the labeling of a patient as difficult or undesirable.

Socioeconomic differences between patient and health professional can surface in values about cleanliness. Most health professionals are from the middle or upper-middle class and hold certain values about cleanliness and other "correct" ways of being in the world. They are not only unfamiliar with the ways of poor people but may also hold them in disdain (Figure 13-1). Persons in lower socioeconomic groups may be so concerned about basic human needs, such as food and shelter, that they have little time or resources for luxuries such as bathing. It may appear that they do not care at all about cleanliness. Middle-class health professionals often,

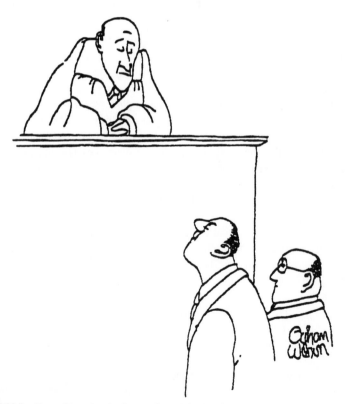

FIGURE 13-1: "You understand you're the sort of person I ordinarily wouldn't even speak to." (From Wilson G: Is nothing sacred? New York, 1982, St. Martin's Press.)

unconsciously, try to impose their values on patients concerning cleanliness. If neither the health professional nor the patient is aware of differences in socioeconomic status that generate values about bathing and hygiene, a struggle can ensue regarding cleanliness that is out of proportion to its importance in most patient care situations. Matters of hygiene are not the only issues that can escalate into battles with patients. Confrontation and power struggles should be avoided at all cost. Tactics for successful negotiation are outlined later in this chapter.

Sources within Interactions with Patients

What makes a patient "undesirable?" Patients who are overly demanding or who do not comply with treatment are generally labeled as problematic, as this family physician notes:

> Let's be blunt. It's hard to care for difficult patients. It's sometimes impossible to actually like them. This species of sick individuals tends to strain time, patience, and resources. They often generate a cascade of phone calls. They sometimes demand a heap of medically unnecessary tests. They occasionally refuse recommended treatment. Many have unreasonable expectations. Some whine and gripe incessantly. A few threaten to sue.[7]

Other types of behaviors that commonly elicit a negative response from health professionals are violence, anger, or self-harm behaviors such as substance abuse. Kelly and May[8] proposed a theoretical framework for the way health professionals conceptualize good and bad patients using an interactionist perspective. According to this view, patients come to be regarded as good or bad not because of anything inherent about them or in their behavior but as a consequence of the interactions between health professionals and patients. Patients are not passive recipients of care but active agents in the interaction process. Kelly and May explain that patients have the power to "influence, shape and reject professionals' attempts to impose a definition on their situation, with profound consequences for nurse-patient relations and the professional task."[8] Even though Kelly and May focused on the nurse-patient interaction, their framework appears applicable to all health professionals and their reaction to withholding affirmation for the health professionals' roles.

As you can see from the list of dislikes that the students in Highley and Norris's study generated, the focus of the dislike easily moved from dislike for the consequences of inappropriate or unacceptable behavior to dislike for the patient. For example, patients with illnesses that are socially unacceptable are often labeled as difficult even if their behavior is a model of compliance. People with addictive disorders such as alcoholism or drug abuse are often viewed as unacceptable or bad patients. Even if a health professional views alcoholism as a disease rather than a behavior a patient should be able to control, the patient who has a problem with alcohol is commonly rejected by most professional personnel.[9] Patients who appear to be responsible in some way for their illness or injury, such as obese patients or smokers, are also labeled as less worthy of respect than patients who are "blameless" for their present health condition. All of these patients have one thing in common: Either because of the nature of their health problems or the way they respond to the health professionals involved in their care and treatment, they withhold the legitimation that makes health professionals feel good about who they are and what they do.

Thus, a large part of the label a patient receives depends on our role expectations of patients in general and of patients with specific characteristics. One of the most basic expectations of patients is compliance with agreed-upon treatment. Noncompliance is largely viewed in health care literature as a problem to be resolved. The problem is located in irrational patient beliefs that contradict scientific evidence or in patients' lack of knowledge or understanding.[10] Thus, we assume patients are not following medical advice because they do not understand or have some misconception that prevents them from understanding. Major efforts, then, are directed toward getting patients to understand so that they will comply. An alternative view of noncompliance implicates the social context of patients' lives as follows, "Within this alternative social view, it cannot be assumed that noncompliance is simply a matter of patients choosing not to follow advice. Instead, it is recognized that choice may be severely constrained by the social circumstances in which patients live their lives."[10]

If health professionals approach the problem of noncompliance by trying to understand the factors in patients' lives that mediate their cooperation, then efforts can be made to change those factors that are amenable to change or adjust treatment to meet the reality of a patient's life.

Sources in the Environment

As we noted specifically in Chapters 8 and 9, the health professional and patient interaction takes place in a particular context. At times the context can be the source of difficulty in an interaction. For example, if the environment is strange and frightening, the patient or health professional may react in a fearful or angry manner. For many patients, a health care facility can be an extremely threatening place. Taken in this context, even a simple activity such as bathing can be viewed as menacing. Rader noted that for a person with apraxia (inability to execute purposeful, learned motor acts despite the physical ability and willingness to do so), agnosia (inability to recognize a tactile or visible stimulus despite being able to recognize the elemental sensation), and aphasia (loss of language function either in comprehension or expression of words)—symptoms often found in patients who have had a cerebrovascular accident—the standard nursing home bathing experience may be perceived as horrific. Consider these limitations, and place yourself in the patient's position.

> A person the resident does not recognize comes into her room, wakens her, says something she does not understand, drags her out of bed, and takes off her clothes. Then the resident is moved down a public corridor on something that resembles a toilet seat, covered only with a thin sheet so that her private parts are exposed to the breeze. Calls for help are ignored or greeted with, "Good morning." Then she is taken to a strange, cold room that looks like a car wash, the sheet is ripped off, and she is sprayed in the face with cold and then scalding water. Continued calls for help go unheeded. Her most private parts are touched by a stranger. In another context this would be assault.[11]

An environment can be equally strange and intolerable to the health professional. For example, we have noted in other chapters that, in community health practice, health professionals may go into the unknown realm of the patient's living environment. One of us recalls a home visit to a small, run-down house literally butted up against the back fence of the holding pens for cattle at the stock market. The smell of manure was overwhelming both outside and inside the house. The elderly woman who lived there (and the subject of the home visit for management of diabetes) seemed oblivious to the odor. In fact, she had just finished hanging a load of clean sheets on the line to dry in her tiny backyard!

Similar stresses can arise in a hectic and crisis-ridden environment. Patients who are kept waiting in an overcrowded emergency department or office are more likely to be frustrated and hostile to health professionals when they are finally seen. Understaffing often leaves health professionals feeling frustrated and dissatisfied as they attempt to meet the needs of too many patients with too little time and resources. Overworked staffs worry about the effect of stretching themselves too thin and the impact this can have on patient care. The physical and psychological exhaustion resulting from excessive professional demands that can drain you have been aptly dubbed "compassion fatigue."[12]

Other environmental factors that make care difficult include the aesthetics of a space, crowding, and climate. One of us worked in a large acute care pediatric setting during the hottest months of the year with no air conditioning. As the temperature rose during the day, so did everyone's irritability; children cried more easily, and co-workers snapped at each other for the slightest offense. Only with the setting of the sun and the resultant drop in temperature did the atmosphere on the unit cool down as well.

Disparities of Power

We have noted several times in this book that patients are placed in a position of diminished power upon entering the health care environment. The content in Chapter 6 specifically discusses numerous losses that patients face because of illness or trauma: Independence, social status and responsibility, and expressions of identity are often taken away from people upon entering a health care institution, and all of these factors contribute to feelings of powerlessness. A common reaction to powerlessness is anger, and a common target of anger is the most accessible and least-threatening health professional involved with the patient.[13] Thus, students are often the target for a torrent of rage from a patient that has little to do with the student or his or her abilities. Few studies have explored patients' perceptions of this inequity in power, but in one study of mental health workers and patients, both groups reported an awareness of the struggle to gain or retain power and control. Patients noted that when health professionals demonstrated respect, took time with them, and were willing to give them some control and choice in their own care, feelings of anger were reduced.[14]

Role Expectations

Because we are socialized not to use negative terms such as "bad," we substitute euphemisms to describe patients with the attributes listed earlier: They are described as disruptive, unmotivated, regressed, maladaptive, and manipulative. Patients who are perceived to be difficult to treat evoke intense negative-affective responses in the health professional that can work against establishing a positive, constructive relationship.[15] Furthermore, there is also a strong possibility that the professional's language exerts a powerful impact on thought and, consequently, action. Negative words lead to negative thoughts and actions regarding difficult patients. An example from rehabilitation medicine highlights the impact of language.

Most rehabilitation staff members have encountered patients who resist their best efforts to engage them in therapeutic activities. These patients seem to not want to be in rehabilitation. They may view therapies as trivial, irrelevant, uninteresting, or too demanding, and they must be constantly coaxed to attend therapy sessions; if they do attend, they do not participate. Staff members become quickly frustrated with patients who do not share the "rehabilitation perspective" that places a high premium on attaining maximal independent functioning. The patient's lack of involvement produces slow progress, proving the patient's point that therapy is valueless. This further antagonizes staff members who, feeling professionally and personally offended, may diminish their efforts to engage the patient, thus producing a hostile standoff and virtually guaranteeing therapeutic failure. This is the fate of the "unmotivated" patient.[16]

Any patient behavior that is inconsistent with expected patient role behavior (read "good patient behavior") could negatively influence the care of the patient. Not only might you be tempted to diminish your efforts in the care of a difficult patient, but you might also resort to distancing yourself from the patient. Unfortunately, avoidance and distancing may result in the reinforcement of deviant behavior as a patient response to nonsupportive care. In extreme cases, health professionals have been known to respond to difficult patients with their own version of negative behavior. In a study of nurses by Podrasky and Sexton,[17] vignettes describing a variety of negative patient behaviors were used to elicit the following responses describing actions these professionals would take or would like to take, including, "I have to keep myself from hauling off and whacking her one," "I would restrain her just a little bit too tight," and "I'd make her stay in the wet bed for a long while." More profound and perhaps life-threatening consequences can result from a health professional's negative reactions to a patient. In a national study of transplant coordinators, a full 62% revealed a belief that a hostile or antagonistic patient should not receive an organ transplantation.[18] The irony and tragedy in such findings are that expressions of anger and frustration (behavior that can be labeled as *hostile*) may be a natural response by patients to chronic illness.

Most health professionals are able to control these kinds of strong emotional reactions and continue, at least marginally, to meet their obligations to the patient. The result is a sort of "grudging attention" (i.e., the patient gets the minimal care that he or she needs and nothing more). Grudging attention occurs because of a combination of factors. Once a negative label is attached to a patient, it is difficult for health professionals to look past it and process other data about the patient. Negative labels often get "passed on" until a patient develops a bad reputation.[19] It is as if we see only one aspect of the patient. Couple these stereotypes about the difficult patient with idealistic role expectations of health professionals as caring, nonjudgmental, and capable of reaching every patient, and the result is an interaction devoid of everything but going through the motions.

Although it is important to work toward the goals of acceptance and constructive problem-solving, sometimes the only solution is to do what you must for the patient and then leave. This is exactly what happened in the case of a sexually aggressive patient who made lewd propositions and repeatedly exposed himself to his caregivers. The health professionals in this case responded with grudging attention as follows:

> By now Mr. Leland was getting only the absolute necessities—no extras. After all, who wants to sit down and chat with someone who talks about nothing but his sex life—or yours? Once our professional responsibilities were met, we avoided Mr. Leland. He couldn't fail to notice this, and as a result his demands for attention become angrier and more disruptive.[20]
>
> ▶ If you were assigned to care for Mr. Leland and he continued to talk explicitly about sex after you asked him not to, what would be your next step?
> ▶ What are some possible negative outcomes of "grudging attention"?

Going through the minimal motions of care is a temporary, and not very effective, solution to a much larger problem. Often it results in guilt on the part of the health professional and can result, as in the case of Mr. Leland, in an escalation of the behavior that led to avoidance in the first place. Although the following quote refers to nurses, the same can be applied to all health professions: "If patients interpret a nurse's manner as uninterested, or if they overhear pejorative comments, they fear that they won't be cared for adequately. It's as valuable to examine staff's behaviors as it is to understand a patient's motivations."[21]

Difficult Health Professional and Patient Relationships

In this section, we introduce you to two patients who share some of the attributes that have been identified as undesirable or difficult by most health professionals. As you examine some of the character traits and behaviors of the two patients and the nature of the relationships with health professionals, perhaps you will gain insight into your own values and attitudes and begin to prepare yourself for how you will respond.

Working with Patients Who Are Self-Destructive

Sometimes the most difficult patient is not the one who commits actions that are outrageous or inappropriate but who shrinks from constructive action and resorts to self-harm behavior such as that encountered in the case of Violet Mercer and Tina Kramolisch.

Tina Kramolisch worked evenings and weekends in a busy, urban emergency department as a technician while she finished her last year of professional preparation. Tina often commented to classmates that you really do not have a taste for what it is like in practice without the experiences you find in an emergency department. In fact, Tina felt as if she had seen it all and was quite proud of her ability to work with different types of patients in various levels of distress. However, after taking care of Violet Mercer, Tina wondered if she was ready to care for all types of patients.

Tina entered the holding area where Violet lay absolutely still on the examination cart under a sheet. When Tina said Violet's name, there was no response, so Tina gently touched the woman's arm. Violet flinched so violently at the touch that it startled Tina as well and she jumped back from the cart. Tina was even more shocked at how Violet looked. Violet murmured, "You scared me." The words were somewhat difficult to understand as Violet's lips were swollen and split in one corner. Violet had lacerations, contusions, and swelling all over her face. Tina had never seen anyone so badly beaten. Tina noticed old bruises and injuries all over Violet's body as she conducted her intake assessment. Tina knew the physician would have to confirm her observation, but she was almost certain that several of Violet's ribs were fractured.

Because Tina had been trained to work with women who had been abused, she knew the right questions to ask and did so. Violet admitted, cautiously, that her husband, Donnie, had lost his temper and done this to her. Tina reported her findings to the nurse and physician, and they set into motion the services and protection the health care and criminal justice systems can offer battered women. In fact, Donnie was being treated down the hall for a scalp laceration that Violet had inflicted as she tried to defend herself. The police who brought both of the Mercers into the emergency department were waiting outside Donnie's room to see if Violet would press charges. Tina was holding Violet's hand as the rib binder was put into place when the nurse entered the room and said, "The social worker can take you to the women's shelter after you talk to the police." Violet did not look up as she said in a flat voice, "I've changed my mind. I don't want to press no charges. I'm going with Donnie." Tina was speechless as she watched every effort to change Violet's mind fail. Tina felt hot tears of frustration and anger run down her cheeks as she watched Violet and Donnie walk out of the emergency department arm-in-arm.

▷ Why do you think Tina felt a combination of frustration and anger with Violet?
▷ What would your reaction be?

In this case, Violet is compliant and willing to accept professional intervention—to a point. In Violet's case, the perception of difficulty rests to some extent on the invalidating effects of Violet's behavior on Tina and the other health professionals caring for her. In the eyes of the professionals, intervention in Violet's case should include more than merely suturing her cuts and bandaging her broken ribs; it should also include offering her a way out of an abusive, potentially life-threatening situation. When Violet fails to accept the help that is offered to her, the primary treatment goal is thwarted and the health professional's role as a therapeutic agent is invalidated.

Working with Patients with a History of Violent Behavior

Many health professionals feel inadequately prepared to deal with patients who have a complex medical condition that is complicated further by a history of violent behavior. The case of Darrin Block and Austin Greder involves a seriously ill patient and behavior that is generally unacceptable in an acute care institution.

Darrin Block was an orderly on the step-down unit at an urban medical center. Because of the medical center's location in a large city, the intensive care unit got more than its fair share of victims of gunshot wounds. Most of these patients were African-American, male, young, and unemployed and knew their assailants. Many were members of gangs and had to be admitted under aliases for their own protection. Austin Greder fit this description exactly. He was a 21-year-old high school dropout who had been shot by a rival gang member. Although he lacked formal education, Austin was bright. His major sources of support were his mother and a girlfriend. He was admitted to the surgical intensive care unit in serious condition but had begun to recover, so he was moved to a medical/surgical step-down unit. His wound was not healing as well as the treatment team expected. Since his admission to the step-down unit, the staff had referred to Austin and his numerous visitors as "nothing but trouble." Large numbers of visitors moved in a steady stream in and out of Austin's room, even though the staff had told them about the restrictions on visitors in the unit. Austin's girlfriend, Alicia, had practically taken up residence in Austin's room. One time, Darrin walked into Austin's room and found him and Alicia involved in what appeared to be sexual activity. Darrin left in confused embarrassment but was somewhat angry, too. He did not expect to walk in on a sexual encounter and did not believe he should have to apologize. After this incident, Darrin asked Alicia to leave whenever he entered the room to provide care. In response, Austin became angry and abusive to Darrin, refusing to let him perform wound care and asking for one of the other staff members to care for him. To make matters worse, Austin told one of his friends what his alias was even though this undermined maintenance of security on the unit. Darrin believed that the right thing to do was set limits on Austin's behavior because things were clearly getting out of control. However, he was fearful of retaliation by Austin's friends outside of the safety of the hospital. He had heard more than one other staff member talk about being confronted in the parking garage by one of "these gang members."
▶ Put yourself in Darrin Block's position. What would you do the next time the patient refused wound care?
▶ What resources might there be in the hospital to assist Darrin in working with Mr. Greder?

These patients challenge the notion of what it means to be a "good" health professional. They make us realize that, although we are generally able to effectively help patients, sometimes we fall far short even with our best efforts. Various techniques may help you in working with difficult patients of all types, and we also share some ideas about changing a difficult working environment.

Showing Respect in Difficult Situations

When patients are uncooperative, manipulative, or angry, or they reject help, this is not a license to show disrespect toward them as persons. You will have to be responsive to your own feelings of disgust, fear, anger, and so forth, as well as manage patients' unacceptable behavior. An appropriate place to start is to show respect by initially refusing to believe that you are dealing with a person whose character is flawed. The behaviors and attitudes may be the result of a treatable or modifiable factor. For example, one of your first determinations is to make certain that the patient has received a thorough, understandable explanation of the treatment or therapy in question. The patient may also be unmotivated or uncooperative if he or she has not been shown the respect of participation in establishing personally meaningful goals. After these more obvious problem areas are explored and resolved and problems still persist, you can turn to the following types of behaviors that have been found to be effective in working with difficult patients.

As a general rule for all types of difficult situations, structure and consistency in communication in every aspect of patient care are important.[22] A key component of a deliberate, consistent approach is "setting limits." Setting firm limits is a part of setting boundaries with all patients but with additional safeguards given the extremity of the situation. By setting forth clear, consistent expectations in a nondefensive manner, you can help strengthen the patient's inner control. Be open to negotiation. Listen for opportunities to find out what is important to the patient.

However, when you are involved in setting limits, respect for the patient must govern. You should ask yourself whether the limits you are setting are arbitrary—that is, do they stem from your need to be in control or to punish the patient—or whether the patient's welfare would indeed be best served by establishing external limits. Any plan to set limits should be agreed upon by all members of the health care team to avoid the potential for a patient to "split" the staff (i.e., divide staff into all good or all bad). To avoid division of the staff, good communication lines between all members of the team are essential. For example, the patient may use charm and flattery to manipulate some staff members but make disparaging and critical comments about their coworkers.[23]

It is also helpful to focus on a patient's unacceptable behaviors rather than on the patient himself or herself. This allows for open communication and avoids negative labeling that tends to stick to patients and obscure the real problem. One way to avoid negative labeling of patients is to be honest with them and tell them exactly how you feel. Again, your honest comments should be directed at the patient's behavior and not at the patient. This way you can share your reactions and still not humiliate the patient. Look for opportunities to give plenty of positive feedback for desired behaviors. Also, focus on the here and now rather than long-term aspects of behavior. If all else fails, a behavioral contract can be developed to focus on specific actions. A contract, sometimes called a *patient care agreement,* "outlines the expectations, plans, and responsibilities of the patient and the consequences for noncompliance."[22]

On a broader basis, you can encourage the development of an environment that is respectful of everyone. Such a setting encourages patients to ask questions and challenge the system's rules and practices. If just a single member of the health care team prompts the patient legitimately to question his or her care, the rest of the team could come to see the patient as "difficult." Having patients ask about the care they receive and make decisions about their care must be considered the normal, desired state. The safety of health professionals should also be encouraged in a respectful environment. There must be practices and policies in place to give staff members basic protection from harassment, abuse, and so forth. You may find yourself in an environment that is amenable to change through education and support for staff. In fact, the support of supervisory staff in the form of validation and insight is an essential component of an environment that fosters positive health professional and patient interactions.

In summary, here are general guidelines for showing respect toward difficult patients, keeping in touch with your own values, and making the system more responsive to both:

1. Avoid the use of derogatory labels as a means of reducing your frustration or anger.
2. Remember that the caring function is as important as other interventions. Make an empathetic statement such as, "I know you must be frustrated or disappointed." This kind of response tells the patient that you understand there is a problem and are sympathetic, which allows the patient to be less defensive.[24]
3. Set realistic expectations of your own power as a health professional to force compliance.
4. Do not expect to change aspects of the patient's situation beyond your control.
5. Take care of your emotional well-being. Select a time to talk to the patient when you are able to be a good listener. Do not try to tackle problems when you are overly tired or busy with other concerns.
6. Try to help change the underlying social and institutional conditions or attitudes that lead to devaluing behavior by health professionals.
7. When interacting with an aggressive patient, "ensure that exit is possible for both you and the patient; monitor your body language and tone of voice; avoid pointing your index finger or putting your hands on your hips in a threatening stance; avoid sarcasm or loudness."[20]
8. Work to affirm policies and practices that encourage the respect of everyone while ensuring their physical and emotional safety.

Although all of your efforts as a health professional should be directed at acknowledging negative biases and keeping them in check, you may find that you cannot operate in the best interest of a given patient, no matter how much you try. If it comes to letting a patient go, be certain that you are referring him or her to a capable professional and not abandoning the person. Respect includes everybody, but as humans we come in all shapes and forms, so the wise health professional recognizes that difficulties with patients and situations will arise.

An additional difficult situation that is unfortunately all too common in health care is dealing with errors in patient care, whether they are the result of individual mistakes or lack of attention to details or system-level problems. Actually, all errors include challenges between the individual health professional and patient involved, as well as within the broader system in which the error occurred.

Professionals' Mistakes and Making Apology

In recent years, a significant literature in the health professions has emerged on the topic of the response of health professionals to a patient when a mistake related to the patient's care is made by individual professionals or due to a systems error in the health care institution. The number of deaths and serious injuries that occur in the United States each year alone is staggering. One major report estimated about 200,000 deaths per year.[25] Errors that have serious negative consequences for the patient must be disclosed to the patient or his or her family, and appropriate restitution must be made. However, disclosure of an error is generally difficult for health professionals.

Reasons why disclosure of errors to a patient and his or her family is so difficult for health professionals are numerous. One reason is that health professionals often believe that they are immune to error, so they find it difficult to admit that an error has occurred. The second reason it is so difficult to disclose an error is that it is seen as a sign of failure. Third, until recently there have been few mechanisms in place for health professionals to talk freely with peers about the circumstances surrounding an error because of shame and irrational legal fears. Finally, disclosing an error to a patient and following the disclosure by apologizing requires a great deal of humility and skill on the part of the health professional. The case of Melanie Lieberman, RN, and Laura Keenan deals with the various facets of disclosure of an error that resulted in harm to the patient.

It was an exceptionally busy night on the medical/surgical floor where Melanie Lieberman worked. To make matters worse, one of the nurses called in sick at the last moment and the supervisor was unable to get a replacement for the first 4 hours of the 7 PM to 7 AM shift. Melanie had to take care of twice the number of patients that she usually would during the beginning of the shift, the busiest time during the 12 hours she would be on duty. One of the patients under Melanie's care was Laura Keenan, who returned to the unit in the late afternoon from surgery for a mastectomy and breast reconstruction. Melanie was able to manage a full assessment of Laura at the beginning of the shift, but after that she was on a dead run with medications, dressing changes, pages, and phone calls from physicians for new orders on a transfer from the emergency department, etc. When Melanie sped past Laura's room, she did look in once or twice to affirm that the patient was resting quietly but she did not have time to complete a more thorough assessment. When the replacement nurse finally arrived at 11 PM, Melanie offered up a quick report to her colleague on the patients he would assume responsibility for the rest of the shift and then went straight to Laura's room. Melanie realized after taking her blood pressure and pulse that something was wrong. A quick look at the dressings covering the reconstruction indicated that Laura was bleeding and likely suffering from hypovolemic shock. Melanie knew that the most common postoperative problem for breast reconstruction patients was bleeding and she had not checked for the most obvious signs of this complication. As Melanie rushed to contact the surgeon and supervisor, Laura's vital signs indicated worsening shock. Melanie increased the rate of the IV and reinforced the dressing, all the while mentally berating herself for missing such an obvious problem. She knew she was overstretched but thought she could handle the workload. Now her lack of monitoring for a predictable problem was going to require another trip to the operating room for Laura and perhaps life-threatening consequences if they did not get the bleeding stopped fast enough. As if things were not bad enough, Melanie knew that she would have to talk to Laura's family and explain what happened. She dreaded this more than anything. Nothing like this had ever happened to Melanie before.

▶ Review the case and indicate where you think the error of lack of monitoring could have been prevented. In other words, would you have handled the situation differently than Melanie given the same set of circumstances?
▶ What are the system-level problems that contributed to the error?
▶ What are the individual-level issues that contributed to the error?

The type of error in the case of Melanie Lieberman and Laura Keenan is a combination of the failure of the individual, in this case the nurse, to meet basic standards of postoperative care and system-level problems including staffing issues. In order to prevent errors from occurring in the future, health professionals must view errors as a learning opportunity that is different from the "shame-and-blame culture that focuses only on individual responsibility or culpability."[26]

Clearly, Melanie's error is not uncommon. Neither is her reaction to the expectations of negotiating the rough terrain of owning up to her share of the responsibility and disclosing what happened in a manner that is meaningful to the patient and her family. However, there are more and more tools and systems to support the health professional when an error occurs and break the silence surrounding such events in clinical practice.

SUMMARY

This chapter makes suggestions about respectful interaction with types of patients whom many health professionals find difficult to treat without negative feelings or behaviors intruding on the relationship. Sources may be the patient's personality and behavior, societal stereotypes, your own countertransference and learned behaviors, or the opinions of your peers. The environment in which the relationship takes place can also cause difficulties and add to frustration, anger, and other negative responses by both parties. The environment often plays a significant role in one of the most difficult health professional and patient situations, the occurrence of an error and its aftermath. Despite such challenges, your responsibility to show respect for the patient as a person remains and can be expressed through attempts to use behaviors that provide an opportunity to minimize the negative aspects of the relationship.

REFERENCES

1. Shaw I: Doctors, "dirty work" patients, and "revolving doors, " *Qual Health Res* 14(8):1032–1045, 2004.
2. Santamaria N: The relationship between nurses' personality and stress levels reported when caring for interpersonally difficult patients, *Aust J Adv Nurs* 18(2):20–26, 2000.
3. Herbert CP, Seifert MH: When the patient is the problem, *Patient Care* 24(1):59, 1990.
4. Highley BL, Norris CM: When a student dislikes a patient, *Am J Nurs* 57(9):1163, 1957.
5. Papper S: The undesirable patient, *J Chron Dis* 22:777, 1970.
6. Larson PA: Nurse perceptions of patient characteristics, *Nurs Res* 26(6):416–420, 1977.
7. Miksanek T: On caring for "difficult" patients, *Health Affairs* 27(5):1422–1428, 2008.
8. Kelly MP, May D: Good and bad patients: a review of the literature and a theoretical critique, *J Adv Nurs* 7:147–156, 1982.
9. Harlow PE, Goby MJ: Changing nursing students' attitudes toward alcoholic patients: examining effects of a clinical practicum, *Nurs Res* 29(1):59–60, 1980.
10. Russell S, Daly J, Hughes E, op't Hoog C: Nurses and "difficult" patients: negotiating non-compliance, *J Adv Nurs* 43(3):281–287, 2003.
11. Rader J: To bathe or not to bathe: that is the question, *J Gerontol Nurs* 20(9):53, 1994.
12. Leon AM, Altholz JAS, Dziegielewski SF: Compassion fatigue: considerations for working with the elderly, *J Gerontol Soc Work* 32(1):43–62, 1999.
13. Staples P, Baruth P, Jefferies M, Warder L: Empowering the angry patient, *Can Nurse* 90(4):28–30, 1994.
14. Breeze JA, Repper J: Struggling for control: the care experiences of "difficult" patients in mental health services, *J Adv Nurs* 28(6):1301–1311, 1998.
15. Gallop R, Lancee W, Shugar G: Residents' and nurses' perceptions of difficult-to-treat short-stay patients, *Hosp Comm Psychiatry* 44(4):352, 1993.
16. Caplan B, Shechter J: Reflections on the "depressed," "unrealistic," "inappropriate," "manipulative," "unmotivated," "noncompliant," "denying," "maladjusted," "regressed," etc. patient, *Arch Phys Med Rehabil* 74(October):1123, 1993.
17. Podrasky DL, Sexton DL: Nurses' reactions to difficult patients, *Image J Nurs Sch* 20(1):19, 1988.
18. Neil JA, Corley MC: Hostility toward caregivers as a selection criterion for transplantation, *Prog Transplant* 10(3):177–181, 2000.
19. Juliana CA, Orehowsky S, Smith-Regojo P, et al: Interventions by staff nurses to manage "difficult" patients, *Holist Nurs Pract* 11(4):1–26, 1997.
20. Stockard S: Caring for the sexually aggressive patient: you don't have to blush and bear it, *Nursing* 21(11):72, 1991.
21. Nield-Anderson L, Minarik PA, Dilworth JM, et al: Responding to the "difficult" patient: manipulation, sexual provocation, aggression—how can you manage such behaviors? *Am J Nurs* 99(12):26–34, 1999.
22. Morrison EF, Ramsey A, Synder B: Managing the care of complex, difficult patients in the medical-surgical setting, *Medsurg Nursing* 9(1):21–26, 2000.
23. Daum AL: The disruptive antisocial patient: management strategies, *Nurs Manage* 25(8):49, 1994.
24. Baum NH: 12 tips for dealing with difficult patients, *Geriatrics* 57(11):55–56, 2002.
25. Kohn KT, Corrigen JM, Donaldson MS, editors: *To err is human: building a safer health system,* Committee on Quality of Health Care in America, Washington, DC, 1999, National Academy Press.
26. Woods A, Doan Johnson S: Executive summary: toward a taxonomy of nursing practice errors, *Nurs Manage* 32(10):45, 2002.

PART SIX

Questions for Thought and Discussion

1. You are in a patient's room performing a procedure. The patient, who has a type of cancer that is always fatal, has been told of his condition. While you are there, a man visiting a patient in the next bed begins to describe the horror of his wife's last days before she died of cancer. Your patient becomes increasingly tense and finally begins to sob.

   a. What can you do to console or reassure this patient?

   b. How could you have helped to prevent this situation?

   c. Should you report this incident? To whom and why?

2. You are working in an outpatient clinic in an economically depressed area of the city. A disheveled woman comes in dragging three young children behind her. One of the children begins to whine that she is hot. You are in the receiving area and see the woman hit the child so hard that the child falls to the floor and begins to scream. The woman looks at you in panic. You are already late for your next appointment. Your next patient is anxiously waiting to be seen and looks with scorn at the woman and you.

   a. What feelings does this scene trigger?

   b. You probably think there are some things you should do in this situation, but what would you really like to do?

   c. What does this teach you about the possible difference between your emotional and "professional" reaction to this extreme situation?

3. What types of patient care situations make you (or, if you are still a student, do you *think* will make you) the most uncomfortable? Identify two or three concrete interventions you would take to effectively deal with the situations you identified.

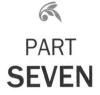

PART SEVEN

Respectful Interaction across the Life Span

Having studied the basic foundational pieces of respectful interaction, you now have an opportunity to apply your learning to several types of patients you will see in the course of your professional career. We have chosen to address them by age group, over the life span, being mindful that individual differences often outweigh the similarities we are emphasizing in these different cohorts.

Life span development encompasses constancy and change in an individual's behavior throughout the life span. Development is not bound by a single criteria—it is multidimensional and multidirectional. Any process of development entails aspects of growth (gain) and decline (loss), and these relate to an individual's adaptive capacity. Each lifetime also presents different paths. Often illness or disability takes patients and families down an unfamiliar path. Your role as a health professional is to help these individuals navigate that path, adjusting and adapting along life's journey.

Part Seven begins with Chapter 14, highlighting the challenges and joys of working with newborns, infants, toddlers, and preschoolers. Understandably, the family is a key element of consideration for these age groups. Chapter 15 moves the focus of your attention to school-age children and adolescents.

In Chapter 16 we discuss your interaction with people who become patients during young and middle adulthood. Only in recent times have these life periods been given more than a cursory glance, and we share some of the insights that researchers and others are finding.

Chapter 17 examines key issues related to working with older adults. Of all age groups this one is increasing more in diversity and size worldwide than any other population.

Throughout the life span, the person who becomes a patient is faced with many of the challenges we have been discussing so far. Injury and/or illness can disrupt a person's life patterns and development, challenging the acquisition of "normal" life skills. You have a substantial role in respectfully helping your client meet these challenges.

Respectful Interaction: Working with Newborns, Infants, Toddlers, and Preschoolers

CHAPTER OBJECTIVES

The reader will be able to:

- Discuss the role of the family as collaborators in respectful interaction with newborns, infants, toddlers, and preschoolers
- Identify five realms of family health that can lend insight into family and patient dynamics
- Make several suggestions that will help support healthy functioning of the family during a child's illness
- Distinguish some basic developmental differences that need to be considered in one's approach to newborns, infants, toddlers, and preschoolers
- Discuss in general terms Erikson's sequential view of the psychological development of infants and toddlers
- List some everyday needs of the infant that may help explain an infant's response to the health professional
- Describe the steps showing how a consistent approach usually builds trust in an interaction with infant patients
- Describe six types of play, and show how each can facilitate respectful interaction with a pediatric patient
- Describe how the young child's developing need for autonomy enters into the health professional and patient relationship

I mean, this is not, you know, a piece of machinery that . . . we want to make work. It's, it's a child and he, you've got all those dynamics of mom and dad, and grandma, and brothers and sisters. And, and you know, all of those things need to be, are, are just as important, just as important as whether that kid is breathing or not. . . . Part of the recovery of the child depends on, and their future depends on, dealing with these issues, too. Because of the attachment that the family has for that child.

—Pinch and Spielman[1]

All health professionals will interact with newborn, infant, toddler, and preschool patients at some time, and some health professionals will work solely with these groups. These small patients must be treated with the respect they deserve as unique individuals like everyone else. Furthermore, the opportunity they are given to experience human dignity and support in their time of illness, injury, or other adversity can become a resource to help them manage future difficulties.

Most of us take for granted that a newborn will live into his or her 7th or 8th decade of life. This has not always been so and is presently not so in many developing countries. Today, the average infant mortality rate is 6.14 infant deaths per 1000 live births.[2] However, the overall infant mortality rate is not shared equally by all groups. Mortality is higher for infants and children in poor families with poor living conditions. The mortality rate for black infants is more than twice that for white infants. Better opportunities for health education and overall longevity in white groups point to deep, internal health disparities, the consequences of which must be reckoned with. As a health professional you will need to call on your skills and knowledge to reach solutions that help close the disparities gap. Being more aware of cultural issues and unconscious biases can enhance the delivery of quality, nondiscriminatory health care.[3]

This is the first of several chapters that will examine your interaction with patients across the lifespan. It begins with the family as a focus of care and then moves to working with new parents and newborns, infants, and toddlers. The section on growth and development includes information that applies across childhood and adolescence as well, although working with each age group has its own challenges. Provided here is a wide range of relevant topics concerning interaction with young patients that should provide a basis for more in-depth exploration in your other coursework during your professional education.

Human Development and Family

In the past, mainstream health care in the United States focused exclusively on the patient as the sole recipient of care. It was not commonplace to attend to families as the focus of care. Today we know how important it is to care for patients, especially children, in the context of their families: The family is implicitly and explicitly recognized as a critical context surrounding and influencing its members and, in turn, being influenced by its members. We will begin by discussing the evolving concept of "family" in contemporary society. If you are to work with families as collaborators in maintaining the health of children and in the care of ill, injured, or disabled family members, then you must understand how families define themselves, how they function, and how best to interact with them.

Family: An Evolving Concept

The term *family* has been defined in a variety of ways. How would you define family? It is safe to say that your notion of what constitutes a family is influenced by your values, culture, upbringing, and professional perspective. For example, a sociologist may define a family in terms of its socioeconomic status, or a psychologist may focus on the interpersonal dynamics of individuals who claim family ties. The most common type of familial bond is through spousal and blood relationships. Families may include several generations of blood kin, a mix of stepparents and children, or a combination of friends who share in household responsibilities and childrearing. However, none of these definitions is sufficient to describe the types of relationships and arrangements that make up the modern family. One area of growth in family units is same-gendered parents with adopted children. As society evolves through scientific and social advances, it must redefine what is meant by "family." The Institute for Patient and Family Centered Care (IPFCC) defines family as "two or more persons who are related biologically, legally, or emotionally."[4]

⊚ REFLECTIONS

- How do you define family? Who are the members of your family?
- Name two ways your family contributes to your health and two ways your family distracts from your health
- If you were acutely ill, which member of your family would you call first and why? How does this family member support you in your day-to-day life?

A definition of family should be inclusive and allow the members of a family to define themselves as a family unit, acknowledging the variety of cultural styles, values, and alternative structures that are part of contemporary family life. In fact, families define a unique culture; that is, a unique behavioral complex that is socially created, readily transmitted to family members, and potentially maintained through generations.[5]

Family structure and function have an important influence on health. Family structure involves the characteristics that make a family unique. This includes family composition and household roles. For example, in one family the parents may be married and living together, whereas in another, the parents may be unmarried and living separately. Some families have two working parents; others have one. According to the U.S. Census Bureau's America's Families and Living Arrangements: 2010, the average household size was 2.59. The percentage of households headed by a married couple who had children younger than 18 living with them was 21%. Of the 74.6 million children younger than 18 in 2011, 69% lived with two parents, whereas another 27% lived with one parent and 4% lived with no parents.[6] Among the children who lived with one parent, 87% lived with their mother. In 2010, 10% of children lived in a household with a grandparent and 23% of children lived in a household with a stay-at-home mom. Of note is that the percentage of children living with two parents varied by race and origin—78% of Asian children lived with two parents compared with 38% of black children.[7]

To work with families, you also must understand how families function. A child's physical and emotional health and cognitive/social functioning is strongly influenced by how well the family functions.[8] There are numerous family theories describing how families operate and how they respond to events both internal and external. Most health professionals use a combination of family theories in their work with children and their families, but all have in common the fact that the focus of health care shifts from the individual member who is ill, injured, or disabled to the family as a unit of care. In this chapter we focus on a particular method of viewing the family—the family health system approach.[9] According to this approach, care is directed toward five processes: (1) interactive, (2) developmental, (3) coping, (4) integrity, and (5) health. The story of Ian will help you by showing how the family health system model applies to a particular child and his family.

Ian was a low-birth-weight infant with short bowel syndrome. Short bowel syndrome is characterized by maldigestion, malabsorption, dehydration, electrolyte abnormalities, and both macronutrient and micronutrient deficiencies. Owing to new medical and surgical treatments, the survival rate ranges from 73% to 89%.[10] Ian will require long-term parenteral nutrition (PN); that is, he will not be able to take food orally and will be dependent on intravenous solution to provide the bulk of his nutritional needs. Ian is the first child of Dylan and Adrianna Chapel, both in their early 30s. After a stay in the neonatal intensive care unit (NICU), Ian was sent home with his parents, who have provided care since that time with the help of a home care agency and a nutritional support company. The Chapels do not have other family members nearby. The majority of Ian's care falls to them.

Ian is now an active 2-year-old. Mrs. Chapel is the primary caregiver during the day and most evenings. She works weekends as a nursing assistant at a local assisted living center to supplement their family income. Mr. Chapel works as a paralegal in a law firm and attends law school at night. The Chapels' insurance coverage is through a group plan at the law firm where Mr. Chapel works.

Assume you are assigned to work with the Chapel family during an on-site educational experience with the home care agency providing primary care. The goal of your interaction with Ian and his family is to help promote family adaptation to his chronic condition (short bowel syndrome) and to empower the Chapels to develop and maintain healthy lifestyles. By reviewing the five processes listed earlier, you can get a picture of the family's functioning and possible areas for intervention.

Interactive Process

The *interactive* process of the family is composed of communication, family relationship, and social supports.[9] In your assessment of the interactive process of the Chapel family, you will explore the types of communication patterns they use; the effect of Ian's illness on the communication of the family both internally and externally; the types of relationships within the family; and the quality, timing, amount, and nature of social support they receive. Open communication should be encouraged. One aspect of care could be to assist the Chapels in mobilizing the informational and emotional support they need to cope with Ian's illness. Because the Chapels do not have family support in the immediate community, they may have to rely on informal support systems, such as friends and co-workers, and formal support systems, such as respite care agencies, to assist them in the care of their child. Perhaps there are other children who have short bowel syndrome or who have to rely on parenteral nutrition in the community. The caregivers of such children may have or could form a support group to help troubleshoot common problems and offer advice.

Developmental Process

Assessment of the *developmental* process includes the family developmental stage and individual developmental stages. The Chapels, as a family, are in the second stage of family development as described by Duvall in his classic work.[11] Stage II of the family life cycle involves integrating an infant into the family unit, accommodating to new parenting roles, and maintaining the marital bond. Ian is moving from infancy to becoming a toddler, and soon he will be increasingly interested in his environment and want to explore it. Ian will become increasingly mobile and develop language during this stage. (You will be introduced to basic development needs of toddlers later in this chapter.) All of this is influenced by the presence of his chronic condition.

Therefore, it would be appropriate for you to assess how well these developmental tasks are being achieved. You will educate the Chapels in the developmental milestones Ian should achieve and the tasks involved. For example, Ian needs freedom of mobility to explore objects in his environment and learn to walk, so his nutritional solution could be placed in a backpack to allow him to move more freely. Children with short bowel syndrome may also require frequent visits to the bathroom throughout the day when the time comes for toilet training. To decrease the Chapels' frustrations, you could plan ahead for this next developmental milestone and work with them to plan a structured routine that is consistently implemented and results in success for all involved, especially the child. There is some evidence that about 10% to 15% of children with short bowel syndrome will experience neurological or developmental delays.[12] Thus, you will also want to watch for possible developmental delays to plan for early therapeutic interventions.

Coping Process

Coping has been identified as problem-solving, adaptation to stress and crisis, and management of resources.[9] Coping helps us lower our anxiety so that we can meet the demands of the day. Each person has a different coping style when dealing with uncertainty. Coping styles can be both problem focused and emotion focused. In general, coping styles depend on what you are like as a person and your role in the family.[13] The uncertainty of illness presents a variety of stressors for families. In your work with the Chapels, you should assess their ability to handle stress and the impact that Ian's illness has on everyday activities.

⊚ REFLECTIONS

Which of these questions would most help you show respect for the Chapels' predicament?

- How do the Chapels conceptualize and manage Ian's diagnosis as a family? What meaning does it have?
- Has Ian's illness caused a change in the family's life plans? For example, did Mrs. Chapel plan on returning to full-time work outside the home after the birth of her son?
- If so, can the family adapt to the loss of income or are support services available to allow Ian to be cared for during the day so that Mrs. Chapel can work?
- Were the Chapels intending to have several children? Have Ian's care needs changed this?
- What else do you want to know in order to care for the Chapel family?

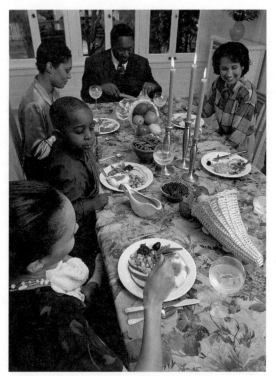

FIGURE 14-1: The process of family life involves family values, rituals, history, and identity. *(© Getty Images/84116)*

Overall, you would want to assess how the family deals with crises in general.

You can support the Chapels' coping processes by offering advice on the progression of the illness, discussing the normal feelings of frustration and guilt that accompany the care of a chronically ill or disabled family member, and offering resources to help the family cope more effectively, such as respite care and other support groups. Can you think of others?

The Chapels will also have to cope with financial difficulties. Even with the best health insurance, there are lifetime limits on coverage; in addition, there are many out-of-pocket expenses related to the care of a child with this diagnosis. Although most children experience small bowel adaptation over time and can be weaned from parenteral nutrition, most children require numerous surgeries, including an intestinal transplantation.[14] Thus, the Chapels may be facing years of out-of-pocket expenses and expensive hospital stays, procedures, and medications. This kind of financial pressure can be stressful for any family.

Integrity Process

The integrity process of family life involves family values, rituals, history, and identity.[9] These aspects of the family process greatly affect its behavior. Family rituals, one facet of the *integrity* process, provide a useful framework for assessing threats to a family's integrity. Family rituals include celebrations and traditions such as activities surrounding birthdays, religious holidays, or bedtime routines for children (Figure 14-1). Suggestions for evaluating family rituals include assessment of the following[15]:

> Does the family underutilize rituals? Families who do not celebrate or mark family changes such as birthdays, deaths, anniversaries, and so forth may be left without some of the benefits that accompany rituals, such as bringing the family together or marking changes in life and family roles.
>
> Does the family follow rigid patterns of ritual? In families who are inflexible, things are always done the same way, at the same time, and with the same people. Families who are rigid do not respond well to necessary changes that disrupt routines and rituals occasioned by illness and injury.
>
> Are family rituals skewed? A family with skewed rituals tends to emphasize only one aspect of family life (e.g., religion) and ignore others. For example, a family might spend all of its time celebrating with the father's side of the family on religious holidays and ignore the different rituals cherished by the patterns practiced on the mother's side.
>
> Has the ritual process been interrupted? For example, the birth of a disabled or chronically ill child may threaten family identity and permanently disrupt family rituals. In the case of the Chapels, they have elected to stay home for traditional family holidays because almost all holidays involve a focus on food. For the foreseeable future, Ian cannot tolerate most food orally, so the Chapels will have to consider what this interruption in ritual means to their life together and may have to develop other rituals at holiday time that do not focus so prominently on food.
>
> Are the rituals hollow? Rituals that are performed just for the sake of performing them have lost their life and may be stressful for the family rather than a source of joy and strength.

In addition to changes in ritual that occur over time in families, many role changes also occur, particularly when chronic illness or impairment is involved. For example, Mrs. Chapel has become the primary caregiver. She may or may not have expected to take on this role. Essential interventions include helping the Chapels redefine major family roles and maintain their new responsibilities.

Health Process

The final process of family experience is related to health. This process includes health status, health beliefs and practices, and lifestyle practices.[9] You would want to assess the family's definition of health and how they define the health of the individual members.

REFLECTIONS

- Besides the responsibilities involved in caring for a child who requires parenteral feedings, what do the Chapels do to maintain their own health?
- How do the Chapels deal with health problems? To whom do they turn?

Interventions in the area of health process include education, encouragement, and counseling regarding the short- and long-term aspects of Ian's care. The situation of Ian and his parents illustrates the family health system as one useful approach to the care of families and children. The family health system applies to all families, whatever the composition and stage of familial development. You are encouraged to explore other models of working with a family and their effectiveness in achieving optimal family health. Regardless of the model you choose, it is clear that family relationships are an important consideration in understanding the conduct of any patient and for developing an effective mode for respectful interaction with that patient. Care can best be accomplished if it is considered a collaborative venture between the family and the health care team. The components of family-centered care in Box 14-1 provide a context for recognizing the family's central role.

BOX 14-1

Core Concepts of Patient- and Family-Centered Care

1. Respect and Dignity.
Health care practitioners listen to and honor patient and family perspectives and choices. Patient and family knowledge, values, beliefs, and cultural backgrounds are incorporated into the planning and care delivery.
2. Information Sharing.
Health care practitioners communicate and share complete and unbiased information with patients and families in ways that are affirming and useful. Patients and families receive timely, complete, and accurate information in order to effectively participate in care and decision-making.
3. Participation.
Patients and families are encouraged and supported in participation in care and decision-making at the level they choose.
4. Collaboration.
Patients and families are also included on an institution-wide basis. Health care leaders collaborate with patients and families in policy and program development, implementation, and evaluation; in health care facility design; and in professional education, as well as in the delivery of care.

From Institute for Patient- and Family-Centered Care website (http://www.ipfcc.org/index.html).

Abuse and Neglect

Legally, the parents or another formally appointed guardian are the voice of the young child, except in rare instances in which the state intervenes to protect the child from caregivers whom the state judges are not acting in the child's best interest. The most grievous situation results when there is growing suspicion or knowledge that the patient is a victim of *child abuse* or *neglect*. In the case of a dysfunctional family in which abuse is suspected, however much you may empathize with the family's suffering, you must turn your attention to the protection of the victimized child. The Child Abuse Prevention and Treatment Act (CAPTA), originally enacted in 1974, has been amended several times. It was most recently amended and reauthorized under the CAPTA Reauthorization Act of 2010 (Public Law 111-320). CAPTA is the key federal legislation addressing *child abuse and neglect.* It mandates reporting and provides support for community-based grants to prevent *child abuse and neglect.*[16] CAPTA defines *child abuse and neglect* as "any recent act of failure to act on the part of a parent or caretaker, which results in death, serious physical or emotional harm, sexual abuse, or exploitation, or an act or failure to act which presents an imminent risk of serious harm."[17] Younger children are more frequently maltreated than older children, with those younger than the age of 1 being at the greatest risk. A good general rule is to be suspicious of maltreatment when reports of the history of the child's injuries do not coincide with physical findings. Furthermore, you must become acquainted with appropriate reporting procedures for persons in your chosen profession. The procedures vary from state to state. Parents and others caregivers who maltreat children are deeply troubled. Your support of policies and practices that address maltreatment of children as a family affair is a valuable contribution to society.

In summary, in spite of the occasional problematic family situation, the family is usually a sound and reliable bridge to building better understanding of the needs of infants, toddlers, and young children. Involving family systems in care is critical because families are the primary social context in which children live and receive care and nurturing. We now direct your attention to the growth and development of the child, another important factor in working with pediatric patients.

Useful General Principles of Human Growth and Development

Growth and development occurs in numerous ways—physical, emotional, intellectual (or cognitive), social, and moral—and all aspects of development affect one another. Some theories are hierarchical models of development, whereas others are dynamic. Although professionals often talk about growth and development simultaneously, growth can be thought of as quantitative (changes in height and weight) and development can be thought of as qualitative (changes in performance influenced by the maturation process). We will address growth first. Human growth proceeds in accordance with general principles of (1) orderliness, (2) discontinuity, (3) differentiation, (4) cephalocaudal, and (5) proximodistal and bilateral. Each is instrumental in helping you understand what occurs in the growth process, when, and why.

Orderliness

Growth and changes in behavior usually occur in an orderly fashion and in the same sequence. Thus, infants can turn their heads before they can extend their hands. Almost every child sits before he or she stands, stands before walking, and draws a circle before drawing a square. Most babies babble before talking and pronounce certain sounds before others. Likewise, certain cognitive abilities precede the next. Children can categorize objects or put them into a series before they can think logically.

Discontinuity

Although growth is orderly, it is not always smooth and gradual. There are periods of rapid growth—growth spurts—and increases in psychological abilities. Parents sometimes speak of the summer that a child grew 2 inches. Many adolescents experience a sudden growth spurt after years of being the ones with the smallest stature in their class.

Differentiation

Development proceeds from simple to complex and from general to specific. An example of differentiation in the infant is seen in an infant's ability to wave his or her arms first and later develop purposeful use of his or her fingers. Motor responses are diffuse and undifferentiated at birth and become more specific and controlled as the child grows. Beginning motor activity in the toddler involves haphazard and unsystematic actions, progressing to goal-directed actions and specific outcomes.[18]

Cephalocaudal

Cephalocaudal development means that the upper end of the organism develops sooner than the lower end. Increases in neuromuscular size and maturation of function begin in the head and proceed to the hands and feet. After birth, an infant will be able to hold its head erect before being able to sit or walk.

Proximodistal and Bilateral

Proximodistal development means that growth progresses from the central axis of the body (the trunk) toward the periphery or extremities. Thus, the central nervous system develops before the peripheral nervous system. *Bilateral development* means that the capacity for growth and development of the child is symmetrical—growth that occurs on one side of the body generally occurs on the other side of the body simultaneously. These principles apply throughout the lifespan, from infancy to old age.

Theories of Human Development to Guide You

Development can be discussed in domains of human performance: cognitive, affective, and psychomotor or through standardized language/classification systems of human function and abilities such as the International Classification of Function, Disability and Health (ICF) developed by the World Health Organization.[19] The ICF dimensions of functioning and disability are body structure and function, activities and participation, and personal and environmental factors. We focus primarily on cognitive development because it entails how a person perceives, thinks, and communicates thoughts and feelings. Time is spent on psychosocial development because of the profound impact this has on the health professional's interactions with patients.

Although this chapter focuses on the cognitive and psychosocial development of the infant through preschooler, the same theories are applicable to the school-age child and adolescent discussed in Chapter 15.

The manner in which a child learns to think, reason, and use language is vital to the child's overall growth and development.[20] Traditionally, health professionals have based their interventions with children on the stages of cognitive development described by Jean Piaget (1896–1980).[21] Piaget's theory is a logical, deductive explanation of how children think from infancy through adolescence. Piaget described the earliest stage of cognitive development as *sensorimotor*. At this stage, infants take in a great deal of information through their senses. Tactile and verbal stimulation and auditory and visual cues can have positive, long-range results. The early beginnings of cognitive development can be stimulated by talking to the infant and by face-to-face interactions.

Piaget labeled the cognitive abilities of toddlers as *preoperational*. Toddlers learn to think and understand by building each new experience upon previous experiences. Miller summarized Piaget's depiction of the cognitive stage of toddlers in terms of egocentrism (seeing the world from a "me-only" viewpoint), rigidity of thought ("Mom is always right"), and semilogical reasoning ("my dog died because I was a bad boy").[22] Children in this stage are confused about cause and effect, even when it is explained to them, and think in terms of magic (e.g., wishing something makes it so). However, more current researchers refute Piaget's beliefs and claim that he may have underestimated the cognitive abilities of toddlers. These researchers suggest that children have far more potential to understand complex illness concepts than they have previously been given credit for.[23] Thus, some toddlers may be capable of appreciating the perspective of another and adapting their behavior accordingly. Others propose that, rather than viewing the toddler as incapable of thinking a certain way, one should view him or her as a novice. Children have much less life experience than adults. Thus, when children gain experience through chronic illness, for example, or perform tasks involving their own expertise, they can demonstrate adult-like performance and more sophisticated thinking and reasoning.[24] The debate in the area of cognitive development is ongoing. For example, evolutionary developmental psychology, which takes into account genetic and ecological mechanisms that affect development, as well as the effect of cultural contexts, has recently added voices in the discussion regarding variability in development.[25,26] The various ideas of developmental theorists are important to explore because they have direct implications for how best to work with young children.

As with cognitive development, there are numerous stage/phase theories about the psychological and social dynamics of child development. Development, seen this way, is a process or movement. "Movement from potentiality to actuality occurs over time and in the direction of growth and progress. It is not surprising, then, that most conceptualizations of development incorporate the notion of improvement—of 'better' more integrated ways of functioning."[27]

Almost all theories stress the importance of bonding or forming attachments as the primary developmental task. No one has done more to promote this idea than Erik Erikson, a psychologist who, in the 1950s and 1960s, proposed eight stages of psychosocial development.[28] According to his theory, the development of trust (shown in Chapter 10 to be fundamental to the effective patient and health professional relationship) is one of the tasks facing the child in all relationships. He or she is engaged in a process that will affect his or her ability to engage in respectful interaction with everyone. During infancy, the child is introduced to trust and begins to experience (or to not experience) its power.

The psychosocial development of the toddler involves acquiring a clearer sense of himself or herself that is separate from that of the primary caregiver, becoming involved in wider social relationships, gaining self-control and mastery over motor and verbal skills, and developing independence and a self-concept. Later in this chapter, we spend time considering specific examples of how you can effectively interact with infants and toddlers by anticipating the developmental tasks specific to their age group. A caveat is warranted at this juncture about developmental stages. All stage models are just that—models—and it is difficult to place a child in a specific stage merely by chronological age. Stages are only a way to describe an ongoing process. It is important to note that behaviors typically occur in context and that the environment or task-specific demands can alter function during that process.

Early Development: Infancy and Early Childhood

Between the first day of life and the first day of kindergarten, development proceeds at a lightning pace like no other. Consider just a few of the transformations that occur during this 5-year period:

▶ The newborn's avid interest in staring at other babies turns into the capacity for cooperation, empathy, and friendship.

▶ The 1-year-old's tentative first steps become the 4-year-old's pirouettes and slam dunks.

▶ The completely unself-conscious baby becomes a preschooler who can describe herself in great detail. Her behavior is partially motivated by how she wants others to view and judge her.

▶ The first adamant "no!" turns into the capacity for elaborate arguments about why the parent is wrong and the preschooler is right.

▶ The infant, who has no conception that his blanket came off because he kicked his feet, becomes the 4-year-old who can explain the elaborate (if messy) causal sequence by which he can turn flour, water, salt, and food coloring into play dough.

It is no surprise that the early childhood years are portrayed as formative. The supporting structures of virtually every system of the human organism, from the tiniest cell to the capacity for intimate relationships, are constructed during this age period.[29]

Normal Newborn

The anticipation of the birth of a child is fraught with emotions ranging from joy to fear. In economically developed countries the birth process has largely moved from the home to the hospital. Many hospitals attempt to duplicate the comforts and familiarities of home by designing birthing suites complete with a DVD player and rocking chair. With the move to shorter lengths of stay for a normal delivery, it is unlikely that you will have much opportunity to work with these tiniest of patients unless you choose to work in labor and delivery or neonatology.

⊚ REFLECTIONS

Picture this . . .

You are pregnant with your first child. You and your partner have been family planning for almost a year and are very excited.

Today is your first prenatal visit. At this visit, the obstetrician (whom you just met for the first time today after waiting six weeks for the appointment) recommends an early ultrasound based on your family history. The ultrasound reveals a "suspicion of cardiac defect". The team informs you that you will need to follow up with a high-risk obstetrician in two weeks for additional definitive testing.

• What is your immediate reaction/feelings in this situation? Do you think you and your partner will respond the same way?

• Your sister calls to ask how your appointment went. What do you say?

The normal newborn is highly vulnerable but also amazingly adaptable to the new environment outside the womb. The newborn period ends at the first month of life. After that, newborns are called *infants*. Newborns have many needs, especially when health problems are present at birth. They are human beings worthy of full respect.

Life-Threatening Circumstances

New technology is changing the possibility for survival in neonates and newborns. Smaller and smaller neonates who have had shorter gestations in the womb are often seen in neonatal intensive care units (NICUs). Many variables enter into survival for these tiny patients.

Newborns in these settings range from those with high-intensity care needs (such as mechanical ventilation) to those with lower-intensity care needs (such as monitoring of oxygen levels). Some babies will be full term, but others will be as young as 25 weeks' gestation. Sometimes a neonate who weighs more than the fragile neonate in the next Isolette is the one who does not survive. Each year tens of thousands of babies are born too early and too small and end up in a NICU. In each case, parents and health professions share a common goal—to make each baby healthy. New medical technologies are saving babies who until only recently would not have survived. Unfortunately for some of these families, the result may be a baby whose future entails chronic health conditions. With little or no preparation, parents often find themselves in times of great uncertainty and are often being asked to decide when the technology is doing more harm than good. It is interesting to note that in retrospect, many parents do not identify involvement in decision-making. In Pinch's longitudinal study of parents' experiences in the NICU, "Parents recalled that possibilities or alternatives were seldom offered to them. They were simply told what the professionals were required to do, what the baby needed, or what was suggested as the best treatment."[30] The NICU can be an overwhelming environment for many families. Thus, respectful interaction with parents and these fragile newborns requires that you take extra care to inform them about the status and progress of their children. Understanding and empathy for the complex stresses and losses parents are experiencing as they cope with their new roles as parents are key.[31]

Moving into Infancy

When working with an infant, you will be in a position to make independent clinical judgments about his or her best interests and to observe the interaction between parents and their new baby. Happily, the parents almost always provide the primary supportive bridge between you and the infant patient, interpreting the baby's expressions, babbles, and postures and providing insight into how continuity of approach to the infant can be maximized. During this time parents have to learn cues from their infants, and sometimes you can teach the parents, as well as learn from the parents' comments and behavior.

The needs of infants are sometimes difficult to determine because these small patients are vulnerable and lack the sufficient verbal skills to express their wants and needs. Professionals who rely solely on a patient's ability to ask for what he or she needs take a narrow view of needs assessment. As with any nonverbal patient, the health professional must learn to read the infant's signals and collaborate with the caregiver to determine the infant's needs.

Infant Needs: Respect and Consistency

There are two contexts by which to view the infant's needs. The first focuses on the stage of psychosocial development that we have already discussed, and the second focuses on immediate concrete needs such as the need for a drink of water, food, pain relief, or a diaper change. You have an opportunity to demonstrate respect for the infant by responding effectively to each type of need.

Remember that parents often have explicit ways of doing things for their infant that can help, too. For example, parents may hold the infant in a certain way or play a favorite game such as pretending to sneeze or rubbing the baby's back that will, at a minimum, help calm the infant while you look for other reasons for the infant's distress.

A primary approach is characterized by the three "C's": consistency in approach, constancy of presence, and continuity of treatment. Consistency is especially important because it builds trust (infant self-confidence) through the following steps:

1. An infant's need exists.
2. The infant exhibits generalized behavior.
3. The caregiver responds.
4. The need is satisfied.
5. The need recurs.
6. The infant predicts the caregiver's response.
7. The infant repeats previous behavior.
8. The caregiver responds in a consistent manner.
9. The need is satisfied.
10. The infant's trust toward the caregiver develops.
11. The need recurs.
12. The infant is confident that the caregiver will respond appropriately.[32]

Of course, all infants have different temperaments, which will create differences in responses to you, the health professional. These individual differences are welcomed by health professionals because they support the belief that humans are unique, each deserving of unique respect.

Everyday Needs of Infants

By now you should have discovered in this book that the "solutions" to challenges during interaction with patients are sometimes concrete and mundane and dictated by common sense. Fussy, irritable, crying infants are in the position of becoming the least liked (and probably least cared for) patients on the pediatrics unit. Crying is one way infants try to communicate distress.

More likely than not, because of the infant's age and stage of development, this distress is related to a concrete, immediate need. Respectful interaction with infants in distress requires careful attention to several types of detail.

Comfort Detail

Small children most often become irritable when they experience physical discomfort. Careful attention to comfort is key to their sense of well-being. This becomes all the more reason to check for factors that could lead to discomfort whenever possible. It is too easy to assume that a baby's crying or other belligerence is because he or she is a fussy or cranky baby. Examine the bed shirt, diaper, and crib sheets.

---

⑤ REFLECTIONS

Which of these comfort detail questions should the health professional ask?
- Is the bed shirt, diaper, or crib sheet wet from urine, sweat, or a spilled medication?
- Are they wrinkled and creating pressure spots?
- Does the baby have abrasions, punctures, or other bodily tenderness that causes contact pain? Is tape pinching the baby or has an intravenous line infiltrated?
- Check the ears, nostrils, and throat. Is there something lodged in one of them?
- Are the infant's throat and mouth dry?
- What did the baby eat and when? Is he or she taking fluids?
- Is he or she hungry or thirsty, perhaps?
- Is he or she having some predictable side effect from a medication?
- What is the environment like? Is it too noisy? Too bright? Too dark?
- What other comfort questions can you name?

Health Professional Detail

Discomfort can also be caused by what you are wearing or doing.

Think about the kind of clothing and adornments such as name tags that you wear in clinical practice.
- Is your uniform scratching the baby? Is the color or design too complex?
- Are you wearing jewelry that scratches, scrapes, or pinches?
- Are your hands clammy and cold?

Think about the number of providers evaluating or treating the infant.
- Is the baby constantly being dressed and undressed?
- Has the baby been evaluated back to back without the opportunity to rest?
- Is the baby overstimulated by machines and mechanical or procedural-based touch (versus the skin contact and loving touch to facilitate bonding with providers)?

Your conduct is like a mirror to the baby. If you are anxious or uncomfortable with caring for an infant, the infant will sense it.

In addition to the immediate discomfort you may cause an infant by inattention to these details, a more persistent negative response could be a sign of deeper discomfort. A good general rule is to remain consistent, approaching the infant similarly in each interaction in hopes that the familiarity itself will be a comfort. Also, watch how the infant interacts with others, especially those who appear to be successful in calming him or her. Try altering your approach to match those that seem to help the infant. Always orient the infant to your presence and provide comforting touch when procedural touch is also required.

Environmental Detail

Like all of us, infants have various comfort zones, which include temperature, space, noise, and other environmental factors. Look about the room that you are currently occupying and imagine it is one that includes an ill infant.

⊚ REFLECTIONS

- Is the room too warm?
- Is the infant sweaty or clammy?
- Are there noises in the area from nearby construction, an open window, or a newly placed monitor?
- Are there different smells in the air because of painting in the hallway or a new disinfectant used by the cleaning staff?
- Where is the crib placed? Try placing it in another position or placing the infant in a different position in the crib. Is he or she exposed to open spaces on both sides of the crib or is one side against the wall? Try alternatives to this arrangement.
- What else do you notice about the environment that could have an impact on an infant's well-being?

In short, you should be attentive to the behavior of the young patient and to the people who are associated with his or her care. One of the primary developmental goals of infancy is social attachment. Attention to comfort of the infant, the environment, and the care provider is essential so that the infant can engage with others.[33]

Early Development: The Toddler and Preschool Child

Much of the material related to respectful interaction with the infant patient and his or her family can be applied to the child past the stage of infancy into other stages of childhood. As a child grows, however, new challenges confront both parents and health care providers. This is especially true of the toddler and preschooler. These years are ones of rapid physical, social, emotional, and cognitive growth. Children begin to walk, run, and climb. They have increased control over feeding and toileting habits and start learning about limits. The early years are also ones during which developmental disabilities are typically diagnosed.[34] Given their effect on early childhood functioning, developmental disabilities (such as autism) are being diagnosed much earlier than in years past. It is not uncommon for diagnosis to occur in the 18-month-old to 3-year-old. The median age of autism diagnosis is 4.5 to 5.5, yet 80% of parents report seeing problems by 24 months.[35]

A review of Erikson's stages shows that the young patient's psychosocial tasks in moving from infancy to becoming a toddler and then an older child focus on becoming one's own "self," separate from others. Unique personalities develop, and respect for a toddler and preschool-age child can be enhanced when the child actually asks for what he or she wants. Of course, sometimes the toddler will have difficulty making himself or herself understood and may be embarrassed by his or her own awkward attempts to act grown up. Especially important to the child is the need to succeed at "adult" tasks (which include anything new, from the early tasks of learning how to walk and to feed oneself, no matter how long it takes).

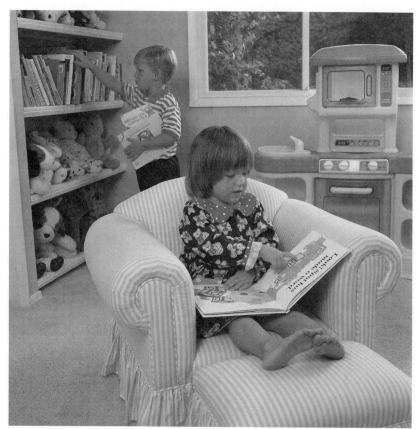

FIGURE 14-2: Parallel play can be encouraged as part of treatment or other aspects of interaction with a child. *(© Corbis.)*

Play is an important vehicle through which a toddler patient's sense of worth can be fostered. According to developmental psychologists, play may be the child's richest opportunity for physical, cognitive, language, and emotional development. Play is the primary tool through which the child learns social and cultural roles and norms. Freiberg describes several types of play, any of which can be encouraged as part of treatment or other aspects of interaction with the child. These include the following:

▶ *symbolic play,* used by children to make something stand for something else, such as when the young patient "becomes" the more powerful health professional by wearing the health professional's clothes or stethoscope

▶ *onlooker play,* which involves watching others, such as when the health professional entertains the child or when the child observes others at play but does not participate

▶ *parallel play,* which is side-by-side play characterized by activity that is interactive only by virtue of another's presence (the participation by observation and side-by-side types of play may help to decrease a young patient's loneliness, even though he or she cannot fully interact with others) (Figure 14-2)

▶ *associative play,* which involves shared activity and communication but little organized activity
▶ *constructive play,* which involved the making or building of things
▶ *cooperative play,* in which rules are followed and goals are achieved (associative
play and cooperative play are generally beyond the capabilities of the toddler)[36]

Toddler Needs: Respect and Security

Attention to personal detail outlined in the section on infants applies to interaction with
the toddler as well. Fortunately, in most cases toddlers can verbalize their basic needs
("Me hungry," "Me go?" "More," or "No") and express their curiosity by pointing to
something and asking, "Dis?" Their illness, the intimidating surroundings, or their shy-
ness, however, may make young children even more reticent than most patients to make
their needs known in this direct manner. They often show their feelings of insecurity
about what is happening to them by being cranky or acting overly fearful and demanding.

Children, like all patients, tend to regress when they become ill. Having so recently
moved out of infancy, toddlers sometimes return to infant-like behavior. You need
to be aware that this is a normal tendency and that you should not condemn young
patients who do not "act their age."

One of the authors recalls hearing a health professional tell a pediatric patient
they were acting "childish," to which the patient confidently responded, "Well, I am
a child!" Remember, even the smallest patients need care providers to validate their
emotions. Tone and cadence of speech matter greatly in respectful interactions with
children. In the following story, a nurse tells of a toddler with Burkitt's lymphoma,
a particularly fast-growing cancer, who was not doing well and was essentially silent:

> . . . I don't know how I knew this, but something said to me that he needed to be held
> right then. I asked him if he would like to rock in the rocking chair, and of course he
> didn't answer but he did not resist when I picked him up. We sat in that rocking chair
> for an hour and a half, and I could feel him settling in. I had on this knit sweater with a
> print, and when he finally sat up I laughed and said, "Jason, you've got waffles on your
> face!" He said, "I know, I've got them on my knees, too." That was the first time he
> spoke, and after that we couldn't shut him up.[37]

A combination of gentle support for age-appropriate behaviors and tender care,
such as holding and rocking, can encourage the young child to feel nurtured and secure.

SUMMARY

This chapter has presented an overview of a variety of theories that seek to explain how
human beings develop biologically, psychologically, and socially over the lifespan. The
progression from infancy to early childhood is shaped by the environment, the most
important element of which is the family. As an infant becomes a toddler, he or she starts
taking steps, literally and figuratively, toward a lifelong journey that is unique to each
child. Recognizing the uniqueness of the child as an individual, as well as the product
of a developmental phase, will help you to better understand the many dimensions in
which respect can be conveyed, and the success of your interactions will be maximized.

REFERENCES

1. Pinch WJE, Spielman ML: Ethics in the neonatal intensive care unit: parental perceptions at four years postdischarge, *Adv Nurs Sci* 19(1):72–85, 1996.
2. Murphy SL, Xu JQ, Kochanek KD: *Deaths: preliminary data for 2010. National Vital Statistics Reports,* vol 60, no 4, Hyattsville, MD, 2012, National Center for Health Statistics.
3. White AA, Seeing patients: unconscious bias in healthcare, Boston, 2012, Harvard University Press.
4. Institute for Patient- and Family-Centered Care: *Frequently asked questions.* http://www.ipfcc.org/faq.html. Accessed March 5, 2012.
5. Sparling JW: The cultural definition of family, *Phys Occup Ther Pediatr* 11(4):17–28, 1991.
6. Census Bureau Reports: More young adults are living in their parents' home, *Newsroom release, CB 11-183,* Thursday November 3, 2011, http://www.census.gov/newsroom/releases/archieves/families_households/cb11-183.htlm. Accessed March 7, 2012.
7. Census Bureau Reports: Families with children increasingly face unemployment, *Newsroom release, CB 10-08,* Friday January 8, 2010. http://www.census.gov/newsroom/releases/archieves/families_households/cb10-08.htlm. Accessed March 7, 2012.
8. Schor E: Family pediatrics: report of the task force on family. American Academy of Pediatrics, *Pediatrics* 111:S1541–S1571, 2003.
9. Anderson KH: The family health system approach to family systems nursing, *J Fam Nurs* 6(2):103–119, 2000.
10. Duro D, Kamin D, Duggan C: Overview of pediatric short bowel syndrome, *J Pediatr Gastroenterol Nutr* 47(S1):S33–S36, 2008.
11. Duvall EM: *Family development,* ed 5, Philadelphia, 1977, Lippincott.
12. Beers SR, Yaworski JA, Stilley C, et al: Cognitive deficits in school-age children with severe short bowel syndrome, *J Pediatr Surg* 35(6):860–865, 2000.
13. Doherty RF, Kwo J, Montgomery P, et al: *Maintaining compassionate care: a companion guide for families experiencing the uncertainty of a serious and prolonged illness,* Boston, 2008, MGH Institute of Health Professions.
14. Neuhaus P, Pascher A: How successful is intestinal transplantation and what improves graft survival? *Nat Clin Pract Gastroenterol Hepatol* 2:306–307, 2005.
15. Imber-Black E, Roberts J, Whiting R: *Rituals in families and family therapy,* New York, 1988, Norton.
16. CAPTA Reauthorization Act of 2010 Public Law 108-36, 111th Cong., 2010, http://www.gpo.gov/fdsys/pkg/PLAW-111publ320/pdf/PLAW-111publ320.pdf.
17. Child Welfare Information Gateway: Definition of child abuse and neglect, state statutes series, Washington, DC, February 2011, U.S. Department of Health and Human Services: Children's Bureau/ACYF.
18. Puskar KR, D'Antonio IJ: Tots and teens: similarities in behavior and interventions for pediatric and psychiatric nurses, *J Child Adolesc Psychiatr Ment Health Nurs* 6(2):18–28, 1993.
19. World Health Organization: International classification of functioning, disability and health: ICF, Geneva, 2002, http://www.who.int/classifications/icf/training/icfbeginnersguide.pdf.
20. Mott S, James S, Sperhac A: *Nursing care of children and families,* ed 2, Reading, MA, 1990, Addison-Wesley.
21. Piaget J: *Six psychological studies,* New York, 1964, Vintage.
22. Miller SA: *Developmental research methods,* Englewood Cliffs, NJ, 1987, Prentice Hall.
23. Rushforth H: Practitioner review: communicating with hospitalized children: review and application of research pertaining to children's understanding of illness, *J Child Psychol Psychiatry* 40(5):683–691, 1999.
24. Yoos HL: Children's illness concepts: old and new paradigms, *Pediatr Nurs* 20(2):134–140, 145, 1994.

25. Geary DC, Bjorklund DF: Evolutionary developmental psychology, *Child Dev* 71(1): 57–65, 2000.
26. Suizzo MA: The social-emotional and cultural contexts of cognitive development: neo-Piagetian perspectives, *Child Dev* 71(4):846–849, 2000.
27. Clark MC, Caffarella RS, editors: *An update on adult development theory: new ways of thinking about the life course: new directions for adult and continuing education*, San Francisco, 1999, Jossey-Bass.
28. Erikson EH: *Identity and the life cycle*, New York, 1959, WW Norton.
29. Shonkoff JP, Phillips DA, editors: *From neurons to neighborhoods: the science of early childhood development*, Washington, DC, 2000, National Academy of Sciences Press.
30. Pinch WE: *When the bough breaks: parental perceptions of ethical decision-making in NICU*, Lanham, MD, 2002, University of America Press.
31. Sweeney JK, Heriza CB, Blanchard Y, Dusing SC: Neonatal physical therapy. Part II: Practice frameworks and evidence-based guidelines, Pediatric Physical Therapy, Special Communication Section on Pediatrics of the American Physical Therapy Association, p 2–15.
32. Schuster CS, Ashburn SS: *The process of human development*, Boston, 1986, Little Brown.
33. Cronin A, Mandich MB: *Human development and performance throughout the lifespan*, Clifton Park, NY, 2005, Thomson Delmar Learning.
34. Boulet SL, Boyle CA, Schieve LA: Health care use and health and functional impact of developmental disabilities among US children, 1997–2005, *Arch Pediatr Adolesc Med* 163(1):19–26, 2009.
35. Centers for Disease Control and Prevention: Data and statistics, autism spectrum disorders. National Center for Birth Defects and Developmental Disorders. http://www.cdc.gov/ncbdd/autism/data/html. Accessed March, 5th, 2012.
36. Freiberg KL: *Human development, a life span approach*, ed 3, Boston, 1987, Jones and Bartlett.
37. Montgomery CL: *Healing through communication*, Newbury Park, CA, 1993, Sage.

Respectful Interaction: Working with Children and Adolescents

CHAPTER OBJECTIVES

The reader will be able to:

- Discuss in general terms the key developmental tasks of children and adolescents
- Distinguish some developmental challenges that need to be considered in one's approach to children beyond the toddler stage into adolescence
- Describe how the five types of play introduced in Chapter 14 are relevant—or not relevant—to respectful interaction with older children
- Describe how a child's developing need for successful relatedness enters into the health professional and patient relationship
- Make several suggestions that will help minimize the disequilibrium of the family during a child's illness
- List some compelling reasons for giving respectful attention to an adolescent's desire to exercise authority in regard to health care decisions and describe legitimate limits on that authority
- Describe high-risk behaviors in adolescence that can lead to long-term health problems

The important thing about you is that you are you. It is true that you were a baby, and you grew, and now you are a child, and you will grow, into a man, or into a woman. But the important thing about you is that *you* are *you.*

—M.W. Brown[1]

Much of the material related to respectful interaction with the infant or toddler and his or her family can be applied to older children. As a child grows, however, some new challenges confront the child, parents, families, and health care providers. Therefore, in this chapter we add some dimensions to the groundwork we laid in Chapter 14 to highlight some of the most important differences, as well as focus on the situation of adolescent patients.

Childhood Self

A young child's psychosocial tasks in moving from infancy to childhood focus on the need to recognize that one has a "self," separate from others, but that ultimately many aspects of that self must survive and thrive in relationships with others. Therefore, much activity and energy are focused on being different from others at the same time that much is invested in learning how to be accepted by others and having some say in relationships. As we address later in this chapter, these tasks become paramount during the adolescent years, but the fundamental building blocks begin much earlier.

Needs: Respect and Relating

Writer Annie Dillard poetically describes the first part of the child's developmental task, that of becoming a "self" different from others. She recalls it this way in her autobiography, *An American Childhood:*

> I woke up in bits like all children, piecemeal over the years. I discovered myself and the world, and forgot them, and discovered them again. … I noticed this process of awaking and predicted with terrifying logic that one of these years not far away I would be awake continuously and never slip back and never be free of myself again.[2]

Children, in general, want to make it alone and have learned not to accept the full dependence of infancy and the toddler years but are not independent yet. When they become patients they regress. The dependence side of the scales tips heavy, and the good fit of selfhood that the child is slipping into suddenly escapes. In this confusing never-never land of being neither infant nor fully child nor adult, children must try to reestablish some sense of equanimity and self-identity during their time of being patients.

Most children beyond the preschool years have learned to communicate verbally and have many more experiences upon which to rely compared with an infant or a toddler. Thus, their resources for effective relating are greater than those in their earlier years. The school-age years open up the child's world to interactions with many new and different people. These are mainly authority figures, such as teachers, coaches, and other role models, with whom the child will interact.

However, for the most part health professionals present types of authority that are often unfamiliar to the child. Family and school authority figures usually do little to prepare him or her for the health professions setting and its unique challenges and choices.

The Importance of Play

Play is a child's primary occupation.[3] Play appropriate to the child's age and social development can be an important vehicle to help ease the tension a child is feeling about relating to people in the health care setting. In Chapter 14 we introduced six types of play. As children develop new motor and cognitive skills, their play changes. Gender is an important contributor to play, as is age, peer group, and play opportunities. In their study of 7- to 11-year-old children, Miller and Kuhaneck[3] found that friends, siblings, and even pets figured prominently in children's descriptions of play and fun. This and other studies remind us that regardless of environment (hospital, school, or home), children *need* to play. Some older children who become patients may regress to an earlier stage of play, but many will be able to assume roles at the higher levels of play, which will allow them to act out their predicament of being in such a new situation. For example, associative play can involve playing "hospital" with a professional or family member and assuming the powerful role of the nurse or someone else in charge, thereby revealing children's own anxieties and how they perceive their situation. Clues to how they think their tension could be eased may be revealed in their attempts to minister to the play partner who has now become the patient. Cooperative play can involve table games, card games, or sports, using their participation and mastery as an effective way of relating.

Young patients often play with toys, too, so a truck, doll, puzzle, or other object may be an effective means of helping to establish a relationship. At the same time, children can be sensitive about being "too old" for certain types of toys, so health professionals and others must think carefully about which toys to offer and how to best integrate family and siblings into their sessions. Health professionals must also be sensitive to the fact that some children may not have access to toys and books. Twenty-one percent of children ages 0 to 17 in the United States live in families with incomes below the poverty level ($22,050 a year for a family of four).[4] These children are vulnerable to environmental, health, educational, and safety risks. They are also at particular risk for developmental challenges. Thoughtful considerations on how to help families modify environments and maximize access can bring about meaningful change in the number of opportunities for children to engage in play (e.g., repurposing everyday use items as toys, accessing library services).

⊚ REFLECTIONS

- When was the last time you engaged in "play"?
- Perhaps it was a board game, card game or sports related activity.
- How did you feel during the activity? After the activity?
- How did it contribute to your mood?

School Issues

When school age children become patients, health professionals are faced with additional challenges. Even a short illness or injury may disrupt school attendance and may not only put the child behind in schoolwork but also have devastating consequences socially. During the school years children organize most of their relational activity around family and school; therefore, they are at risk of being "out of the action" in every way when removed from the educational environment. At the very least you should be aware of this loss and show interest in his or her school-related activity if, indeed, any is being carried on at the moment.

Most children with chronic illnesses or long-term disabilities will receive special attention regarding education through the school system itself. Over the past 30 years, the definition of disability has changed. In the 1970s and 1980s, the concept of a disability referred to an underlying physical or mental condition that reduced one's abilities. Today, disability is seen as a complex interaction between a person and his or her environment. The development of the international classification of functioning, disability, and health (ICF) by the World Health Organization (introduced in Chapter 14) reflects this new perspective. In this classification, *disability* is an umbrella term for impairments, activity limitations, and participation restrictions. This perspective acknowledges that any individual can experience a decline in health at various points in his or her lifespan, hence experiencing disability. It is a biological, individual, and social perspective of health rather than a diagnosis or label.[5] A significant portion of children, estimated to be 6% of all those 17 years or younger, have experienced some degree of disability.[6] The number of U.S. children with developmental disabilities is on the rise. Developmental disabilities were reported in approximately one in six children in the United States in 2006-2008. The prevalence of any developmental disability in 1997 to 2008 was 13.87%.[7] This increase is significant because it will have a direct bearing on the need for health, educational, and social services for this population and their families.

The Americans with Disabilities Act (ADA) and the ADA Amendments Act of 2008 (P.L. 110-325) prohibits discrimination on the basis of disability in employment, state and local government services, public accommodations, commercial facilities, transportation, and telecommunications.[8] You can find out about the different components of the ADA at http://www.ada.gov/. The Individuals with Disabilities Education Act (IDEA) (formerly called *Public Law 94-142* or the *Education for all Handicapped Children Act of 1975*) is the federal law that governs the provision of special education services. It requires public schools to make available to all eligible children with disabilities a free, appropriate public education in the least restrictive environment appropriate to their individual needs.[9] However laudatory this is, the law does little to address the accompanying problems that sometimes arise: Able-bodied children may be cruel toward peers who have medical conditions, parents may believe that their child is not getting care as good as they would like or disagree with the individualized education program that has been developed for their child, teachers may feel that they do not have enough time to devote to the needs of all the children in their classrooms, and children with serious but not permanent conditions may not qualify.[10] When you come into contact with families who are trying to work through some of these issues, you can often encourage them and direct them to the appropriate resources when problems arise. For example, if parents disagree with the individualized education program, they can request a due process hearing and a review from the state educational agency if applicable in their state.

In short, during the school-age years a child's feelings of self-worth and experiences of relatedness usually are tied to school. Any means by which you can convey empathy for the child's predicament and respect for his or her capacities will enhance the child's self-esteem and help ensure success in the relationship.

Family—A Bridge to Respectful Interaction

All of the family dynamics described in Chapter 14 apply as the child grows older. The growing child, however, does present some additional challenges to the family and health professional working with the family. The needs of the school-age child revolve around tasks, hobbies, and activities. It is during this stage that 7- to 12-year-olds develop a sense of values to guide decision-making and interests.

It has been noted that the child's desire to become more independent is one of the major developmental tasks of this growth period, while at the same time he or she may feel extremely lonely and insecure when illness strikes. The family is often torn between wanting to support the child as an independent "big girl" or "big boy" while being attentive to his or her needs. They may also be dismayed by the child's obvious regression or respond to their own feelings of guilt for the child's illness with overprotectiveness. Your awareness of their struggles and needs is essential if you are to be successful. Remember, you must always show family members the due respect they deserve. They are the people who are most knowledgeable about the child and are key collaborators in clinical decision-making. Lawlor and Mattingly[11] put this best when they stated: "Collaboration is much more than being nice. It involves complex interpretive acts in which the practitioner must understand the meanings of illness or disability in a person and family's life and the feelings that accompany these experiences."

Children as Active Participants in Care

Respect for the child's input, especially when his or her opinions seem to differ from those of parents, is essential, too. Although developmental psychology has often used age as an indicator of competency, this view is being challenged and replaced by the principle that social experience is a more reliable marker of maturity and decision-making ability.[12,13] Although the legal age of consent is 18 in the United States, many policies now acknowledge the importance of listening to children and having them *assent* to care decisions. Assent in children honors respect for persons and should be sought from the age of 7 upwards. It ensures that they can communicate a choice and have a say in what happens.[14] Children often express their preferences through body language and actions. However difficult the discussion may be, many children should be invited to be active participants in the care planning process. It is through this participation that they learn the life skills necessary for decision making and illness management. Children often are aware of their parent's anxiety, opposition, or denial, and they try to act as referees among family members or between health professionals and family. Children can participate in a meaningful way in discussions about their health care (Figure 15-1). "The challenge is to provide appropriate techniques that neither exclude nor patronize children. Notions of children's incompetence are reinforced by methods that oversimplify and 'talk down' to them."[13]

In studies where children themselves are asked to identify the characteristics of a good health care provider, the following themes present[15,16]:
1. Good communication—using terms of endearment, sitting down to meet children at their eye level, having good body language (e.g., hands visible)
2. Professional competence—being organized, knowledgeable, skilled, and prompt
3. Safety/Appearance—following good hygiene practices, wearing a hospital identification badge
4. Virtues—being honest, trustworthy, polite (particularly toward family and visitors)
5. Fun—someone who does not forget that kids still need to play, laughing or using humor when performing care activities

In addition, brothers and sisters of the ill child are also affected by the stress such illness creates in the family. In a study of the siblings of hospitalized children, the

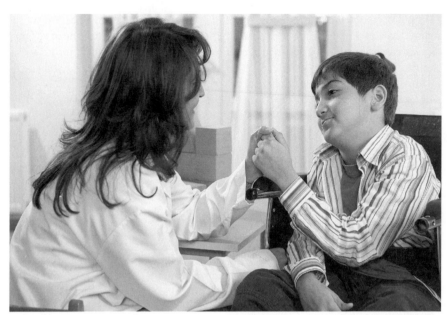

FIGURE 15-1: The health professional must listen to what the child has to say during an exam. (© *iStock-photo.com.*)

brothers and sisters noted stress that included feelings of loneliness, resentment and fear, and positive feelings of resilience, such as lessons learned and independence.[17] You can help siblings cope by providing support and information. Anything the health professional can do to keep the supportive context for siblings alive is well worth the effort. You can also help by trying to keep family disequilibrium at a minimum while acting primarily as an advocate for the child.

This balancing act is sometimes easier said than accomplished. The following story from one of the author's experiences highlights how such a dilemma can arise. As you read this case, think about your reasons for wanting to share the information about this child's condition with him or wanting to withhold it.

When John was 6, he fell from a swing, had some joint pain of the lower left extremity, and was unable to fully extend his knee. Numerous radiographic studies were completed, and results were largely normal. However, John could still not fully extend his knee and continued to complain of tenderness. Finally, a magnetic resonance image (MRI) revealed a lesion that turned out to be non-Hodgkin's lymphoma (NHL). John received combination chemotherapy and appeared to be in remission for several years. As John has gotten older the physician who has followed John and his family has grown somewhat concerned about his mother's overprotectiveness. Although it was less noticeable when he was younger, it has been the topic of conversation among the professionals when he and his mother have come to the clinic. For instance, she mentioned that she still dresses John and accompanies him almost everywhere.

John is now 9, and during a follow-up visit to the oncologist, it is discovered that he has a recurrence of NHL. Although the prognosis for children with NHL has improved, the outcome for children with recurrent NHL remains bleak.[18]

John is readmitted to the hospital for treatment. John had always asked many questions about his treatment, and so it seems odd to the nurses and others that he is uncharacteristically silent on the matter of his illness now, even though his condition continues to worsen. His mother visits for a minimum of 6 hours every day and warns everyone that John is not to be told that he has a recurrence of cancer.

During the last week, John has had several serious episodes. Last night he had a cardiac arrest and was resuscitated. The resident physicians and nurses would like to put him on a "no code" or do not resuscitate (DNR) status so that if his heart stops again he will be able to die peacefully. They would also like him to know the seriousness of his illness and that he has cancer, because they think he has a right to know he is going to die.

Today the physician approached John's mother about the team's desire to talk with him about his life threatening diagnosis. She flew into a rage and threatened to move John to another hospital immediately if they did not promise to never tell him under any circumstances. Although the health professionals know she has a legal right to remove him from the hospital, few of them think she actually will. Their opinions on whether he should be told are now divided.

Ⓢ REFLECTIONS

- If you were a member of the health care team treating John and his family, what would you do at this point?
- What would telling John about his illness accomplish?

Several suggestions may help you to decide what to do when you are faced with dilemmas concerning how much information to share with child patients:

1. *Make your own position clear* to yourself and to the patient's parents. Do you believe the child is able to handle information about his or her condition? Why or why not? What is in the best interests of the child? The family as a unit? Under what conditions would you feel morally bound to disclose relevant health information to this child? Under what conditions would you withhold such information, even if you believed that doing so could increase the child's distrust in you?

2. *Explore the resources available in your health care setting* to support families as they work out their anxieties and difficulties. As one author notes, "The purpose is ... to support, not supplant, the family. An atmosphere of acceptance and assurance allows each family to manage their own lives and to arrive at a solution most adequate for them."[19] Social workers and ethics committees are two

examples of the many supports available to families and teams of care providers in these types of situations.

3. *Present information in a way the child can understand* with ample opportunity for questions and explanations from the child in his or her own words about what has been discussed. Assent in children should help the pediatric patient achieve a developmentally appropriate awareness of the nature of his or her condition, while informing them about what to expect.[20]

4. *Implement strategies to lower family stress.* Two major tasks can help lower family stress and ensure that they are involved. The first is providing information. As collaborators in the care process, families need ongoing information. Structured communication such as a daily phone call, family meetings, or simply involvement in team rounds can help the family understand and cope with their child's prognosis.[21] The second is involving families in the care of their family member. Family involvement in various patient care tasks may help reduce the sense of powerlessness.

In summary, a child brings to the health care interaction hopes, fears, and dreams that reflect his or her need to establish autonomy and initiative as a "self" while maintaining the security of relationships with family, friends, and others. The delicate balance between being an individual and being part of relationships that are difficult under the best of circumstances is further challenged by illness or other incapacity. The efforts of health professionals and family alike are required for successful adaptation or recovery. The benefit is that within a context of respect for the child as a unique individual, the health professional and family will be able to work together to meet the patient's best interests.

Adolescent Self

The word *adolescent* means literally "to grow into maturity or adulthood." During the later stages of child development, all children are thrust into the difficult position of having to show industry and individuality in the larger world, to assert who they are, to command authority in some areas, and to explore the mysteries of developing sexuality. "Adolescence typically is defined as beginning at puberty, a physiological transformation that gives boys and girls adult bodies and alters how they are perceived and treated by others, as well as how they view themselves." [22]

Early and Late Adolescence

Most psychologists and others writing about adolescence divide it into two stages: early and late, each with developmental tasks. Early adolescence lasts for about 2 years and is characterized by growth spurts, maturing of reproductive functions and sex organs, increased weight, and changes in body proportions. These profound changes understandably may have profound psychological results.

Anyone who is around early teens knows that their self-images govern everything they do. The teen years are a time of intensely seeking one's "self." In its extreme form, the self is the way the body looks and nothing more. However, for many teens the absorption with the self goes beyond bodily appearance alone. Adolescents are generally concerned with fitting in with their peers. They will try various roles in an attempt to integrate their developing social skills with goals and dreams.

This early period of adolescence is so unsettling that psychologists and others have described it as a period of adolescent turmoil. However, other researchers indicate that adolescence may not be as fraught with emotional issues as has been previously thought. In an ethnographic study of early adolescent girls, both popular and not so popular, the findings revealed a close relationship with parents and certainly not the trauma and stress suggested by common discourses (or myths) about adolescence. Teachers, parents, and health care professionals may expect trouble from adolescents due to or attributed to "raging hormones," but in this study the trauma did not materialize.[23] At a minimum, there is clearly a disconnect between physical development and psychosocial maturation that may be the source of some conflict and also in part offers an explanation for the number of teen pregnancies and instances of sexually transmitted diseases.

⊙ REFLECTIONS

You walk into your co-worker's office and she is distracted and teary. You ask her what is wrong, and she says, "I am so upset. I found a bag of marijuana in Emma (her daughter's) backpack this morning. She is only 13. I don't understand what she could be thinking!"
- What advice would you give your colleague?
- Are there resources you would recommend?
- How would you feel if this was your daughter?
- How does your knowledge as a health care provider inform this scenario?

After this period of rapid and profound change, young people move into late adolescence. Here self-identity fully emerges as they practice the various roles and responsibilities they will assume as adults. Some adolescents do not move on to this stage of development because they literally do not survive. Teens 12 to 17 years old were, on average, more than twice as likely as adults (18 years and older) to be victims of violent crimes. Among this group, blacks were five times as likely as whites to be homicide victims.[24] The difference in the leading causes of death between white and black adolescents is one indication of the profound impact disparities can have on an adolescent's health and mortality. For example, adolescents in developing countries have to contend with poverty, starvation, and infectious diseases. Those in developed countries contend with obesity, sedentary lifestyles, violence, and eating disorders. Adolescents tend to spend less time with family and more time in new environments such as work settings, peer relationships, and romantic relationships. They move toward a more mature sense of themselves and start to question old values without losing their identity.

The impact of a peer's behavior on an adolescent is significant (Figure 15-2). In a study of 527 adolescents in grades 9 through 12, substance use (cigarette, marijuana, and alcohol use); violence (weapons and physical fighting); and suicidal behavior (suicidal ideation and attempts) were related to their friends' substance use, deviance, and suicidal behaviors, respectively. On the positive side, the more prosocial behavior of friends had a negative correlation with violence and substance abuse.[25] Other factors, such as family function, depression, and social acceptance, influenced adolescents' health-risk behavior as well.

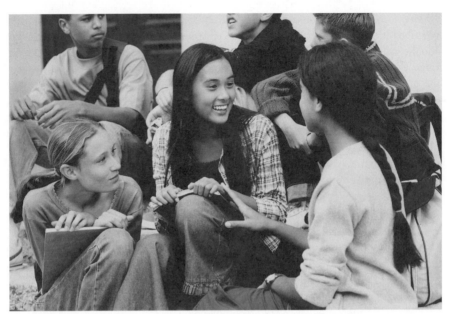

FIGURE 15-2: An adolescent's behavior is influenced by that of his or her peers. *(© Getty Images/590044.)*

Many adolescents who experience injury, illness, or disability find themselves halted in their progression to adulthood. The quote below by a parent sums this up nicely.

"Jeffery's accident struck him like a bomb as he was crossing the bridge to manhood. He was approaching independence. … Quadriplegic paralysis steals legs, arms, hands, fingers —and the future. Jeffery's paralysis stole our future … because no dream included paralysis. Not one."[26]

Needs: Respect, Autonomy, and Relating

Autonomous decision-making raises some delicate questions for health professionals who work with adolescent patients because adolescents often want to aggressively assert their authority in decisions. It is not always clear whether adolescents are capable of making wise authoritative decisions. Only in recent years has there been an attempt to address the legal rights of adolescents. The most prominent view, referred to as the *Mature Minors Doctrine,* allows for parents or the state to speak on behalf of a minor's interests only as long as the minor is unable to represent himself or herself. Thus, the level of the young person's development emerges as a decisive factor. In keeping with the legality of the Mature Minors Doctrine, you can try to assess the maturity of an adolescent patient in regard to his or her ability to cope effectively with illness or injury. The question whether an adolescent is a "mature minor" must be decided by health care professionals independent of parental judgment.[27]

There are some compelling reasons to give decision-making authority to mature adolescents. Some adolescents would never consult a health care provider with a problem if they knew it would require parental consent before treatment. Also, in their developing autonomy, they would never share delicate information with the provider if they thought confidentiality would be violated. Coupled with the reluctance of adolescents to speak about risky behavior or other health issues, they often do not receive recommended and preventive counseling or screening services appropriate to their age group.[28]

Adolescence was often viewed as a relatively healthy time in a person's life. However, behavior patterns can change rapidly in adolescence and can include irregular dietary habits, lack of sleep, inactivity, experimentation with drugs, alcohol and tobacco use, sexual activity, and reckless driving. The connection between these behaviors and long-term consequences for health is being increasingly recognized:

> ... [A] degree of experimentation and risk taking seem to be an integral part of the transition from childhood to adulthood, and most young people come through this phase of life relatively unscathed. So the challenge to researchers and clinicians alike is to be able to identify those at most risk of adverse consequences, without interfering with normal development, and to evaluate possible interventions that will result in improved long-term outcomes.[29]

Programs to promote healthy lifestyles for adolescents should include information on nutrition, activity, stress management, family planning, prevention of smoking, alcohol and substance abuse, safety (particularly personal computing and motor vehicle safety), and the spread of sexually transmitted diseases. Adolescents should be involved in the design of such health promotion programs so that they are both age and culturally relevant.

Family and Peers—Bridges to Respectful Interaction

Families and friends should not be excluded from the health care interaction process for adolescent patients. The aforementioned emphasis on the importance of the adolescent's autonomy and authority should in no way be seen as undermining the importance of treating the patient as a part of a family unit when one exists.

Most adolescents like to argue about adult rules, even those they accept. Listening to family exchanges about rules that the adolescent disagrees with often will provide insight into the conduct of the adolescent toward you, too. Also, the health professional should not assume that the adolescent's attitude toward parents means there is not a deep dependence on them or heartfelt caring from the family. Although adolescents always challenge authority figures, they need or want limits. Limits provide a safe boundary for teens to grow and function.[30]

⊚ REFLECTIONS

- What does it mean to "set limits"?
- Is limit setting easy or hard for you?
- How do you envision setting limits with clients and families in your professional practice?
- Do you anticipate that limit setting will be an easy or hard task for you?

It is important to note that families, like individuals, also develop over time. The family system changes as children and parents age. Normal life events such as job changes, relocations, changes in schools, changes in the family structure (e.g., loss of a grandparent), and changes in support systems all impact family function. Contemporary trends in family systems, such as divorce and remarriage, may also require additional developmental tasks to reestablish family cohesion. These types of families may exhibit higher levels of conflict during a child's illness because individuals who typically do not interact with each other may need to come together around care.[21]

Health professionals often benefit from including an adolescent patient's close friends and peers in interactions. Peer group activity is essential for identity formation, and all illnesses or injuries are jolts to the adolescent's identity. Getting to know an adolescent patient's friends by name, seeking their support, and trying to understand their feelings about the patient's condition can be helpful to all.

SUMMARY

In this brief overview of children and adolescents, the theme of respect revolves around at least two ideas—patient autonomy and effective relatedness. There are numerous ways in which the young patient will try to exert autonomy and find a way of relating with you effectively. By showing imagination—and at times, patience—you will have an opportunity to build a close and rewarding relationship.

One of the greatest challenges for you as a health professional is to think of the development of people from birth to adulthood as a continuum, with some moving along it faster than others. We have provided some guidelines that will help you think generally about people as they pause—then continue to pass through—older childhood and adolescence. The individual patient will present himself or herself as a unique individual still in the process of forming and refining an identity. You have a responsibility to be sure that, in the midst of activities such patients may engage you in, their health care needs are met. Having said that, we move ahead to the next chapter and the unique challenges associated with treating people in the adult years.

REFERENCES

1. Brown MW: *The important book*, New York, 1949, HarperCollins Publishers.
2. Dillard A: *An American childhood*, New York, 1988, Harper & Row.
3. Miller E, Kuhaneck H: Children's perceptions of play experiences and play preferences: a qualitative study, *Am J Occup Ther* 62:407–415, 2008.
4. Federal Interagency Forum on Child and Family Statistics: *America's children: key national indicators of well-being, 2011*, Washington, DC, 2011, U.S. Government Printing Office.
5. World Health Organization: *International classification of functioning, disability and health (ICF)*, Geneva, 2002, WHO. http://www.who.int/classifications/icf/training/icfbeginners-guide.pdf.
6. U.S. Census Bureau: *2010 American community survey*. http://www.census.gov/acs. Accessed February 29, 2012.
7. Boyle CA, Boulet S, Schieve LA, et al: Trends in the prevalence of developmental disabilities in US children, 1997-2008, *Pediatrics* 127:1034–1042, 2011.
8. *Americans with Disabilities Act of 1990 and ADA Amendments Act of 2008 (PL 110-325)*, January 1, 2009. http://www.ada.gov/pubs/ada.htm. Accessed March 29, 2012.

9. U.S. Department of Education: *Office of Special Education Programs: IDEA 04. Building the legacy.* http://idea.ed.gov/explore/home. Accessed March 29, 2012.

10. Sullivan PM, Knutson JF: Maltreatment and disabilities: a population-based epidemiological study, *Child Abuse Negl* 24(10):1257–1273, 2000.

11. Lawlor MC, Mattingly C: Understanding family perspectives on illness and disability experiences. In Crepeau EB, Cohn ES, Schell BA, editors: *Willard and Spackman's occupational therapy,* ed 11, New York, 2008, Lippincott Williams & Wilkins, pp 33–43. 2008.

12. Christensen P, Prout A: Working with ethical symmetry in social research with children, *Childhood* 9(4):477–497, 2002.

13. Kellett M, Forest R, Dent N, Ward S: "Just teach us the skills please we'll do the rest": empowering ten-year-olds as active researchers, *Children Soc* 18:329–343, 2004.

14. Purtilo RD, Doherty RF: *Ethical dimensions in the health professions,* ed 5, St Louis, 2011, Elsevier.

15. Brady M: Hospitalized children's views of the good nurse, *Nursing Ethics* 16:543–560, 2009.

16. Forsner M, Johnson L, Soerlie V: Being ill as narrated by children aged 11-18 years, *J Child Health Care* 9:314–323, 2005.

17. Fleitas J: When Jack fell down Jill came tumbling after: siblings in the web of illness and disability, *MCN Am J Matern Child Nurs* 25(5):267–273, 2000.

18. Kobrinsky NL, Sposto R, Shah NR, et al: Outcomes of treatment of children and adolescents with recurrent non-Hodgkin's lymphoma and Hodgkin's disease with dexamethasone, etoposide, cisplatin, cytarabine, and L-asparaginase, maintenance chemotherapy, and transplantation: Children's Cancer Study Group CCG-5912, *J Clin Oncol* 19(9):2390–2396, 2001.

19. Fleming SJ: Children's grief: individual and family dynamics. In Corr CA, Corr DM, editors: *Hospice approaches to pediatric care,* New York, 1985, Springer.

20. Committee on Bioethics: Informed consent, parental permission, and assent in pediatric practice, *Pediatrics* 95(314):314–317, 1995.

21. Leon AM, Knapp S: Involving family systems in critical care nursing: challenges and opportunities, *Dimens Crit Care Nurs* 27(6):255–262, 2008.

22. Call KT, Riedel AA, Hein K, McLoyd V, Petersen A, Kipke M: Adolescent health and well-being in the twenty-first century: a global perspective, *J Res Adolesc* 12(1):69–98, 2002.

23. Finders MJ: *Just girls: the hidden literacies and life in junior high,* New York, 1997, Teachers College Press.

24. Office of Justice Programs Press Release: *Nation's younger teens experienced largest decrease in crime victimizations between 1993 and 2003, Department of Justice.* http://www.ojp.usdoj.gov/archives/pressreleases/2005/jvo03pr.htm. Accessed April 1, 2012.

25. Prinstein MJ, Boergers J, Spirito A: Adolescents' and their friends' health-risk behavior: factors that alter or add to peer influence, *J Pediatr Psychol* 26(5):287–298, 2001.

26. Galli R: *Rescuing Jeffery: a memoir,* New York, 2000, St. Martin's Griffin. 48.

27. Cook R, Dickens BM: Recognizing adolescents' "evolving capacities" to exercise choice in reproductive healthcare, *Int J Gynaecol Obstet* 70(1):13–21, 2000.

28. Bethell C, Klein J, Peck C: Assessing health system provision of adolescent preventive services: the young adult health care survey, *Med Care* 39(5):478–490, 2001.

29. Churchill D: The growing pains of adolescent health researRch in general practice, *Prim Health Care Res Dev* 4:277–278, 2003.

30. U.S. National Library of Medicine, National Institutes of Health: *Adolescent development: MedlinePlus medical encyclopedia.* http://www.nlm.nih.gov/medlineplus/ency/article/002003.htm. Accessed March 27, 2012.

Respectful Interaction: Working with Adults

CHAPTER OBJECTIVES

The reader will be able to:

- Compare unique challenges of development in young and middle adulthood
- Discuss the meaning of work for adults
- Discuss "responsibility" as it applies to the middle years of life and how it may affect the patient's response to health professionals
- Describe at least three social roles that characterize life for most middle-age persons and consider ways in which showing respect for a patient requires attention to those roles
- Discuss how stress enters into attempts to carry out the responsibilities of each of the aforementioned roles and some health-related consequences of negative responses to stress
- List basic challenges facing health professionals who are working with an adult going through a midlife transition

"From a young 30- or 40-year-old, I turned into an old 30- or 40-year-old. But once I was 59 I wasn't too certain that the same magic as had been wreaked once I became a novice in other decades would continue to exert its power once I reached 60. Like Doris Day, I thought that "the really frightening thing about middle age is the knowledge that you'll grow out of it."

—V. Ironside[1]

Who Is the Adult?

It may be true that of all the life periods, adulthood has been the least understood and least studied. A stereotype about adult life is that it is only a waiting period or holding place made up of work, establishing a family, or dealing with menopause or other physical changes on the way to retirement and old age. In reality, there is a wide variation in the type and timing of transitions and activities in adult life that is far richer than this stereotype suggests. For these reasons, it is important to examine some vital issues concerning life as an adult in today's society.

Adulthood can be legally defined by chronological age or at the time a person begins to assume responsibility for himself or herself and others.[2] It can also be defined by achievement of certain developmental tasks such as being independent; establishing long-term relationships; establishing a personal identify in a reflective way; finding a meaningful occupation; contributing to the welfare of others or making a contribution to family, faith community, or society at large; and gaining recognition for one's accomplishments. Finally, adulthood can be defined in psychological terms, that is, by the level of maturity exhibited by a person. Mature persons are able to take responsibility, make logical decisions, appreciate the position of others, control emotional outbursts, and accept social roles. What it means to be an "adult" is a combination of many factors, the most important of which you will be introduced to in these pages.

Needs: Respect, Identity, and Intimacy

Adult development is not marked by definitive physical and psychomotor changes such as those seen in toddlers (e.g., learning how to walk), but it is full of challenging and largely unpredictable experiences. Adult life is marked by concepts such as independent life choices, midlife physical and emotional challenges and changes, generativity, facing the empty nest, the return of adult children, and the expansion of generations through the addition of grandchildren, although not every adult has these experiences. We would be better able to predict the response of a 5-year-old to a major illness than we would that of a 30-year-old. In addition, there may be differences in the way adulthood is experienced by men and women. Also, the specific point in history that a person enters adulthood may have profound implications for adult life. For example, many women who entered adulthood during the women's movement of the 1960s and 1970s had more opportunities regarding work and sexual freedom than the previous generation of women. Finally, development may also differ because of sexual orientation, race and ethnicity, socioeconomic status, and education, to name a few differences.

Biological Development during the Adult Years

From adolescence on, human beings continue to grow and mature. *Aging* can be defined as "the sum of all the changes that normally occur in an organism with the passage of time."[3] Demographers, social scientists, and developmental psychologists consider young adulthood to be roughly between ages of 21 and 40 and middle adulthood to be between the ages of 40 and 65.[4] Aging, like adulthood itself, is complex and varies from one person to another. The rate at which individuals age is highly variable, but so is the way they adapt to age-related changes and illness. Aging also gives rise to feelings of anxiety in a way no other area of human development does. Failing intellectual or biological functions in the middle years can become a preoccupation for your patient. For example, during this period the pure joy of physical activity experienced in younger years may acquire a sober edge. One of us overheard a man who for years has enjoyed running just for the sport of it tell his friend, "Yeah, my running will probably guarantee that I live 5 years longer, but I will have spent that 5 years running!"

Adults may also worry about the age-related changes that begin to take place in their body structures and functions. Suddenly, forgetfulness is no longer something to be taken lightly but could portend more serious problems generally associated with age. Perhaps the anxiety that aging provokes is due to the close relationship most of us believe exists between biological development and illness, decline, and death.[5] Rather than view aging in this way, gerontologists have proposed the concept of *compressed morbidity,* which suggests that people may live longer, healthier lives and have shorter periods of disability at the end of their lives. The focus of health care then becomes one of prevention, health improvement for chronic disease, and postponement of disability or death rather than cure.[6] In Chapter 17 we will discuss different views of aging and their impact on your interactions with older patients

In human beings the lifespan is thought to be about 110 to 120 years. In Western nations the average life expectancy is said to be 78.7 years, although this varies according to race and other variables (Black females, 78 years; Black males, 71.8 years; White females, 81.3 years; and White males, 76.5).[7] The 10 leading causes of death for all age groups in the US are listed in Table 16-1.[7] Cause of death varies according to race and sex, but this table provides a general idea of the types of illnesses you will encounter most often with adult patients. You will note that many of these causes of death are chronic diseases. Chronic disease is a major health problem in the United States. One in four Americans has multiple (two plus) chronic diseases, and the burden of chronic disease among racial and ethnic minorities is notably disproportionate.[8] Conditions such as diabetes, depression, and cardiovascular disease are now being diagnosed and treated earlier in adulthood than ever before.

As science progresses we learn more about how individual genes, biology, and behaviors interact with the social, cultural, and physical environment to influence health outcomes. Targeting prevention, illness management, and lifestyle modification in young and middle adulthood can increase quality of life and prevent the development and severity of chronic disease in older adulthood. Young adulthood is often referred to as the *healthy years and the hidden hazards.* Individuals in early and middle adulthood tend to underestimate the impact that poor lifestyle choices may have on their overall health span.

TABLE 16-1 Cause of Death

Causes of Death	Total Number of Deaths in the U.S. Population
1. Diseases of the heart	595,444
2. Malignant neoplasms	573,855
3. Chronic lower respiratory diseases	137,789
4. Cerebrovascular diseases	129,180
5. Accidents (unintentional injuries)	118,043
6. Alzheimer's disease	83,308
7. Diabetes mellitus	68,905
8. Nephritis, nephrotic syndrome, and nephrosis	50,472
9. Influenza and pneumonia	50,003
10. Intentional self-harm (suicide)	37,793

From U.S. Department of Health and Human Services, Centers for Disease Control and Prevention, National Vital Statistics Report January 11, 2012: Deaths: preliminary data for 2010, *Natl Vital Stat Rep* 6(4):1-69. Retrieved from: http://www.cdc.gov/nchs/data/nvsr/nvsr60/nvsr60_04.pdf.

Early Adulthood

As discussed in Chapter 15, it is during late adolescence that self-identity begins to form. These processes of identity exploration and consolidation continue in the beginning of early adulthood (generally between the ages of 17 and 24). Adulthood is not defined by a single factor, rather an integration of cognitive development, physical development, and societal experience. How individual's transition through adulthood is heavily influenced by experiences in previous stages of life.

⊚ REFLECTIONS

The transition from adolescence to adulthood is a process.
- Can you identify two to three factors that influenced your own transition to adulthood?
- How did your family or peers influence your transition?
- If you could go back in time, would you do anything differently? If so, why?

In the span of a few generations, the path to adulthood has changed dramatically. Today's young people are taking longer to leave home, attain economic independence, marry, and form families than did their peers half a century ago.[9] These longer transitions put strains on families and institutions (such as health care systems) that work with young adults. For example, adults who have children might believe that they have moved through an adult developmental task of parenting children, only to find their children returning home after a divorce or unemployment. Therefore, a parent or parents who might have been rejoicing in an empty nest and time for each other may find their adult children under their roof once again and with grandchildren in tow.

Thus, the societal context of delayed acquisition of independence, earlier physical maturation characteristic of modern cultures, pressures on young people to grow up fast, return of adult children to their parents' home, and delayed childbearing all complicate the traditional views held about progression through adulthood.

Even if we hold several variables constant (e.g., age, gender), it is still difficult to predict how two adult patients would react to the same diagnosis. Consider the example of Ms. McLean and Ms. Jeon, both of whom have just learned that they have in situ cancer of the cervix.

Sara McLean, age 34, has a family history positive for cervical cancer. Her maternal aunt and older sister both died of cervical cancer. Ms. McLean has recently become engaged and plans to be married in 6 months. She put off committing to a permanent relationship and starting a family until she completed graduate work in clinical psychology. With the support of her husband-to-be, she had planned on balancing a career as a private therapist with raising a family. She is devastated when the oncologist presents information about the treatment of choice for her condition—a total hysterectomy.

Continued

Eunice Jeon, age 33, also has in situ cancer of the cervix. She has no family history of cancer and has always prided herself on her "hearty" family stock. All of her grandparents are alive and well. Mrs. Jeon married her high school sweetheart the weekend after graduation. The Jeons have four children aged 5, 8, 10, and 12. Mr. Jeon is an emergency medical technician and plans someday to enroll in medical school after he finishes his bachelor's degree. Mrs. Jeon works as a secretary/receptionist at the Catholic grade school her children attend. She is troubled by the diagnosis, but when presented with treatment options merely asks, "When can we schedule the surgery? I want to get this taken care of as soon as possible."

Both of these women's feelings and reactions are the result of their life experiences to this point, which in turn, are determined by their roles and familial contexts. In Ms. McLean's case, her response to the diagnosis is influenced by her roles as daughter, sister, niece, fiancée, and psychologist. Mrs. Jeon's response is influenced by her roles as mother, wife, daughter, granddaughter, and receptionist. These life roles are only a few that we can ascertain on the basis of the information presented in the brief cases. It is highly probable that both women have many more roles. Ms. McLean planned her life around finishing her education. Mrs. Jeon's has revolved largely around her family. In short, just looking at their ages, it would be impossible to predict how Ms. McLean and Mrs. Jeon would interpret this crisis.

Illness and injury invariably result in changes in the patient's identity, as described more fully in Chapters 6 and 7. Identity provides continuity over time and across problems and changes that arise in life. So there is a sense of maintenance of self through identity and yet room for change to accommodate the vicissitudes of life. Adult patients are generally more capable of entering into a professional relationship as an equal partner than younger people. Even though adult patients are better able to protect their own interests and make their wishes known, they are still worthy of the respect that we accord to younger, generally more vulnerable, patients. Respect continues to be one of the hallmarks of effective interaction as we work our way through the lifespan.

Intimacy is another developmental task of the adult. According to Erikson, adult development is marked by the ability to experience open, supportive, and loving relationships with others without the fear of losing one's own identity in the process of growing close to another.[3] You were introduced to the difference between personal and intimate relationships in Chapter 5 illustrating that the type of intimacy a patient will experience with family members, lovers, and friends is deeper and more involving than personal caring relationships the patient and you will engage in. It is that deeper intimacy that Erikson is talking about. The major developmental facets of adult life are referred to repeatedly as we explore the social roles, meaning of work, and the challenges of midlife.

Psychosocial Development and Needs

Maturity requires the acceptance of responsibility and empathy for others. The concept of achievement central to adult life can be defined in a number of ways. Some midlife challenges discussed later in this chapter seem to stem from a person's having adequately assumed responsibility and realized his or her achievement potential, whereas others arise when the individual has failed to do so.

A profile of a person in the adult years of life will necessarily involve a consideration of his or her sense of "responsibility." When we ask if someone is willing to "assume responsibility," we are concerned with acts that the person can do and has voluntarily agreed to do. Given these conditions of ability and agreement, we want to know whether the person can be trusted to carry out the acts, regardless of whether the agreement was explicit (i.e., a promise to abide by the terms of a contract) or implicit (i.e., a promise to provide for one's own children or parents).

REFLECTIONS

Describe an activity you currently participate in.
- What are the environmental, personal and family or societal factors that facilitate your participation?
- How has this activity helped you find purpose/meaning in your life?
- How does this activity related to those you were exposed to as a child or young adult?
- Do you project that you will still be doing this activity in middle adulthood? Late adulthood? Why or why not?

Underlying the idea of acting responsibly is an assumption that the individual is a free agent (i.e., one who is willing and able to act autonomously). Thus, a person coerced into performing an act is not considered to have accepted responsibility for it.

During adulthood, there is another aspect to acting responsibly: it involves having a high regard for the welfare of others. The adult must find a way to support the next generation by redirecting attention from him or herself to others. In other words, the adult learns to care.[10] This involves empathy for the predicaments that befall others in life. The acts may flow from a free will, but the will must operate in accordance with reasonable claims and justifiable expectations of other people. The claims of society on a person peak during the middle years, so "acting responsibly" must be interpreted in terms of how completely the person fulfills the conditions of those claims.

For instance, in Hindu culture, one stage of acting out one's karma involves active engagement in the affairs of family and business. Only when an individual has successfully completed these tasks may he or she move on to higher, more contemplative levels of existence.

One way to view the matter in our culture is to review the discussion of self-respect in Chapters 4 and 5. Although our discussion there was on you, the same principles apply to adult patients. This basic value is among the most essential ingredients of "the good life." During the adult years, most people perceive their self-respect as being vulnerable to the judgments of others: One's self-respect at least partially depends on the extent to which he or she commands the respect of employer, family, and friends. This idea is related to our concept of "reputation": One commands respect by giving due consideration to society's claims. Hiltner notes, correctly we believe, that, to a large extent, even the personal values of the middle years must include a regard for others. For most, it is a highly social period when interdependencies are complex and pervasive.[11]

Adulthood sometimes involves people going back to previous developmental tasks such as establishing an identity if they did not resolve these issues previously in late adolescence or early adulthood. For example, in a study of gay males in middle adulthood, the researcher found that "these men were facing issues befitting their chronological age (nongay issues that had been worked on while leading a double life), as well as unresolved identity issues from the past."[12] The key point of this study is that the subjects were initially working through the earlier stage of development rather than reworking earlier developmental issues that can occur throughout adult development.

Social Roles in Adulthood

Several social roles most fully characterize this period involving primary relationships, parenting, care of older family members, and involvement in the community in the form of political, religious, or other social or service organizations and groups.

Primary Relationships

It is almost always during adulthood that a person decides with whom lasting relationships will be developed. Fortunately, an increasing number of older people are also developing new relationships, but they are usually people who were able to sustain deep and lasting relationships in the middle years as well.

The primary relationship takes priority over all others, the most common type being the relationship with a spouse. Choosing a spouse or other permanent companion and becoming better acquainted (i.e., learning to know the person, discovering potentials and limits, similarities and differences, and compatibilities and incompatibilities) are processes interwoven with the more basic activities of eating, sleeping, acquiring possessions, working, worshipping, relaxing, and playing together.

Those who do not enter into a marriage relationship sometimes develop a deep and lasting involvement with a partner, often a friend or sibling. One of your first tasks of respectful interaction with an adult patient is to find out if there is a key person in his or her life and, if so, who that person is. This can be accomplished without unnecessary probing into the person's private life. Particularly in times of crisis the patient looks to that key person for comfort, sustenance, and guidance. However, sometimes the person you assume would be the most supportive is not. Consider the case of Mary Ogden and Pam Carlisle.

> Mary Ogden, age 52, is a, single teacher who is hospitalized for treatment related to severe diabetes. The entire small community where she has resided and taught for 25 years adores her. Through the years she has received numerous awards for community service. She is a cheerful person, who, in spite of her illness, continues to be an inspiration to everyone. She is especially fond of Pam Carlisle, the head nurse on the unit where Mary is being treated.

On the afternoon before Mary's planned hospital discharge, an unscheduled visitor comes to the nursing desk insisting to speak to Pam about a highly personal matter. The visitor is Agnes Ogden, an elderly lady who informs Pam that she is the older sister (and only living relative) of Mary. The visitor seems sincere and asks that Pam provide details of her sister's condition so that she might be better prepared to aid her with both her physical illness and personal affairs. Pam complies with her request, actually feeling relieved that there is someone to share this burden with her. The following morning Pam visits Mary's room and finds her profoundly irate for the first time. She informs Pam that she has not been on speaking terms with her sister for many years, that she considers her sister to be untrustworthy, and that she thoroughly resents her sister's having the knowledge of her personal affairs and illness. Mary feels betrayed and develops a distrust of Pam as her health care provider. She becomes depressed, agitated, and uncooperative.

▶ What could Pam have done differently to foster Mary's trust rather than to destroy it? What would you have done when Agnes came to you requesting information?

▶ Besides violating HIPAA regulations that protect Mary's privacy and confidentiality, Pam has also broken the trust that once existed between them. How might you rebuild the trust that once existed between you and a patient should such a breakdown occur?

Parenting

Caring for children is often a part of adult life. The gender role stereotypes traditionally assigned to mothering and fathering are breaking down in many families so that both parents share the whole range of parenting skills. The concept of parenting is being expanded, too: There is the "single parent," who provides the full care usually shared with another; same-sex couples are parenting; and many children live within extended family situations in which parenting is shared by several persons.

⟳ REFLECTIONS

Parenting is often a part of adult life.
- What are some of the advantages and disadvantages of parenting children today?
- Is it one of your life goals to be a parent? Why or why not?
- If you are already a parent, how did you transition into this role?

Whatever the challenges of each model, all share the assumption that the child's welfare depends on the quality of parenting. The age-old recognition that a child's physical and emotional well-being depends on adult care is now buttressed by more recent assertions that the child's potential for fulfillment and satisfaction in later years is also determined in the earliest years of life that are strongly influenced by the parent. The least that can be said of parenting relationships is that they are among the most enduring and complex of human interactions (Figure 16-1). The health professional who fails to consider them respectfully neglects an integral part of the patient's identity.

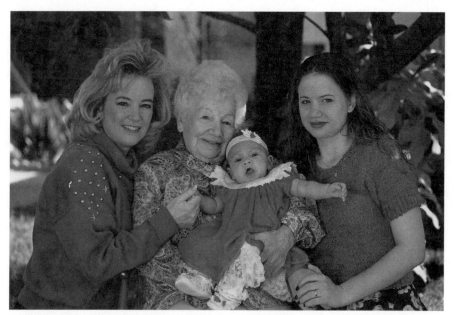

FIGURE 16-1: Parenting relationships are among the most enduring and complex of human interactions. (© Corbis.)

Care of Older Family Members

Not only do many adults care for children as a part of their daily responsibilities, but they also care for their parents, parents-in-law, and other older friends and relatives. Middle-age adults are often referred to as the "sandwich" generation because they are responsible for care of both the young (children) and the old (aging parents/ family members). The move toward supporting the older adult to age in place often increases the demands placed on adult children who support aging parents. A study by the national alliance for caregiving and the American Association of Retired Persons (AARP) found that one in four households in the United States provides care to someone 50 or older.[13] The average caregiver in the United States is a female in her late 40s. More than half of all caregivers are employed full or part time, and many care for their children at the same time. Caregivers often put the needs of their care recipients ahead of their own, placing them at high risk for poor physical and emotional health, as well as decreased quality of life. The responsibilities of caregiving can disrupt employment, health maintenance, leisure, and social participation.[14]

It is important to remember that just as family structure and functions differ from culture to culture, so do caregiving roles and expectations. For example, in a study of Mexican-American families and elder care, it was found that there is a clear sense of responsibility to care for the elder members of one's family.[15] Thus, women in this culture may go about readjusting their work obligations in different ways than women in other cultures. The cultural lens is essential for accurately viewing this role of adult life.

Political and Other Service Activities

Involvement in political and social organizations has traditionally been at a peak during the adult years. Responsibilities stemming from membership in such organizations are often second only to those of work if measured in terms of energy consumption and personal commitment. A sense of identity in adulthood depends heavily on belonging to such groups whether they be a political party, religious group, or service organization. These service activities are not only a source of identity but also a vehicle for contributing to one's profession or community.

In summary, there are other sources of claims on adults, but attending to primary relationships such as spouses, friends, children, and parents and contributing to public initiatives constitute some highly significant ones.

Work as Meaningful Activity

Work, like family and adulthood, is a concept that can be variably defined. Work as meaningful activity can occur in a variety of settings and assumes many patterns. Therefore, the meaning of work and the responsibilities it requires will depend on the person's value system, expectations, and aspirations, as well as the specific environment, job title, and position within a hierarchy. For some, work is performed primarily in the home; for a great many others, it entails a significant amount of time away from home. Adults are judged to spend about half of their waking hours engaged in work. The average U.S. employee works 7.5 hours a day. Women have a greater likelihood of working part time compared with men.[16] The kind of work they do largely determines their income, lifestyle, social status, and place of residence. Because of the amount of time and energy expended, the type of factual information one acquires over a lifetime is often influenced by the working situation (Figure 16-2). Studies of professional socialization suggest that, at least for white-collar and professional workers, the kind of work done also defines their worldview.

Work-related responsibilities still differ generally for men and women. You have undoubtedly observed what most women experience in their work roles: expectations on them include not only doing a job in the labor force as well as men but also maintaining the quality and amount of work performed in the home. Women respond to these various needs or demands by trying to balance their impulse to care and the level of personal support available.[17] When the limits of caregiving are reached, something else has to give. In many cases, women make changes and adjustments in their employment in order to continue in the caregiving role.[18]

Two types of responsibilities are associated with the work role: (1) to do one's job well and (2) to fulfill the reasonable expectations of others (e.g., employer, peers, family members). The professional relationship has the added dimension of caregiving: One is expected to help those who seek professional services.

Work relationships are different from simple friendships in a number of ways, although the former can be lasting, deep, and complex. Moreover, there is not always clear separation of the two. The carpool phenomenon is an intriguing combination of how work and friendship roles become intermingled; here people who are grouped together for the purpose of getting to and from their workplace also usually engage in camaraderie over minutes or hours each week and sometimes more regularly than

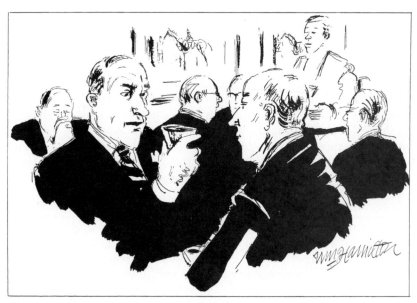

FIGURE 16-2: "I've learned a lot in 63 years. But, unfortunately, almost all of it is about aluminum." *(From The New Yorker, November 11, 1977, p. 27. © The New Yorker Collection 1977 William Hamilton from cartoonbank.com. All Rights Reserved.)*

with their own family members. We have known some carpool members who interact as friends or acquaintances during the commute, then assume their "proper" workplace role with each other when work begins.

Your task as a health professional is to assess how the patient views his or her work situation, what work means, and particularly the responsibilities and relationships in it. Whether a patient's work involves providing quality child care, laboring on the section crew to replace railroad ties, or presiding over a meeting in the executive suite, the work entails responsibility toward both a job to be done and other human beings. Treatment goals must be tailored to help the patient carry out these responsibilities, modify them, or accept that work may no longer be possible.

Those who work with adult patients in the areas of occupational health are keenly aware of the relationship among health, injury, or illness and the worker's role. Consider the following case:

> Masie Baldwin has worked as a nursing home aide for the past 15 years. She is the sole provider for her three children, one of whom has just started college. Although Ms. Baldwin has attended the mandatory in-service sessions on proper body mechanics and lifting of patients, she has not always followed the proper procedure. Ms. Baldwin stated to her fellow workers more than once, "I'm big and strong. I don't like waiting for help or lugging out the lift to get patients up. I can get them up and out of bed without help." Unfortunately, while getting Mr. Collins out of bed, Ms. Baldwin injured her lower back and neck.

Ms. Baldwin has been on workers' compensation leave for the past month and is now involved in a "work-hardening" program to determine if she is capable of returning to work in the nursing home. The health professionals working with Ms. Baldwin observe that she is highly motivated to return to work but frightened of reinjury. Her confidence in her strength and sense of invulnerability has been badly shaken. During a particularly trying day in the work-hardening program, she tells her therapist, "If I can't work in the nursing home, I don't know what I'll do. It's the only kind of work I've ever done. All my friends are there."

⑨ REFLECTIONS

- What "meanings" do you think Ms. Baldwin gives to her work?
- How does her identity tie to her work roles?
- What are some of the challenges you might face in working with Ms. Baldwin?

We have emphasized responsibility in terms of relationships and work roles in the adult years and that self-respect during this period is determined in large part by meeting the justifiable expectations of others. However, self-respect unquestionably also depends somewhat on believing in and being true to oneself. Thus, adults who meet all of society's expectations can still be unfulfilled.[19] That, in fact, is precisely the plight of many people today who have not pursued personal interests and goals at all or minimally. This situation can be viewed as an inability or unwillingness to assume responsibility toward oneself, and it contributes to the challenges of midlife that are discussed in this chapter. Accepting the consequences of one's own behavior is vital; all of us share, to some extent, the problem expressed by the motto on President Truman's desk, "The buck stops here." The sense of "being somebody," such an integral part of adolescence, must become more fully defined in the young and middle adult years. By middle adulthood, individuals are expected to be able to show more clearly who they are and what they are able to contribute to the welfare of loved ones and to society.

Stresses and Challenges of Adulthood

"In terms of social roles, adulthood is described generally as a time when the individual is a responsible member of society under pressure to coordinate multiple roles (e.g., spouse, worker, parent, caregiver)."[20] The more responsibilities a person assumes, the more vulnerable he or she becomes to the symptoms associated with stress. Stress is recognized as a potential threat to well-being and its negative effects will increase if steps are not taken to respond positively. Major problems associated with negative responses to stress in adult life are finally gaining the attention of investigators, health professionals, workplace counselors, and religious groups.

Chapter 4 addresses some sources of stress in students, and Chapters 6 and 7 suggest types of challenges faced by patients likely to produce stress at any age. The specific sources differ, but the means by which a young person has learned to cope and deal with stress will be carried into adulthood. One significant difference is that, in the middle years, no clearly defined end to some sources of stress—no "gracious exit" from an impossible situation—may be in sight. The stress attending next week's exam can be more easily managed than that arising from the realization that one has a stressful lifestyle in general.

Some stresses result from personal life choices. The responsibilities assumed in marriage and other primary relationships (e.g., childrearing, parent care, work) all create stress, as do unemployment and some factors in the social structure itself. Each is discussed separately.

Primary Relationship Stresses

Marriage relationships during the middle years have been studied more extensively than other types of primary relationships, but it is reasonable to believe that all such intimate relationships produce stressful situations. Common sources of stress in the marriage relationship include nonfulfillment of role obligations by a spouse, lack of reciprocity between marital partners, and a feeling of not being accepted by one's spouse. Illfeld maintains that sources of stress that are damaging to the marital relationship are those of an ongoing nature instead of those of a discrete event. He further proposes that these common, mundane stressors in everyday life take more of a toll in suffering than does the impact of a dramatic life crisis.[21] Couples with children often experience stress around the departure of their children, leaving both (and not only the woman, as is often thought) with the "empty nest syndrome." The empty nest has traditionally been a gendered approach to theorizing about changes in midlife. In addition to the empty nest, women's middle age is often discussed in terms of menopause and new opportunities for activity and self-expression. Also, menopause is not universally viewed as the critical event of middle age that many popular authors once claimed it to be.[22]

A more violent expression of stress, the primary source of which may not arise from the relationship itself but is acted out within it, is spousal domestic violence. This includes both physical and emotional abuse. Some persons involved in situations of domestic violence receive attention from self-help groups and other organizations, but not all do. They may well be present among your patients, exhibiting symptoms that deserve attention. For generations they have remained hidden and silent, victimized by the fear of stigmatization and having no place to go.

Refuges, or safe houses, exist in many cities and sometimes in rural areas. An increasing number of health professionals are volunteering their services for the treatment and rehabilitation of these women and men and their abusers.

Parenting Stresses

The tremendous responsibility associated with parenting also leads to stress situations in young and middle adulthood. Parenting is socially constructed, and there are both burdens and benefits to parenting. Because there is no "instructor's manual" on how to manage the twists and turns of parenthood, many of your patients may turn to you for advice. As a health professional, you may be the first to recognize the signs of parent stress. Providing a listening ear and care for the caregivers are key first steps in helping parents cope with stress. This supports the health of the family as a unit. Child abuse and neglect (discussed in Chapter 14), which are increasing (or, perhaps, are being reported more systematically), are tragic examples of what can happen when stress is not controlled. Most stress related to childrearing leads to less deplorable results, but nonetheless, it does take an immense toll on both parent and child.

Stress in Care of Elderly Family Members

Growing numbers of baby boomers will experience the struggles of an aging parent. Assuming the parents of baby boomers bore an average of two children, there are about 76 million parents of baby boomers who are dealing with the acute and chronic disabilities of old age.[23] As previously mentioned, the majority of the burden for parent care falls on adult women. Many quit their jobs to fulfill the responsibility of caring for one or more elderly family members. The stress is often borne with considerable grace as adult children express the desire to care for their parents and the satisfaction and joy it brings them in concert with the burdens. Unfortunately, elder abuse, like spousal and child abuse, is on the rise. Much needs to be done in the way of effective social policy development to assist families in caring for their frail family members so that they do not reach the limits of their endurance.

Work Stress

For many individuals in the middle years, stress related to work is their primary stress, manifesting itself in a wide range of disorders. The source of stress may be job dissatisfaction in general, coupled with the notion that there is nowhere else to turn. The job may be basically satisfactory but some component is an ongoing source of stress, such as a coworker who is a continual "thorn in the flesh." Some jobs are in themselves highly stressful. One of the highest-stress jobs is an enlisted soldier. Others are working in an airport control tower or a medical intensive care unit. Studies have demonstrated that a job with high responsibility in which the consequences for a mistake are dire creates the highest stress. Boredom and repetition also create stress. Work-related stress can be a key factor in the development of serious health problems such as cardiovascular disease and alcoholism or other substance abuse.

A particular form of stress related to the work role is caused by the inability to hold a job or find one. In a society that rewards its members for paid work, the stress of working can be less threatening to health and well-being than the stress of being unemployed.

Thus, it becomes evident that the middle years, in which a person is in many ways at his or her prime, are also years of responsibility and stress. The burdens, although each taken alone may be a small constraint, sometimes have the overall effect of making the middle-age person feel exhausted and overwhelmed. Although these years are sometimes characterized as a plateau or holding pattern, they are much more varied than that: They are filled, instead, with alpine meadows, treacherous cliffs, cool blue pools, and swift undercurrents.

⊚ REFLECTIONS

Think about all your current life roles.
- Did you choose these roles, or were they assigned to you?
- What are the behaviors expected by you in these individual roles?
- How do your roles influence your use of time? Do they conflict?
- How have you shaped this role? How has the culture in which you live shaped the role?
- What are the stressors associated with this role?

Doubt at the Crossroads and Midlife Challenges

The task of assuming responsibility and its attendant stresses, the great desire to achieve, or transitions in career, family life, and health condition may at some critical moment trigger an opportunity to take stock. The feeling accompanying the experience is most clearly expressed as doubt. It differs from the vacuous zero point of boredom and lacks the volcanic fervor of other types of stress. Doubt allows no rest; indeed, it is a relentless churning that nakedly reveals almost all the dimensions of one's life. The masks that have allowed the masquerade to go on, the clatter that has accompanied the parade, and the walls that have kept fearful monsters from view all suddenly evaporate and leave a pregnant silence. The self stands alone. Middle-age adults may wonder "Is this all there is?" and feel that "something is missing." Also, the focus on worldly aspirations may start to shift to more spiritual aspects of life and their place in the bigger scheme of things. Middle-age adults make more informed decisions about their futures.

The various transitions that are a part of adult life allow people to come to terms with new situations. Bridges conceptualize a transition as a three-phase psychological process people go through: ending, neutral zone, and new beginning.[24] A transition begins with an ending. Something must be left behind to move to the next phase. A transition may be sought or thrust upon a person.

⏀ Consider the case of Tanya Zorski, who worked as a claims processor at an insurance company for the past 10 years. Recently, Tanya's employer merged with another company, resulting in "downsizing" or firing of many people in the claims department, including Tanya. Tanya's transition begins with the ending of her job. The next phase of transition is the neutral zone. After letting go, willingly or unwillingly, she must examine old habits that are no longer adaptive.[21] As Tanya begins to look for another position, she will discover that the computer skills that had been adequate at her old job are not marketable. Employers want people with experience in leading-edge computer programs, and Tanya does not possess these skills. During the neutral zone phase, people start to look for new, better-adapted skills or habits. People may take this opportunity to pursue a long-held dream. The final phase is the new beginning. Tanya decides to move into a new beginning in her life by pursuing a degree in nursing. She reasons that if she is going to invest the energy, time, and financial resources in learning new skills, she might as well do it in a profession that she has wanted to join since she was young.

> ⊙ **REFLECTIONS**
>
> • Do you anticipate working in the same job for your entire career?
> • What would make you "shift gears" in your work, living arrangements, or location?

Although changes in midlife have often been labeled as a "crisis," perhaps the language is too strong. "Instead, perhaps, many individuals make modest 'corrections' in their life trajectories—literally, 'midcourse' corrections."[25] These corrections to one's life course are often the opportunity for growth and learning along the lifespan. As is the case with Tanya Zorski, the more life changing an event, the more likely it is to be associated with learning opportunities. "In fact, learning may be a coping response to significant life changes for many people."[26]

Regardless of whether a vision is being claimed or reclaimed, the adult's task is to prepare for the adjustments and challenges still to come.

Working with the Adult Patient

This chapter deals almost exclusively with the psychosocial processes people face in their young and middle adult years.

The patient you encounter in his or her adult years who arrives at the health facility may be working to maintain health or may be experiencing an illness-related symptom. Because these years are not "supposed to be" characterized by painful or other troubling physical symptoms, patients may feel especially angered or confused by this physical intrusion into their work of being a responsible person and pursuing goals. A woman of middle years who was being interviewed recently in a seminar reported that "being an adult was overrated!" Her father was in hospice for end-of-life cancer care, two of her three sons required special education services for attention deficit hyperactivity disorder and learning disorders, and she was just told by her primary care physician that she needed to follow up with an oncologist for a positive mammogram. The idea of being struck down in one's prime and that of the "untimely" accident or death are often applied to this age group. The denial, hostility, and depression that patients feel about being so attacked are factors to which you should give your attention, whether your interaction occurs only once or extends over a long period of time.

Because psychological and social well-being are preeminent for adults, treatment must be attuned to both. Of all the challenges described in Chapter 6, the loss of independence most epitomizes the overall loss experienced by the adult patient. Of course, the person's former self-image is threatened, too, but this is almost a direct outgrowth of the loss of independence. A patient who can no longer go about meeting the responsibilities expected of him or her and pursuing the numerous life goals now established may feel trapped, vulnerable, and frustrated. The primacy of these concerns in middle life should help you to understand why a patient seems overly concerned about having to get a babysitter for an hour or having to be home at a given time or why he or she is willing to forego treatment rather than to take time from work for a trip to the health facility.

Furthermore, an adult patient experiencing acute stress poses special problems and challenges. Each one must be treated according to the particular manifestations of the stress. Part of the respect you must express is to assess physical or psychological symptoms that may be arising from stress. This, of course, must often be done with a psychiatrist or psychologist, but not always. As you learned in Chapter 8, the skills of listening to the patient's narrative are tools to help you discern what is on a patient's mind. Listening may not only help to decrease his or her anxiety at the moment but may also enable you to make adjustments in schedule, routine, or approach that will further diminish it.

Many of the suggestions given throughout this book apply to all age groups. However, if you are alert to some of the central concerns and roles of young and middle adulthood, you may well find that your success in achieving respectful interaction with the adult patient is heightened. In the next chapter you have an opportunity to examine some changes that are faced by the person who has successfully lived through the middle years. As you will see, these changes involve some of life's greatest challenges, both positive and negative.

SUMMARY

Even though biological capacities begin to diminish in adulthood, adults have sufficient capacity for personally satisfying and socially valuable participation. The major life tasks for adults are to establish personal identity, develop intimate relationships, and feel and act on the desire to make a lasting contribution to the next generation through parenting, work, and public service activities. Although some people never resolve the issues that are brought into focus during the transitions of midlife, fortunately most do. Some emerge from the process with a new job, a new mate, or a new life view. The various aspects of adult development that were presented in this chapter are a sampling of the ways you can look at the complex process of how people grow and develop as adults with an eye to how these observations can help you to be respectful in your relationships with adult patients and their families.

REFERENCES

1. Ironside V: *You're old, I'm old … get used to it! Twenty reasons why growing old is great*, New York, 2012, Plume—The Penguin Group.
2. Erikson EH: *Childhood and society*, ed 2, New York, 1963, WW Norton.
3. Matteson ES, McConnell ES, Linton AD, editors: *Biological theories of aging in gerontological nursing: concepts and practice*, ed 2, Philadelphia, 1996, WB Saunders.
4. Brim OG, Ruff CD, Kessler RC, editors: *How healthy are we? A national study of well-being at mid-life*, Chicago, 2004, University of Chicago Press.
5. Mott VW: Our complex human body: biological development explored. In Clark MC, Caffarella RS, editors: *An update on adult developmental theory: new ways of thinking about the life course: new directions of adult and continuing education*, San Francisco, 1999, Jossey-Bass.
6. *U.S. Department of Health and Human Services Healthy People.* (website) , 2010. http://www.health.gov/healthypeople. Accessed July 12, 2006.
7. U.S. Department of Health and Human Services: *Centers for Disease Control: National Vital Statistics Report*, January 11, 2012. http://www.cdc.gov/nchs/data/nvsr/nvsr60/nvsr60_04.pdf. Accessed April 3, 2012.
8. IOM (Institute of Medicine): *Living well with chronic illness: a call for public health action*, Washington, DC, 2012, The National Academies Press.

9. Settersten RA, Ray B: What's going on with young people today? The long and twisted path to adulthood, *Future Children* 20:19–41, 2010.
10. Reeves PM: Psychological development: becoming a person. In Clark MC, Caffarella RS, editors: *An update on adult developmental theory: new ways of thinking about the life course: new directions of adult and continuing education*, San Francisco, 1999, Jossey-Bass.
11. Hiltner S: Personal values in the middle years. In Ellis EO, editor: *The middle years, Acton, Mass*, 1974, Publishing Sciences Group.
12. Peacock JR: Gay male adult development: some stage issues of an older cohort, *J Homosex* 40(2):13–29, 2000.
13. National Alliance for Caregiving: Caregiving in the United States, *Press Release*, December 8, 2009. http://www.caregiving.org/pdf/research/CaregivinginUS09Release12309.pdf. Accessed April 3, 2012.
14. Piersol CV, Earland VT, Herge EA: *Meeting the needs of caregivers of persons with dementia: an important role for occupational therapy, OT practice*Bethesda, MD, March 26, 2012, AOTA Press. p 8–12.
15. Clark M, Huttlinger K: Elder care among Mexican American families, *Clin Nurs Res* 7(1):64–81, 1998.
16. U.S. Department of Labor Bureau of Labor Statistics: *American Time Use Survey—2010 Results. News release,* June 22, 2011. http://www.bls.gov/news.release/pdf/atus.pdf. Accessed April 3, 2012.
17. McGrew KB: Daughters' caregiving decisions: from an impulse to a balancing point of care, *J Women Aging* 10(2):49–65, 1998.
18. Pohl JM, Collins CE, Given CW: Longitudinal employment decisions of daughters and daughters-in-law after assuming parent care, *J Women Aging* 10(1):59–74, 1998.
19. Moos RH, Billings A: Conceptualizing and measuring coping resources and processes. In Goldberger L, Breznitz S, editors: *Handbook of stress: theoretical and clinical aspects*, New York, 1982, Free Press.
20. Helson R, Sato CJ: Up and down in middle-age: monotonic and nonmonotonic changes in role, status and personality, *J Pers Soc Psychol* 89(2):194–204, 2005.
21. Illfeld FW: Marital stressors, coping styles and symptoms of depression. In Goldberger L, Breznitz S, editors: *Handbook of stress: theoretical and clinical aspects*, New York, 1982, Free Press.
22. Gergen MM: Finished at 40: women's development within the patriarchy, *Psychol Women Q* 14:471–494, 1990.
23. Sherman FT: This geriatrician's greatest challenge: caregiving, *Geriatrics* 61(3):8–9, 2006.
24. Bridges W: *Managing transitions: making the most of change*, Reading, MA, 1991, Addison-Wesley.
25. Stewart AJ, Ostrove JM: Women's personality in middle age: gender, history, and mid-course corrections, *Am Psychol* 53(11):1185–1194, 1998.
26. Zemke R, Zemke S: Adult learning: what do we know for sure? *Training Magazine* 32:31–40, 1995.

Respectful Interaction: Working with Older Adults

CHAPTER OBJECTIVES

The reader will be able to:

- Discuss in general terms the developmental tasks in the later years of life
- Describe the roles of friendship and family ties among older people and how these ties can have an impact on an older patient
- Compare and contrast at least two psychological theories of aging
- List some basic challenges to well-being that present themselves in old age and some ways to help older people meet such challenges successfully
- Summarize the reasons an established time for treatment and a regular routine may be signs of respect toward older patients
- Discuss appropriate and inappropriate responses to a patient who has acute or permanent cognitive impairment
- List some values that may become highly prized among many older people, and suggest approaches that the health professional can use to optimize those values

John Quincy Adams is well. But the house in which he lives at present is becoming dilapidated. It is tottering upon its foundation. Time and the seasons have nearly destroyed it. Its roof is pretty well worn out. Its walls are much shattered and it trembles with every wind. I think John Quincy Adams will have to move out of it soon. But he himself is quite well, quite well.

—*John Quincy Adams in a response to a query regarding his well-being on his 80th birthday[1]*

One of the challenges confronting anyone who attempts to speak of the older adult is to earmark exactly when old age begins, even though it is a phase of life everyone will enter if they are fortunate enough to live past middle age. According to many statements on social policy, eligibility for financial and other supportive benefits begins at age 65, but the usefulness of this age as a distinguishing line largely ends there. In fact, people's feelings that they are "old" are usually determined by the presence (or absence) of sickness, disability, or other factors rather than simply by their chronological age. For the purposes of this chapter, terms such as "elder," "old," and "aged" will refer to individuals in later adulthood—age 65 or older. Late adulthood can be divided into the young old, age 65 to 75; the middle old, age 75 to 85; and the old old, age 85 and older.

The older population numbered 40.3 million in 2010 (the latest census year for which data are available). They represented 13% of the U.S. population. By 2050, there will be about 88.5 million older persons, more than twice their number in 2010.[2] The baby boomer generation is largely responsible for this increase in the older adult population. A "baby boomer" is an individual born between 1946 and 1964. Boomers comprise one of the largest generations in U.S. history. The boomers began crossing into the older adult (65+) category in 2011, and they will continue to do so until 2030, shifting the U.S. age structure from 13% of the population in 2010 to 19% of the population in 2030. Geographically, the South contains the greatest number of people age 65 and older, while the Northeast has the largest percentage of people in older ages.[3] Even though not all older Americans are sick, it is true that the average patient in a health care facility is likely to be older than 75 years of age. Additionally, the older population—the heaviest users of the health care system—will be far more diverse and will be women, especially among the oldest old, or people older than 85.[3] Thus, if you work in an inpatient health care facility you will probably encounter older patients who will likely be women from diverse backgrounds.

Almost every generality advanced about the older person is quickly countered by an individual's personal experience with a chronologically older man or woman. However, many processes that take place in a person as he or she advances in years differ from one individual to another. This chapter provides an overview of physiological and psychosocial changes, with a special emphasis on the psychosocial aspects of aging as they are relevant to respectful interaction. We urge you to study the burgeoning literature of aging further because the questions and clinical issues surrounding care of older patients are complex.

⊚ REFLECTIONS

Close your eyes and imagine yourself at age 85.
• What do you imagine you will be like? Look like?
• What roles will you have? How will they differ from your roles today?
• When you tell your life story – what will the highlights be?

The days of "over the river and through the woods to grandmother's house" have disappeared in large segments of today's society. Indeed, grandmothers may be actively involved outside of the home in a work setting or in voluntary community work. She may be raising grandchildren while mom or dad works.

Older persons are among us in a variety of roles. The rapid societal changes taking place around older people give them greater opportunity for divergent roles than ever before. If they are unable to take advantage of these opportunities, as many are, then they are burdened with greater insecurity and more complex problems than were any of their predecessors. However, if they can make the best of these opportunities, their potential for an active and meaningful old age is excellent.

Views of Aging

"Aging is a highly individualized process that affects each person in unique ways. Aging is the result of the interaction among genetics, environmental influences, life-styles, and the effects of disease processes."[4] This definition of aging is fairly straight-forward, but there is much more to aging than mere physiological changes. Cultural and societal views of aging influence how you understand the aging process and how you work with older patients. The following are various views of aging, with some examples involving older patients.[5]

Unwelcome Reminder of Mortality

Death is more common in old age in the United States than it is in younger age groups. Thus, it is often seen as an expected part of older age and more "natural." "The effect of this view is that the more natural and acceptable mortality is thought to be for 'the elderly,' as they are sometimes called, the more unthinkable it is for the non-elderly, and the more elderly people are avoided as symbols of the unthinkable."[5] Thus, one of the major problems of working with older people is that we have not come to terms with our own aging and mortality. The presence of the aged is an uncomfortable reminder of the future that is in store for all of us. Health professionals sometimes react to this discomfort by trying to avoid such patients whenever possible.

Underprivileged Citizens

Ageism as a type of discrimination and demeaning behavior was addressed in Chapter 3. "Most people, including healthcare professionals, are more familiar with path-ological aging than with healthy aging and tend to generalize and project expectation of pathology. Ageism is thus the composite of stereotypical beliefs and attitudes held about a group of people based on their advanced age."[6] In this view, old adults are not readily accorded the respect they deserve but are forced often to rely on the benevo-lence of society in an attempt to make up for past and continuing discrimination. Programs such as Medicare and Medicaid, "senior discounts," and special services for "senior citizens" are examples of programs designed to redress shortcomings in society's treatment of older people as full citizens. Because we live in a youth-oriented society, older people may seem to have little importance. What young people see or read in the media or hear from adults plays a critical role in shaping their perceptions of older people.[7] Thus, it is important to promote representations of elderly people in the full range of activities and health states that comprise old age.

Aging as a Clinical Entity

This view of aging sets it apart from other life experiences shared by all human beings. Aging is seen as a clinical entity in its own right, something to be studied and analyzed through research. The subspecialties of *geriatrics* in health care and *gerontology* in the social sciences bear witness to the trend of separating out the unique features of aging. Although considerable positive developments have come from this view of aging, such as recognizing the special strengths of older patients, as well as deficits, the risk remains that older patients will be treated differently from younger ones merely because they are old. An example of this can be found in a study of the recommendations medical students give to older (≥59 years) and younger (≤31 years) women regarding breast-conserving procedures. Although research has determined equivalent results between breast-conservation therapy and modified radical mastectomy, the medical students ($N = 116$) were biased by patients' ages when making recommendations. "They recommended breast-conservation therapy for a significantly higher percentage of younger patients than older patients (86% vs. 66%)."[8] When age is inappropriately used to determine treatment options, it is a form of ageism. Fortunately, new theories of social and psychological development show that some aspects of development can continue throughout the life span.

Older People as a Cultural Treasure

The most positive view of aging is to see people who have lived a long time as a source of wisdom and experience. Recent interest in obtaining oral histories from elders who have witnessed great and mundane historical events is evidence of this view. The past experience of elderly people is of value to younger generations and fits well with Erikson's theory about the later stages of adult development.

⊚ REFLECTIONS

Historic events in our society and culture greatly influence our lives. You often hear older adults reminisce about these events. For example, they may say –
"I remember exactly where I was the day JFK was shot" or "it was a historic day when man landed on the moon".
Name a historic event that influenced you and/or your family.
- you participated in your life roles?
- How did your family talk about this event?
When you recount this event to the next generation, what will you say?

Needs: Respect and Integrity

Several basic psychological and social processes are evident in the widely divergent lifestyles of today's older people. Erikson proposes that the success with which an older person can make psychological and social adjustments will depend on his or her ability to meet the most basic psychosocial developmental challenge of old age— that of integrity. In this last stage of human development, the person "understands, accepts, and loves the life he [or she] has led."[9] The person "possesses wisdom" and is willing to share this wisdom with the younger generation.[9] The little girl and older man in Figure 17-1 perfectly illustrate this sharing of expertise across generations.

Health professionals are delighted, and sometimes awed, by an older person who expresses the breadth and depth of acceptance described by Erikson. These older people readily accept the psychological and social adjustments that confront them. However, some older persons despair of being old, the psychological and social adjustments of old age overwhelm them, and they find little from their past to support them in their present situation. Key psychological and social processes assist or deter older persons from achieving a sense of wholeness and integrity in old age. Some of these are discussed on the following pages.

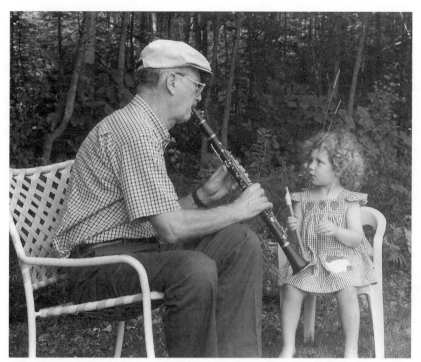

FIGURE 17-1: Shared expertise across generations (© 1995 Joan Beard, from Family: a celebration, edited by Margaret Campbell, Peterson's [USA].)

Psychology of Aging

One theory of aging, the disengagement theory, suggests that, even before their friends die, some people contribute to their own isolation. In Elaine Cumming and William Henry's 1961 book, *Growing Old: The Process of Disengagement,* the following broad points were made:

> Starting from the common-sense observation that the old person is less involved in the life around him than he was when he was younger, we can describe the process by which he becomes so, and we can do this without making assumptions about its desirability. In our theory, aging is an inevitable mutual withdrawal or disengagement, resulting in decreased interaction between the aging person and others in the social systems he belongs to … [The individual's] withdrawal may be accompanied from the outset by an increased preoccupation with himself; certain institutions in society may make this withdrawal easy for him.[10]

They view disengagement as a normal process that occurs earlier for some than for others, depending on the person's physiology, temperament, personality, and life situation. Retirement, they propose, is society's permission for men to disengage, whereas widowhood serves the same purpose for women; the disengaged person eventually develops a high morale. Some of the postulates of the disengagement theory appear dated, such as the one regarding gender roles.

Many critics, beginning in the 1970s, have questioned whether disengagement theory is a true or desirable indication of successful aging. The theory views the elder as less important in the nuclear family, business, and social arena, which can lead to the dangerous outcome of dependency. It was, however, one of the first attempts at a "grand theory" of aging and, as such, remains of interest to the field of gerontology.[11]

Contemporary theories of aging include the socioemotional selectivity theory (SST), the continuity theory, the activity theory, and the gerotranscendence theory. The SST states that as people age, they become increasingly selective of their social partners in order to conserve energy and to regulate emotions.[12] The continuity theory states that the personality, habits, and preferences that people develop throughout their life experiences are brought into old age. In this theory, how the elder engages in the social environment and the magnitude of this engagement varies according to the person's established lifelong patterns.[13]

The activity theory has also received much attention given the societal focus on aging well. In this theory older people must stay active and involved in activities to maintain their own integrity and life satisfaction.[14] The nature of activities changes over time. They can be informal, formal, or solitary activities. You often hear older adults state, "I never knew when I retired I would be so busy." The engagement in leisure, community, and family activities supports the older adult in health and wellness through participation in meaningful roles.

Another new theory of aging is gerotranscendence, a shift in perspective from a materialistic and rational vision to a more cosmic and transcendent one. Gerotranscendence is the final step in individual maturation and toward achieving wisdom, a new construction of reality for the aged individual.[15]

Recently, healthy aging has been described as a lifelong process optimizing opportunities for improving and preserving health and physical, social, and mental wellness; independence; quality of life; and enhancing successful life-course transitions.[16] This definition of healthy aging requires that older adults work to overcome the natural losses that occur with age. As you can see, there is still considerable disagreement about what counts as successful old age. Older adults have defined healthy aging more simply as having the physical, mental, and financial means to go and do something worthwhile.[17]

⊚ REFLECTIONS

- Can you think of some problems that could occur clinically if you and a colleague differed in your definition of "good" old age?
- What if your idea of healthy aging differs from that of your elderly patient? Identify some of the elderly people that you know.
- What theory best describes the attitudes of your elderly patients toward relationships, gains or losses, etc.?

Friendship and Family Ties

The amount of contact older people maintain with their families and friends varies greatly. Many persons lose a valuable source of natural physical contact and companionship with the diminution of friendship and family ties, whereas others remain actively integrated into family and community circles. If you take time to assess how many of your patients' needs for physical contact are still being met by friends and family, you will understand a lot about their conduct during their time with you. It is not unusual for people to transfer their needs to health professionals once they have lost other contacts.

Friendships

Until the present ultramobile way of life in the United States, the acquisition of a single set of friends continued throughout early life and tapered off when one settled down in a community.

One's job seldom changed during the entire period of employment, and, as a result, the community (and the friends therein) remained the same up through old age. In one sense, this is a secure mode of existence, but reliance on lifelong friendship carries with it the risk that, if these friends all die, the person will be left alone. Many people who have depended on lifelong friendships find it difficult to make new acquaintances at 70 or 80 years of age. Friendships have been demonstrated to influence a person's psychological well-being. An older person's attitudes toward friendships and the makeup of the physical environment play a role in the maintenance and development of friendships in old age.[18]

The older person's ability and desire to make new friends depend partly on the extent to which friendship has been considered an important individual value throughout life and therefore on the extent to which friendship skills have been cultivated. Another important determinant is the types of friendships the person established in younger years.

There are basically four types of friendships, which vary in number and importance over the years:

1. *Fusion* friendships, which are fused to or an integral part of other roles, such as those involving family or occupation, increase or decrease in importance according to the person's present situation.
2. *Substitution* friendships are those into which the person channels energies that formerly were directed toward someone or something else.
3. *Complementary* friendships develop from situations in which another role (such as that related to occupation) and the friendship are mutually supportive.
4. *Competition* friendships are those that compete with another role.[19]

Therefore, an older person whose fusion or complementary friendship, made at an early age and, centered on his or her occupation, may find that after retirement the friend is very much alive, but their friendship is dead. Conversely, a substitution or competition friendship may thrive after retirement because energy directed elsewhere can now be devoted to the friend. In this sense, the basis of a friendship is an important determinant of its longevity. In working with patients, you can understand some important things by exploring who the person's friends are and how the friendships were generated and sustained.

Family

As we discussed in Chapter 14, the family structure is changing. Participation in families is one of the most lasting and significant roles a person assumes.

In married relationships or other long-term couple relationships, the history is that the couple usually had an opportunity to spend much time alone together. When children become a part of the relationship, attention is transferred to them, and in many families much of the communication for many years takes place in the presence of at least one child. For persons with no children, jobs often become the center of attention. Only after the children have left home or the working years end is the couple alone again. Their attempts to reestablish direct communications are sometimes futile, causing them to withdraw, literally or symbolically, from the family. Other couples find this to be an opportunity to engage in activities together that they put off in their younger years.

In the present oldest population, those 85 years and older, there are many married or formerly married people. Older men are more likely to be married than older women are. You may work with elderly women who are not prepared to cope with financial and other business affairs because in their youth it was considered improper for women to be thus involved. You may work with elderly men who have never had to prepare a meal or wash clothes because it was considered improper for a man to do "woman's work." There is generally a balance of tasks that most married couples maintain. In the examples given earlier, the husband did the bills and the wife cooked. When a spouse can no longer perform his or her essential role due to illness or injury, the partner may become overwhelmed by the need to complete additional tasks. The death of a spouse or partner can be extremely difficult for older adults. Sometimes they turn to children, nieces, or nephews for help. Elderly people often turn to siblings when they find themselves alone. A sibling has the added benefit of a shared history, as is evident in the following poem:

HOMECOMING

I
after 45 years
of writing letters
& calling, Estelle sent word
to find a contractor—
she wants a home
built next to her sister
the house, brick & modern,
is an oddity—
sits prominently among shotgun houses,
cows, chickens, fish ponds, bait shops
& trailer homes
Celeste walks the clay red road
to her Oakland-California-sister—
they have forty-five years to catch up on

II
Estelle & Celeste talk of the other two sisters
who died in their early 70s—
bring out boxes of black & white worn photos
Estelle rakes arthritic fingers
through Celeste's hair
conjuring memory
she parts the white/yellow-stained strands—
braids her sister's hair.
    —Andrea M. Wren[20]

A discussion of aging and family relationships must include a look at who is most likely to provide support for older people in times of illness. Social support systems for people who are ill include both family caregiving that exceeds normal care or help and informal ones (friends, neighbors, or members of a religious or other type of community). As we discussed in Chapter 16, families provide the majority of care for older relatives. Many families struggle to provide this care, as is evident in the following example.

> Dad may be desperately ill, demanding constant attention and unable to join the family and guests at dinner. Mom may be afflicted with Alzheimer's and can't follow a conversation. Grandma may be bedfast. And in as many cases as not, the woman of the house does the caretaking even though she is poor, busy with a job to stay above subsistence level, preoccupied with her own children, and untrained. In such circumstances—God forbid—there is no extra room for the ill or aged, and little patience or reason for hope. Caring in the home is still the great overlooked medical-social problem among all classes in the United States.[21]

High levels of caregiver stress can sometimes lead to elder abuse. *Elder abuse* can take several forms:
1. Rights violations—denial of basic rights to adequate medical care or decent housing
2. Material abuse/exploitation—monetary or material theft, fraud, or undue influence as a level to gain control over an older person's money or property
3. Physical abuse—covers a variety of practices from omission (leaving a nonambulatory person in bed for long periods of time) to commission (beating or injuring the person)
4. Psychological/emotional abuse—a situation in which the person is debased and intimidated verbally, threatened, isolated, or belittled
5. Sexual abuse—sexual contact that is forced, tricked, threatened, or otherwise coerced upon a vulnerable elder (including one who is unable to grant consent)
6. Neglect/abandonment—a caregiver's failure or refusal to provide for a vulnerable elder's safety, physical needs, or emotional needs; the desertion of a vulnerable elder by anyone with a duty of care[22,23]

Elder abuse is often not reported because the older person (or others) fear retaliation or believe that nothing will be done to change the situation. Just as with a child whom you suspect is being abused or neglected, you are legally responsible in all 50 states for reporting suspected elder abuse. It is important to add, unfortunately, that elder abuse is not isolated to the home setting. Elder abuse can occur in institutional settings as well, such as domiciliary homes, nursing homes, adult day care, or even hospitals.

Where "Home" Is

A major challenge for older people is to decide where to make their homes. Key components of independent living for older adults include physical health, functional ability, and social ability (including driving and access to the community).[24] Security, accessibility to services, transportation, and physical considerations due to bodily changes in aging are important variables in elder housing decisions. Reduced income and the desire to be near friends or relatives also often weigh heavily for people who have a choice of location. Senior apartment communities and naturally occurring retirement communities such as assisted living facilities are housing resources that allow the older adult resident to age in place.[25] For older persons with functional disabilities or those who need more assistance with daily living activities than can be provided at home by family or professional caregivers, an assisted living or nursing home may become their last place of residence. Primary reasons for admission to nursing homes include Alzheimer's disease and osteoporotic hip fractures. About 90% of nursing home residents are older than 65, but only 3.1% of the total 65+ population (approximately 1.3 million people) lives in a skilled nursing facility.[3] Of this population, there were about 2.5 times the number of women than men in this setting. It is important to remember that not all admissions to skilled nursing facilities are for the rest of a patient's life. Some elderly patients are admitted only for a short time for rehabilitation so that they can regain strength and function and return to independent living. Chapter 6 addresses how changes associated with illness or injury are a challenge for any patient.

⊚ REFLECTIONS

Imagine you are suddenly injured and told that you must live in a nursing home for a minimum of one year.
- What would you miss most about your current home? Why?
- What about the move would be hardest for you to cope with?
- What supports would make such a move easier for you?

You will benefit from bearing in mind that these may have already occurred for the older person simply because he or she is old rather than because of illness or injury. The loss of a long-established place of residence, of consequence to anyone, is felt deeply by the older person because self-respect and the power to command the respect of others depend, in part, on independence. Although many patients experience the loss of independence as temporary, older people usually realize that each loss is a one-way street to more dependence. Moving out of one's home permanently symbolizes dependence with a capital D.

Each move of residence may have greater significance for old people than for those of any other age group. For example, a woman who has been forced to move into her daughter's home and who then requires admission to the hospital for elective surgery that results in placement in a nursing home for rehabilitation certainly has grounds for feeling completely "undone" by the number of moves she has had to make in a short period of time. Thoughtful health professionals take these factors into consideration and are patient in helping the older person adapt accordingly. In fact, a key to respectful interaction with an older person is to promote as much stability in the place of residence as possible.

Challenges of Changes with Aging

In the following section, some major challenges described in Chapter 6 are discussed as they present themselves to many older people today.

Challenge to Former Self-Image

Ample evidence supports that we have the potential to continue to develop throughout our lifespan, and our self-esteem can remain high or even grow stronger in the older years. Some recognize talents they never knew they had or refocus their energies on other hobbies or projects. Consider the following poem and the various transformations of the older adult.

> **THE LAYERS**
>
> *I have walked through many lives,*
> *some of them my own,*
> *and I am not who I was,*
> *though some principle of being*
> *abides, from which I struggle*
> *not to stray.*
> *When I look behind,*
> *as I am compelled to look*
> *before I can gather strength*
> *to proceed on my journey,*
> *I see the milestones dwindling*
> *toward the horizon*
> *and the slow fires trailing*
> *from the abandoned camp-sites,*
> *over which scavenger angels*
> *wheel on heavy wings.*
> *Oh, I have made myself a tribe*
> *out of my true affections,*
> *and my tribe is scattered!*
> *How shall the heart be reconciled*
> *to its feast of losses?*
> *In a rising wind*
> *the manic dust of my friends,*
> *those who fell along the way,*
> *bitterly stings my face.*
> *Yet I turn, I turn,*
> *exulting somewhat,*

with my will intact to go
wherever I need to go,
and every stone on the road
precious to me.
In my darkest night,
when the moon was covered
and I roamed through wreckage,
a nimbus-clouded voice
directed me:
"Live in the layers,
not on the litter."
Though I lack the art
to decipher it,
no doubt the next chapter
in my book of transformations
is already written.
I am not done with my changes.
     —*Stanley Kunitz*[26]

⊚ REFLECTIONS

- What is this poet saying about adulthood?
- What is the significance of the poem's title – "The Layers"
- What transitions are highlighted in the verses?
- How would you characterize the poet's view of aging?

Some persons do not even notice the changes in how they look, seeing only what they want to see in the mirror (Figure 17-2). Unfortunately, other people cling to a former visual image and also begin to reject the changes brought about by aging. They see themselves as has-beens who are no longer valuable to society and cannot perform as they did in the past.

Retirement from a long-held job often poses a threat to self-image (and, subsequently, to self-esteem) in many older men and women. With almost all adults employed in the workforce at some time in their lives, more people than ever before will face the challenge of retirement. However, many predict that the baby-boomer cohort, which is steadily moving into older adulthood may not retire at the traditional age of 65 because of concerns about funding shortfalls in Social Security and Medicare, possible cuts in government programs for elderly people, and cuts in traditional benefit pension plans which previously provided a fixed income in old age. For most, retirement not only involves a substantial reduction in income but also signals a change in daily activity.

As the person looks forward in time to retirement, a central issue becomes replacing time spent in work with other productive activities. Although work is only one part of the person's whole landscape of activities, it is a large part. The disappearance of work potentially leaves much of his or her landscape unfilled. At a minimum, retirement precipitates change in the person's whole activity pattern.[27] Four basic

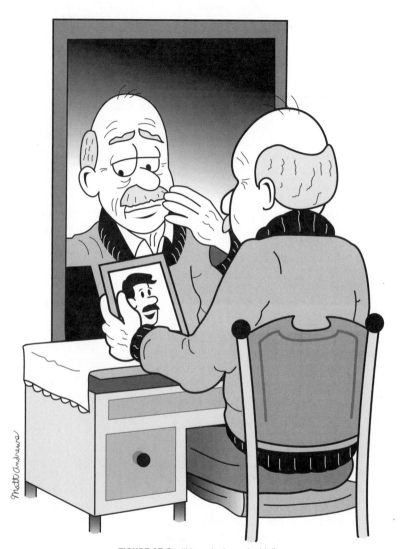

FIGURE 17-2: "I haven't changed a bit."

tasks seem to comprise essential postjob satisfaction: social activity, play, creativity, and lifelong learning.[28]

To maintain their status as useful members of society, almost all older adults need to be engaged in some kind of ongoing activity. This may be a job, a hobby, a volunteer service, or a club. In fact, the majority of volunteer hours are contributed by Americans beginning in midlife and continuing into old age in many areas that U.S. social policy fails to address adequately, such as the provision of basic human services.[29] Regardless of the activity chosen, they do need to have something to look forward to and to know that they are needed in a certain place at a certain time. Research suggests that involvement in volunteer activities may significantly improve the health and well-being of older people themselves through lower rates of depression, increased life satisfaction, retention of functional abilities, improved physical activity, and cognitive activity.[30-32] However, not all older people are able to be involved in such activities, and there are some good reasons why:

▶ They may be shy about meeting new people, particularly if they have maintained one set of friends and acquaintances for many years.
▶ They may possess too many physical or mental health impairments to participate in ongoing activities.
▶ They may have no way to get to them.
▶ They may not be able to afford to go.
▶ They may be afraid to go out alone or at night.

One or more of these reasons may also prevent them from seeking ongoing health care!

Fortunately, as the average age of our society grows, older people will become involved in continuous activities. For example, politics is one area in which the older-than-65 population has gained a powerful voice. Political involvement facilitates progress in legislation regarding personal interests and provides a broader perspective for legislation regarding society as a whole.

Physical Changes of Aging

A high percentage of older adults are remaining in good health longer than ever before; however, all adults will experience physical changes over the lifespan. Their three most common functional problems are reduced strength and endurance, joint problems, and increased safety problems (falls and greater incidence of household accidents). These functional problems are often associated with both physiological and cognitive changes. Examples of physiological age-related changes include bone loss, cartilage thinning, decreased cardiac reserve capacity, loss of muscle mass, sensory changes, and changes in touch, temperature, and pain perception.

Examples of cognitive changes include neuroanatomic changes in the brain that lead to decreased memory, attention, and a general decline in fluid intelligence (the ability to process novel information). With aging, the pattern of intelligence changes. The older adult demonstrates improvements in his or her crystallized intelligence (the ability to apply knowledge gained over time), and this balances the loss in fluid intelligence, which aids the elder in deciding how to respond to certain situations.[33] Visual changes include declines in acuity, speed of focusing, and accommodation in vision. With aging, adaptation to darkness usually declines, too. Hearing losses are greatest in the high-frequency range. There is a steady loss in perception of body movement, or kinesthesia. The older person may "adjust" to the losses gracefully. An example is an exchange that one of the authors had with her 92-year-old neighbor. As she walked into his living room, where the television announcer was blaring the Red Sox's latest play, she was surprised to see Tom planted in front of a blank screen. "Tom!" she shouted above the clamor, "There's no picture!"

"Picture went about a month ago!" he shouted back. "Can't see the screen anyway!" Tom, in spite of his good humor, would probably concede that the savings on the television was not worth the price of failing eyesight. For people with sensory impairment, the start of each day must seem like, as Shakespeare put it, the "Last scene of all/That ends this strange eventful history … /Sans teeth, sans eyes, sans taste, sans everything" (*As You Like It*, II, vii, 139). Your sensitivity to a patient's feelings about these losses can have profound effects on the extent to which the patient feels respected by you.

Understandably, attention to a patient's sensitivity about such matters and attempts to help an older person with sensory deficits prepare for the day are critical components of showing respect.

⊚ REFLECTIONS

Think about an older adult in your family or circle of friends.
• How has that person changed as he or she has aged?
• Has the person aged well? If so, in what ways? If not, why?
• Do you ever talk with this person about the "aging process"? What are his or her views on getting older?

We will not discuss musculoskeletal or neurological changes in the aging process in further detail because many health professionals learn this elsewhere. Posture, balance, strength, endurance, and other physical expressions of aging will vary, but overall wear and tear on the body will affect everyone in their later years. Your role as a health professional is to recognize normal aging versus pathology. An older adult or family member may mistake a clinical condition for normal aging and think "oh, I am just getting older," when in reality there may be a treatable condition that can be managed clinically helping the patient avoid disease and disability. For example, depression is often underidentified in the older adult. It is commonly mistaken for apathy related to age.

Multiple studies demonstrate that exercise has a positive impact on human beings of almost any age. Regular activity can reverse the decreased mobility that contributes to disease and disability in old age.[34] Furthermore, exercise has been shown to promote modest positive changes in cognitive functioning in this phase of the life span.[35] Given demonstrated improvements in so many areas, a prescription for activity seems indicated for most elderly patients. *Self-efficacy* (conviction to organize and implement effective strategies to deal with potential stressors) is also a positive predictor for aging well. Self-efficacy when linked with activity helps maintain cognitive function and social engagement.[36,37]

One way of dealing with all of the physical changes that are a normal part of aging, as well as those that accompany chronic and acute illness and injury, is to share experiences with others who understand what the person is going through. A wonderful example of this can be found in the field study of older women in a neighborhood beauty shop by Furman. Because few of us get to interact with older people who are not related to us, this glimpse into the social life of elderly women is particularly enlightening.

Customers exhibit a capacity for laughing at themselves, at their aches and pains, and at their intense engagement in such matters. For example, Blanche and Carmela, along with Claire, find themselves discussing various surgeries that they've had, stimulated by the fact that Blanche recently had cataract surgery. They first compare notes on that type of surgery; Blanche then talks about the hysterectomy she had years back, and so forth. Rather spontaneously, Blanche breaks into this discussion by saying, "Look at us, talking about cataracts, hysterectomies, hospitals!" They all laugh in this moment of self-recognition and amusement at themselves.[38]

Your sensitivity to changes, offering the person opportunities to talk about illness and loss and especially what changes mean for his or her feeling of well-being, is an avenue to respectful interaction, too.

Mental Changes of Aging

A few minor differences in mental capacity and functioning among all who are older are noteworthy. If attended to they can enhance the health professional's success in working with older people.

All patients benefit from the security of a set schedule, and this may be especially true for many older persons. The security arises from the knowledge that, at least in this one small area, he or she is in control of the environment. Some older people continue to exercise complete control over the details of their existence, whereas others gradually lose this opportunity. Even if this control extends no further than the patient's telling the taxicab driver to hurry because he or she is scheduled to be in speech therapy in 13 minutes, that person's self-respect will have been bolstered by exercising this type of control.

Being able to count on an established schedule also is a way for an older person to maintain a proper orientation to the environment. Some institutionalized older people become confused about the time of day and the date because they have few clues to orient them compared with the person who works 5 days a week or a peer who has more ongoing routine activity.

An older person's sense of security, control, and orientation can be further enhanced if, in addition to being treated at the same time each day, the routine of a treatment or test is kept reasonably stable from one day to the next. If the treatment or testing situation varies significantly every day, the patient may feel that nothing about it is familiar; it may be an anxiety-producing experience every time the person reports to the health professional. Anxiety can greatly decrease the person's performance and have a detrimental effect on both the relationship with you and the patient's progress.

The ideal situation is to create a balance between the patient's need for stability and his or her continuing interest in life and need for stimulation.

Caring for Older Adults with Cognitive Impairments

Cognitive impairment in the aged person can take many forms, and it is important that you study them in more depth than is appropriate to address in this book. However, impairment in one particular aspect of an elderly person's life, instrumental activities of daily living (IADLs), has been shown to be correlated with the presence of dementia and may be one of the early signs of cognitive changes.[39] If there is impairment in one the following four IADLs, a thorough mental status evaluation should be performed: (1) medication/health management, (2) money/financial management, (3) telephone management/communication device use, and (4) transportation management. We engage you in a general discussion about cognitive impairment and provide some general guidelines for respectful interaction with people suffering from brain syndromes that directly affect thought and speech processes.

Acute confusion or disorientation can be caused by a variety of factors, such as an infection, a fluid or electrolyte imbalance, or a cerebral vascular accident. It is important to determine the cause of confusion in an elderly patient and not just ascribe it to "being old." The following case illustrates how critical it is to understand the genesis of a change in mental status in an older patient.

> Family members brought an 81-year-old man, Abraham Steinman, who was in an acutely agitated and confused state, to the emergency department. The family stated that Mr. Steinman had gradually been getting more and more confused over the past few weeks and finally became violently disturbed earlier in the evening. He was admitted to the adult psychiatric unit because he was physically violent to the staff in the emergency department. The distraught family said he had never had an emotional outburst in his life and could not understand his behavior. The next day a careful physical examination revealed that Mr. Steinman had bilateral pneumonia and some signs of kidney failure. His confusion and agitation had only been a symptom of his physical illness.

⑤ REFLECTIONS

- What action might have prevented the admission to psychiatry?
- Would the assessment and treatment have been the same if Mr. Steinman were 40 years old? If he were 20 years old?
- How would you feel if this was your dad? What can the team caring for Mr. Steinman learn from his case to improve the care of future clients?

For such patients, acute confusion can be continual and may be increasingly profound, although you can help diminish the patient's suffering from disorientation at any given moment. Often, a useful approach is to not support the older person's constantly confused ideas, unless correcting them causes him or her to become violent, further disoriented, or deeply agitated. If an old man thinks he is in a hotel, you should try to correct him using a gentle reassuring voice and manner.

If he confuses you with someone else, his mistake can be corrected by showing him your name badge and repeating your name. Chances are that he will be less frightened if the people around him are willing to help him clear up his mind, if only for a few minutes. It is a good general rule of respectful interaction to correct the person. However, you should also remember to listen with interest and politeness to the patient. Listening will help you to determine the depth of the confusion, ascertain the wisdom of trying to correct it, and, in some cases, discern that the patient is making sense within a context not immediately evident.

The seemingly confused person should be treated kindly. Such treatment should never be condescending, but it should reflect the gentle authority that gives the patient a sense of security.

If the confusion is the result of a disease such as Alzheimer's disease or another form of dementia, many of the same principles apply. Some additional strategies for communicating with patients with dementia are as follows: use broad opening statements or questions, try to establish commonalties, speak to them as equals, and try to recognize themes in what the patient is trying to share with you.[40]

Sometimes medications can help the patient relax or in other ways be more comfortable, although with elderly patients it is best to be cautious with the use of drugs. Goals must be adapted according to what patients can comprehend. Some patients may be unable to remember the simplest tasks from one testing or treatment period to the next and may never grasp the most elementary verbal instructions. Others, however, will be able to follow astonishingly complex procedures. It is your responsibility in such situations to approach each person as an individual and to not take for granted that all confused utterances are signs of organic brain changes. In some cases, the confusion will increase no matter what is done. However, none of these complications should deter you from first attempting, in a kind way, to correct the inaccuracies. With a great number of patients, this humane act is the key to respectful interaction.

Assessing a Patient's Value System

The mechanics of adjusting a hearing aid, setting a schedule, or correcting a confused-sounding statement must all be done in a way that supports the older person's value system. Otherwise, the person is reduced to nothing more than an object to be efficiently manipulated. Chapter 1 listed some of the primary societal and personal values cherished by people in this society. Older people as a group can be expected to hold the same range and variety of values; no particular value can be ruled out automatically on the basis of age. However, the topics treated in this chapter can help you understand why so many older people adhere to some values more than others.

For instance, the primary good of self-respect will often be a more consciously prized value for older people because they perceive, correctly, that they are subject to loss of self-respect in an ageist society. Security, both financial and physical, may also be highly prized by older people because, again, for many of them the hold on it is more tenuous. Further, continued independent functioning is valued dearly when transition to a nursing home is a threat or when activities that can be performed alone become increasingly limited. Listening for which values the older patient expresses as his or her most precious and then trying to set treatment goals accordingly will greatly enhance your success. This will also help you understand the patient (and family member's) experience/expectations and build partnerships for shared decision-making. In working with older people, the most important challenge confronting you is resisting the tendency to stereotype them. Society's expectations of older people, many of which are inaccurate and outdated, are propagated through literature, television, and other popular media.

REFLECTIONS

Some states have instituted mandatory age based testing for older drivers. This testing varies from state to state, but ranges from vision exams to on-road assessments.

Your patient is seeing you today for his well visit and states, "I am 75 in a few weeks, so I will have to pass the registry test to keep my license. It's really not fair. That is age discrimination!"

• What do you say?
• How do you feel about the issue of age related mandates?

In thinking about this topic, consider the link between driving and independence in American society.

• How do limitations in this instrumental activity of daily living support or restrict participation for the older adult?

You can learn to appreciate individual differences among aged persons by increasing your contact with people who are older. Programs sponsored by churches, private organizations, and the government offer volunteer opportunities ranging from transportation to recreational activities to providing hot meals for home-bound persons. In some cities, foster care facilities and other institutions where older persons live welcome young people who are interested in volunteering their services or visiting older people. Whether through volunteer services, organizations, or contact as a health professional, your challenge is to develop an acutely discriminating eye for individual differences.

SUMMARY

Care of older adults must be based on a sound understanding of the physiological and psychosocial aspects of aging. The major developmental tasks of old age are to find meaning and satisfaction with life as it becomes more and more difficult to keep up with everything that goes on in a busy world. The chief goal of care is to maintain and support the patient's self-esteem by affirming his or her strengths and discovering hidden resources. By keeping in mind a patient's emotional and social needs, you can help him or her retain dignity and self-respect. The secret to respectful interaction with older adults is to keep their age-related problems in mind while concentrating on their individuality.

REFERENCES

1. John Adams as quoted in Wallis CL, editor: *The treasure chest: a heritage album containing 1064 familiar and inspirational quotations, poems, sentiments, and prayers from great minds of 2500 years*, New York, 1965, Harper and Row Publishers, p 12.
2. Vincent GK, Velkoff VA: *The next four decades: the older population in the United States: 2010 to 2050, Current Population Reports*, Washington, DC, 2010, U.S. Census Bureau. pp. 25–1138.
3. Werner CA: *The older population: 2010. 2010 Census Briefs C2010BR-09*, Washington, DC, 2011, US Census Bureau.
4. McConnell ES: Conceptual bases for gerontological nursing practice: models, trends, and issues. In Matteson ES, McConnell ES, Linton AD, editors: *Biological theories of aging in gerontological nursing: concepts and practice*, ed 2, Philadelphia, 1996, WB Saunders.
5. Gadow S: Medicine, ethics and the elderly, *Gerontologist* 20(6):680–685, 1980.

6. Rosowsky E: Ageism and professional training in aging: who will be there to help? *Generations* 29(3):55–58, 2005.
7. Wircenski M, Walker M, Allen J, et al: Age as a diversity issue in grades K-12 and in higher education, *Educ Gerontol* 25:491–500, 1999.
8. Madan AK, Aliabadi-Wade S, Beech DJ: Ageism in medical students' treatment recommendations: the example of breast-conserving procedures, *Acad Med* 76(3):282–284, 2001.
9. Erikson EH: *Childhood and society*, ed 2, New York, 1963, WW Norton.
10. Cummings E, Henry WE: *Growing old: the process of disengagement*, New York, 1961, Basic Books.
11. Achenbaum WA, Bengston VL: Re-engaging the disengagement theory of aging: on the history and assessment of theory development in gerontology, *Gerontologist* 34(6): 756–763, 1994.
12. Frederickson BL, Carstensen LL: Choosing social partners: how old age and anticipated endings make people more selective, *Psychol Aging* 5:335–347, 1990.
13. Atchley RC: The continuity theory of normal aging, *Gerontologist* 29(2):183–190, 1989.
14. Menec VH: The relationship between everyday activities and successful aging, *J Gerontol Soc Sci* 58(2):S74–S82, 2003.
15. Tornstam L: Transcendence in later life, *Generations* 23(4):10–14, 2000.
16. *Health Canada. Workshop on healthy aging*, (website) http://www.hc.sc.gc.ca/seniors-aines/pub/workshop_healthyaging. Accessed August 24, 2006.
17. Bryant LL, Corbett KK, Kutner JS: In their own words: a model of healthy aging, *Soc Sci Med* 53:927–941, 2001.
18. McKee KJ, Harrison G, Lee K: Activity, friendships and wellbeing in residential settings for older people, *Aging Ment Health* 3(2):143–152, 1999.
19. Riley MW: Friendship. In Riley MW, editor: *Aging and society: a sociology of age stratification*, vol 3, New York, 1972, Russell Sage Foundation.
20. Wren AM: Homecoming, *Afr Am Rev* 27(1):157, 1993.
21. Marty ME: The "god-forbid" wing, *Park Ridge Center Bull* 11:15, 1999. (Sept/Oct).
22. Benton D, Marshall C: Elder abuse, *Clin Geriatr Med* 7(4):831–845, 1991.
23. National Center on Elder Abuse: *Why should I care about elder abuse?* Fact Sheet. Accessed April 18, 2012, at http://www.ncea.aoa.gov/Ncearoot/Main_Site/pdf/publication/NCEA_WhatIsAbuse-2010.pdf.
24. Baker MW: Creation of a model of independence for community-dwelling elders in the United States, *Nursing Res* 54(5):288–295, 2005.
25. Beitman C: Wellness interventions in community living for older adults, *OT Pract* 14(3):1–7, 2009.
26. Kunitz S: *The collected poems*, New York, 2001, WW Norton Company.
27. Jonsson H, Kielhofner G, Borell L: Anticipating retirement: the formation of narrative concerning an occupational transition, *Am J Occup Ther* 51(1):49–56, 1997.
28. Vaillant GE: *Aging well: surprising guideposts to a happier life from the landmark Harvard study of adult development*, Boston, 2002, Little, Brown.
29. U.S. Department of Labor, Bureau of Labor Statistics: *Volunteering in the United States*, 2006, (website) http://www.bls.gov/news.release/volun.nr0.htm. Accessed November 12, 2006.
30. Moen P: Reconstructing retirement: careers, couples, and social capital, *Contemp Gerontol J Rev Crit Discuss* 4(4):123–125, 1998.
31. Fried LP, Carlson MC, Freedman M, et al: A social model for health promotion for an aging population: initial evidence on the experience corps model, *J Urban Health* 81(1):64–78, 2004.
32. Yuen HK, Huang P, Burik JK, Smith TG: Impact of participating in volunteer activities for residents living in long-term-care facilities, *Am J Occup Ther* 62:71–76, 2008.

33. Baltes PB: Theoretical propositions of life-span developmental psychology: on the dynamics of growth and decline, *Dev Psychol* 23(5):661–626, 1987.
34. Buckwalter JA, DiNubile NA: Decreased mobility in the elderly: the exercise antidote, *Physician Sportsmed* 25(9):126–128, 130-133, 153–155, 1997.
35. Van Sickle TD, Hersen M, Simco ER, et al: Effects of physical exercise on cognitive functioning in the elderly, *Int J Rehabil Health* 2(2):67–100, 1996.
36. Robnett RH, Chop WC: *Gerontology for the health care professional*, ed 2, Burlington, MA, 2009, Jones & Barlett Learning.
37. Schepens S, Sen A, Painter JA, Murphy SL: Relationship between fall-related efficacy and activity engagement in community-dwelling older adults: a meta-analytic review, *Am J Occup Ther* 66:137–148, 2012. http://dx.doi.org/10.5014/ajot.2012.001156.
38. Furman FK: *Facing the mirror: older women and beauty shop culture*, New York, 1997, Routledge Press.
39. Barberger-Gateau P, Commenges D, Gagnon M, et al: Instrumental activities of daily living as a screening tool for cognitive impairment and dementia in elderly community dwellers, *J Am Geriatr Soc* 40(11):1129–1134, 1992.
40. Tappen RM, Williams-Burgess C, Edelstein J, et al: Communicating with individuals with Alzheimer's disease: examination of recommended strategies, *Arch Psychiatr Nurs* 11(5):249–256, 1997.

PART SEVEN

Questions for Thought and Discussion

1. If you are asked to propose policies and plans for a waiting room area for families of high-risk newborns in your institution, what will you suggest to the architects, decorators, and administrators? Why? What sorts of support services will you recommend for families in this situation?

2. You are approached by a parent of a child in the elementary school setting where you work. The parent is concerned that her daughter is falling behind in her schoolwork, and she is concerned that "no one appears to be listening to her." Her two older sons have learning disorders, and she is worried that her daughter may be at risk as well. How would you respond to this parent's concern?

3. You are the supervisor of an adolescent unit in a hospital. The patient, a 16-year-old named Sam, is mature for his age, and you have found him to be very thoughtful. Sam has cancer that you know has metastasized. His parents have decided with the surgeon that he should have an amputation, although all agree that the hope of saving him completely from the spread of the disease is negligible. One evening you notice that Sam is withdrawn. He says, "My parents and the doctor are going to cut off my leg, and they haven't even asked me what I think about it. I'd rather die than lose my leg."

    a. What should you do?

    b. To whom should you speak about this conversation? Why?

4. You are hurrying down the hospital corridor when you notice an acquaintance of your family, a bricklayer in his middle 50s. You express surprise at seeing him there because he has always been the picture of good health. He tells you that he has had a heart attack. Suddenly he begins to pour out a blow-by-blow description of the incident. As he talks, he becomes increasingly agitated and finally bursts into tears, sobbing, "It's all over. I'll never be able to go back to my job or anything. What am I going to do?"

    a. What can you say or do right then to calm this man's immediate anxious state?

    b. Will you report this interaction? To whom and why?

    c. How can health professionals work together to treat the middle-age person's anxiety about the long-term effects of illness on family, job, and self-esteem?

5. Young adulthood is often referred to as "the healthy years and the hidden hazards." What does this mean? What are the implications for the life span?

    What do you dread most about growing old? Why? What do you look forward to most? How do you think an older person's role in society will have changed by the time you grow old?

6. An alert 92-year-old patient who has been in your care for several days arrives late for treatment one morning at your ambulatory care clinic. She explains that she missed her usual bus and had to wait in the rain and cold for the next bus to arrive. You begin to converse with her in your usual manner and quickly realize that something is wrong; she does not answer your questions appropriately. Once or twice, she mentions her son (whom you know was killed years ago in the service of his country), but her sentences are disconnected and incomplete.

   a. What possible reasons may there be for her apparent confusion?

   b. Where will you start in your attempt to diagnose her problem?

Index

Page numbers followed by *f* indicate figures; *t*, tables; *b*, boxes.